Pacemakers and Implantable Cardioverter Defibrillators

Editor

THEOFANIE MELA

CARDIOLOGY CLINICS

www.cardiology.theclinics.com

Consulting Editors
ROSARIO FREEMAN
JORDAN M. PRUTKIN
DAVID M. SHAVELLE
AUDREY H. WU

May 2014 • Volume 32 • Number 2

ELSEVIER

1600 John F. Kennedy Boulevard • Suite 1800 • Philadelphia, Pennsylvania, 19103-2899

http://www.theclinics.com

CARDIOLOGY CLINICS Volume 32, Number 2

May 2014 ISSN 0733-8651, ISBN-13: 978-0-323-29701-1

Editor: Adrianne Brigido
Developmental Editor: Susan Showalter

Cardiology Clinics (ISSN 0733-8651) is published quarterly by Elsevier Inc., 360 Park Avenue South, New York, NY 10010-1710. Months of issue are February, May, August, and November. Business and Editorial Offices: 1600 John F. Kennedy Blvd., Ste. 1800, Philadelphia, PA 19103-2899. Customer Service Office: 3251 Riverport Lane, Maryland Heights, MO 63043. Periodicals post-age paid at New York, NY and additional mailing offices. Subscription prices are $320.00 per year for US individuals, $530.00 per year for US institutions, $155.00 per year for US students and residents, $390.00 per year for Canadian individuals, $665.00 per year for Canadian institutions, $455.00 per year for international individuals, $665.00 per year for international institutions and $220.00 per year for Canadian and international students/residents. To receive student/resident rate, orders must be accompanied by name of affiliated institution, data of term, and the *signature* of program/residency coordinator on institution letterhead. Orders will be billed at individual rate until proof of status is received. Foreign air speed delivery is included in all *Clinics* subscription prices. All prices are subject to change without notice. **POSTMASTER:** Send address changes to *Cardiology Clinics*, Elsevier Health Sciences Division, Subscription Customer Service, 3251 Riverport Lane, Maryland Heights, MO 63043. **Customer Service: 1-800-654-2452 (U.S. and Canada); 314-447-8871 (outside U.S. and Canada). Fax: 314-447-8029. E-mail: journalscustomerservice-usa@ elsevier.com (for print support); journalsonlinesupport-usa@elsevier.com (for online support).**

Reprints. For copies of 100 or more, of articles in this publication, please contact the Commercial Reprints Department, Elsevier Inc., 360 Park Avenue South, New York, NY 10010-1710. Tel.: 212-633-3874; Fax: 212-633-3820; E-mail: reprints@elsevier.com.

Cardiology Clinics is also published in Spanish by McGraw-Hill Interamericana Editores S. A., P.O. Box 5-237, 06500, Mexico D. F., Mexico; in Portuguese by Reichmann and Alfonso Editores Rio de Janeiro, Brazil; and in Greek by Dimitrios P. Lagos, 8 Pondon Street, GR115-28 Ilissia, Greece.

Cardiology Clinics is covered in *MEDLINE/PubMed (Index Medicus), Excerpta Medica, The Cumulative Index to Nursing and Allied Health Literature* (CINAHL).

Contributors

BRADLEY P. KNIGHT, MD, FACC, FHRS
Division of Cardiology, Department of Medicine; Director of Cardiac Electrophysiology, Bluhm Cardiovascular Institute of Northwestern; Professor of Medicine, Feinberg School of Medicine, Northwestern University, Chicago, Illinois

MARK S. LINK, MD
Professor of Medicine, Department of Medicine, The Cardiac Arrhythmia Center, Tufts Medical Center, Boston, Massachusetts

JAMES A. MERRIAM, MD
Medical University of South Carolina, Charleston, South Carolina

SUNEET MITTAL, MD
Director, Electrophysiology Laboratory, The Valley Hospital, Ridgewood, New Jersey

COLIN MOVSOWITZ, MBChB
Director of Cardiac Electrophysiology; Cardiology Consultants of Philadelphia, Einstein Medical Center Montgomery, East Norriton, Pennsylvania

SAMAN NAZARIAN, MD, PhD
Section for Cardiac Electrophysiology, Department of Medicine, Johns Hopkins University School of Medicine; Department of Epidemiology, Johns Hopkins Bloomberg School of Public Health, Baltimore, Maryland

OWEN A. OBEL, MD
Associate Professor of Medicine, Division of Internal Medicine, University of Texas Southwestern Medical Center; Director of EP and Pacing, Division of Cardiology, Veterans Health Administration (VA) North Texas Healthcare System, Dallas, Texas

THOMAS M. O'BRIEN, MD
The Heart and Vascular Center, The Christ Hospital, Cincinnati, Ohio

VICTOR G. PRETORIUS, MBChB
Assistant Professor of Surgery, Division of Cardiothoracic Surgery, University of California San Diego Health System, La Jolla, San Diego, California

KUSHWIN RAJAMANI, MD
Section of Cardiac Pacing and Electrophysiology, Robert and Suzanne Tomsich Department of Cardiovascular Medicine, Sydell and Arnold Miller Family Heart and Vascular Institute, Cleveland Clinic Foundation, Cleveland, Ohio

ANIL B. RAJENDRA, MD
Medical University of South Carolina, Charleston, South Carolina

JOHN RHYNER, MD
Division of Cardiology, Department of Medicine, Northwestern University, Chicago, Illinois

ANDREA M. RUSSO, MD, FACC, FHRS
Director, Electrophysiology and Arrhythmia Services, Cooper University Hospital; Professor of Medicine, Cooper Medical School of Rowan University, Camden, New Jersey

EDWARD J. SCHLOSS, MD
Electrophysiology Director, The Heart and Vascular Center, The Christ Hospital, Cincinnati, Ohio

DANIEL SOHINKI, MD
Division of Internal Medicine, University of Texas Southwestern Medical Center, Dallas, Texas

NIRAJ VARMA, MA, DM, FRCP
Heart and Vascular Institute, J2-2 Cardiac Pacing and Electrophysiology, Cleveland Clinic, Cleveland, Ohio

BRUCE L. WILKOFF, MD
Section of Cardiac Pacing and Electrophysiology, Robert and Suzanne Tomsich Department of Cardiovascular Medicine, Sydell and Arnold Miller Family Heart and Vascular Institute, Cleveland Clinic Foundation, Cleveland, Ohio

PAUL D. ZIEGLER, MS
Medtronic Caridac Rhythm Diesease Management Division, Medtronic Inc, Mounds View, Minnesota

Contents

Preface: Pacemakers and ICDs   xi

Theofanie Mela

Erratum   xiii

Newer Indications for ICD and CRT   181

James A. Merriam, Anil B. Rajendra, and Michael R. Gold

The first implantable pacemaker was developed about 50 years ago. Since that time, cardiac implantable electronic device therapy (CIED) has undergone dramatic changes. Two of the most significant advances are the development of implantable defibrillators (ICDs) to treat ventricular tachyarrhythmias and prevent sudden death and left ventricular–based pacing to achieve cardiac resynchronization therapy (CRT). In this article, the authors review the current indications for ICD and CRT, with particular emphasis on recent updates in guidelines. Many countries and regions of the world now have guidelines for CIED use. In this article, the authors only focus on US guidelines.

Shock Avoidance and the Newer Tachycardia Therapy Algorithms   191

Kushwin Rajamani, Adam S. Goldberg, and Bruce L. Wilkoff

Sudden cardiac death is a leading cause of death in the United States and Europe. Implantable cardioverter defibrillators (ICDs) are a cornerstone of therapy for patients at risk of first occurrence of ventricular arrhythmia, or secondary prevention in those who have previously suffered cardiac arrest or life-threatening arrhythmias. Despite their efficacy, ICD shocks are associated with significant physical and psychological adverse effects. As technology has progressed, newer device programing methods have allowed for arrhythmia suppression and termination without the need for high-energy defibrillation, thus improving patient satisfaction, health, and outcomes.

Lead Extractions: Indications, Procedural Aspects, and Outcomes   201

Ulrika M. Birgersdotter-Green and Victor G. Pretorius

As a result of more cardiac implantable electronic devices being placed, a trend toward increasing device infections, and concerns regarding lead malfunction, there is an increased need for lead extraction skills and comprehensive lead management programs. This review discusses the current indications for lead extractions as well as the training requirements and tools and technology needed to create the foundation for a successful lead management program.

Is Defibrillation Testing Necessary?   211

Andrea M. Russo and Mina K. Chung

With advancements in implantable cardioverter defibrillator (ICD) technology, the practice of performing defibrillation threshold (DFT) testing at the time of implantation has been questioned. With availability of biphasic waveforms, active cans, and high-output devices, opponents claim that DFT testing is no longer necessary.

Clinical trials demonstrating the efficacy of ICDs in prevention of sudden cardiac death have, however, all used some form of defibrillation testing. This debate is fueled by the absence of data from randomized prospective trials evaluating the role of DFT testing in predicting clinical shock efficacy or survival. This review discusses both sides of the argument.

The Totally Subcutaneous Implantable Defibrillator   225

John Rhyner and Bradley P. Knight

 A video of the S-ICD implantation procedure accompanies this article

The subcutaneous implantable cardioverter-defibrillator (S-ICD) is a new therapeutic option for patients at risk of sudden cardiac arrest. The device uses a pulse generator implanted in the lateral thoracic region and a tunneled subcutaneous electrode. Benefits of this configuration include the preservation of venous access and reduction in the risk of systemic infection, vascular injury, and lead failure. Clinical trials suggest that the device effectively senses, discriminates, and converts both spontaneous and induced ventricular tachycardia and ventricular fibrillation episodes with minimal complications. The S-ICD represents a novel implantable cardioverter-defibrillator configuration that may provide reliably effective therapy for malignant tachyarrhythmias.

The Modern EP Practice: EHR and Remote Monitoring   239

Suneet Mittal, Colin Movsowitz, and Niraj Varma

Cardiac implantable electronic devices (CIEDs) store clinically valuable, time-sensitive information regarding system integrity, arrhythmias, and heart failure parameters. Remote monitoring has impacted clinical practice by reducing scheduled office visits, providing protocols for device recalls and advisories, and facilitating the management of unscheduled encounters. The successful implementation of remote monitoring into clinical practice requires a new work flow and additional staff; the use of the electronic medical record to manage the data emanating from CIEDs poses an additional challenge. Solutions to these issues are discussed, and projections are made regarding the management of CIEDs in a modern electrophysiology practice.

The Role of the Wearable Cardioverter Defibrillator in Clinical Practice   253

Mina K. Chung

The wearable cardioverter defibrillator (WCD) is an option for external monitoring and defibrillation in patients at risk for sudden cardiac arrest caused by ventricular tachycardia or ventricular fibrillation and who are not candidates for or who refuse an implantable cardioverter defibrillator (ICD). WCDs provide monitoring with backup defibrillation protection. WCDs have been used when a patient's condition delays or prohibits ICD implantation, or as a bridge when an indicated ICD must be explanted. WCDs are used for primary prevention of sudden cardiac death during high-risk gap periods early after myocardial infarction, coronary revascularization, or new diagnosis of heart failure.

Does Atrial Fibrillation Detected by Cardiac Implantable Electronic Devices Have
Clinical Relevance?   271

Taya V. Glotzer and Paul D. Ziegler

The precise role atrial fibrillation (AF) plays in increasing the risk of stroke is not well understood; this is especially true for the implanted device population. Current cardiac implanted electronic devices have a very high sensitivity and specificity for true AF detection. It does not seem to matter if the AF episode is proximal to the stroke event, and risk seems to be increased by relatively brief AF episodes. The appearance of new atrial high-rate episodes increases thromboembolic event rates. Until larger trials or registries are conducted, it is important to follow established guidelines regarding anticoagulation.

Newer Algorithms in Bradycardia Management   283

Daniel Sohinki and Owen A. Obel

Permanent cardiac pacemakers (PPM) are effective in the treatment of bradycardia in a growing number of clinical scenarios. An appreciation of the capacity of PPMs to result in negative hemodynamic and proarrhythmic effects has grown alongside clinical experience with permanent pacing. Such experience has necessitated the development of algorithms aimed at optimizing device functionality across a broad spectrum of physiologic and pathologic conditions. This review highlights recent device-based algorithms used in automated threshold testing, reduction of right ventricular pacing, prevention and treatment of pacemaker-mediated tachycardia, mode switching for atrial tachyarrhythmias, rate-modulated pacing, and advances in arrhythmia storage and remote monitoring.

Indications for Cardiac Resynchronization Therapy   293

Thomas M. O'Brien, Edward J. Schloss, and Eugene S. Chung

Initial studies established patient selection criteria for cardiac resynchronization therapy (CRT) as left ventricular ejection fraction less than or equal to 35%, QRS greater than or equal to 120 ms, and New York Heart Association 3–4. Based on newer data, post hoc analyses, and meta-analyses, these criteria have been refined and guidelines updated, highlighting left bundle branch morphology and QRS greater than 150 ms in selecting patients with a likelihood of favorable outcomes. Guidelines will change as more data become available; the decision to apply CRT should be based on patient clinical profile and the balance of risk tolerance and likelihood of benefit.

MRI for Patients with Cardiac Implantable Electrical Devices   299

Grant V. Chow and Saman Nazarian

MRI has become an invaluable tool in the evaluation of soft tissue and bony abnormalities. The presence of a cardiac implantable electrical device (CIED) may complicate matters, however, because these devices are considered a contraindication to MRI scanning. When MRI is performed in patients with a CIED, risks include reed switch activation in older devices, lead heating, system malfunction, and significant radiofrequency noise resulting in inappropriate inhibition of demand pacing, tachycardia therapies, or programming changes. This report reviews indications and risk-benefit evaluation of MRI in patients with CIED and provides a clinical algorithm for performing MRI in patients with implanted devices.

Implantable Defibrillators in Long QT Syndrome, Brugada Syndrome, Hypertrophic Cardiomyopathy, and Arrhythmogenic Right Ventricular Cardiomyopathy   305

Mustafa Dohadwala and Mark S. Link

Sudden death is often the first manifestation in inherited cardiac arrhythmia syndromes. Patients with long QT syndrome who have an episode of syncope while on beta-blockade should be offered an implantable cardioverter-defibrillator (ICD).

In Brugada syndrome and hypertrophic cardiomyopathy, ICDs are often the most effective treatment of primary and secondary prevention of cardiac arrest. Risk stratification is crucial in identifying those at greatest risk to provide lifesaving therapy with an ICD while avoiding complications in those unlikely to receive benefit.

Index   **319**

CARDIOLOGY CLINICS

FORTHCOMING ISSUES

August 2014
Coronary Artery Disease
David Shavelle, *Editor*

November 2014
Atrial Fibrillation
Hakan Oral, *Editor*

RECENT ISSUES

February 2014
Heart Failure
Howard J. Eisen, *Editor*

November 2013
Cardiovascular Intensive Care
Umesh K. Gidwani, Samin K. Sharma, and
Annapoorna S. Kini, *Editors*

August 2013
**Catheter Interventions for Structural
Heart Disease**
Ray V. Matthews, *Editor*

ISSUES OF RELATED INTEREST

Cardiac Electrophysiology Clinics, September 2013 (Vol. 5, No. 3)
Remote Monitoring and Physiologic Sensing Technologies
Samuel J. Asirvatham, K.L. Venkatachalam, and Suraj Kapa, *Editors*
Available at http://www.cardiacep.theclinics.com/

NOW AVAILABLE FOR YOUR iPhone and iPad

Preface
Pacemakers and ICDs

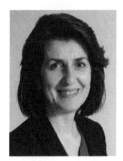

Theofanie Mela, MD
Editor

Technology evolution has contributed to an unprecedented advancement in cardiac rhythm management devices over the past 50 to 60 years. This advancement is multidimensional. It involves the engineering aspect of the device, with more efficient batteries, remote monitoring, functional designs, and new materials. It also involves the clinical evolution of indications for which these devices are being used.

Following the pioneering idea of pacing the heart and the first implantable pacemaker in 1958, pacing has evolved over the years. Contemporary pacemakers carry a number of intelligent functions that make them provide more physiologic performance while avoiding the negative effects of unnecessary pacing.

The revolution in saving lives from arrhythmic death came with the implantable cardioverter defibrillator in the 1980s. Today, ICD technology provides us with the ability to collect a remarkable amount of information for the heart failure patient, retrospectively, but also in real-time, on a day-to-day basis. Being able to utilize this information should be one of the priorities of the Electrophysiology and Heart Failure Clinics, as this is an effective way of providing quality care to the patients and limiting hospitalizations.

Following the implantation of the first ICD in 1980 and for the following two decades, progress was made in small but significant steps, until cardiac resynchronization therapy (CRT) took place. Not only did cardiac rhythm management devices support/correct the rhythm and rate, but they provided advanced therapy for the heart failure patients who had exhausted their medical options.

After the initial effort to prove its significance and improve the ability to implant these devices, CRT indications have significantly expanded. In this issue, we assemble the most recent indications for ICD and CRT implants, as well as recommendations for more sensible use of the CRT, with the goal of increasing the therapeutic response. There will also be a discussion about potential new CRT indications that have not made it yet into the guidelines.

One of the greatest concerns after an ICD implant is that of an inappropriate shock. A number of studies have shown the detrimental effect of shocks to the patient. The ICD technology has advanced significantly over the years, with a big effort directed toward the avoidance of inappropriate shocks. There are also techniques to avoid inappropriate shocks by special device programming; this should be the standard of care nowadays.

It is debatable whether testing a patient for defibrillation threshold (DFT) after an ICD implant has a place in our current practice. Although DFT testing has been routinely used for decades, there are significant arguments against this strategy. The debate is ongoing and we read more about it in this issue.

One concern with cardiac rhythm management devices is that of a component failure. Lead failure has become a common problem in recent years with significant implications for the patient. As the number of indications for ICD implantation increases, the number of devices implanted and the number of leads eventually failing increase. We have also been witnessing a major failure of the

Cardiol Clin 32 (2014) xi–xii
http://dx.doi.org/10.1016/j.ccl.2014.02.001

lead technology in the names of the Medtronic Fidelis and the St. Jude Riata leads and an additional reason for laser lead extraction considerations.

A significant advancement in eliminating the problems that transvenous leads create is the development of the completely subcutaneous ICD. This is a brand new technology that seems to be quite promising, but still bears a number of limitations, by the luck of the ability to pace in bradycardia or ventricular tachycardia, anti-tachycardia pacing.

Another significant advancement in sudden cardiac death prevention is the development of the wearable defibrillator, LifeVest, by Zoll. It has found great use for patients who are not immediate candidates for an ICD, as a recovery is anticipated, or for patients who have had their ICD removed due to infection. The results of ongoing trials may further expand the use of this technology.

Remote monitoring of cardiac rhythm management devices has entered most electrophysiology practices and has brought an unequivocal improvement in the quality of patient care, both due to the ease, but mostly, due to the prompt availability of data that may occasionally be critical. It has become the paradigm for the benefit that remote monitoring may have in the rate of readmissions as well as the transfer of patient data directly into the electronic medical record system.

Overall, we are witnessing a very dynamic change in the way medicine is being practiced. Cardiac rhythm management devices appear to be in the forefront of this evolution. It is exciting to follow along and be prepared for the changes to come.

Theofanie Mela, MD
Pacer and ICD Clinic
Massachusetts General Hospital
75 Fruit Street
Boston, MA 02114, USA

E-mail address:
tmela@mgh.harvard.edu

Erratum

An error was made in an article published in the November 2013 issue of *Cardiology Clinics* (Volume 31, Issue 4) on page 581. "Durable Mechanical Circulatory Support in Advanced Heart Failure: A Critical Care Cardiology Perspective" by Anuradha Lala, MD, and Mandeep R. Mehra, MD, should have included the following disclosure:

MRM is a consultant with Thoratec, chair of the REVIVE-IT DSMB (a National Heart, Lung, and Blood Institute-sponsored trial with Thoratec as the device sponsor) and editor of the *Journal of Heart and Lung Transplantation*. In addition he consults for Boston Scientific, Medtronic, St. Jude Medical, Baxter, the American Board of Internal Medicine, and the National Institutes of Health.

Cardiol Clin 32 (2014) xiii
http://dx.doi.org/10.1016/j.ccl.2013.11.004
0733-8651/14/$ – see front matter © 2014 Elsevier Inc. All rights reserved.

Newer Indications for ICD and CRT

James A. Merriam, MD, Anil B. Rajendra, MD,
Michael R. Gold, MD, PhD*

KEYWORDS

- Implantable cardioverter defibrillators • Sudden cardiac death • Primary prevention
- Cardiac resynchronization therapy • Secondary prevention

KEY POINTS

- Device-based therapy has progressed greatly since the days of the first pacemakers.
- With the advent of the implantable defibrillator, sudden cardiac death can now be aborted successfully.
- With cardiac resynchronization therapy, heart failure symptoms and mortality are improved; in addition, left ventricular remodeling can actually be reversed.
- Patient selection continues to be an imperfect science for many reasons, including a lack of data or a lack of complete understanding of the underlying mechanisms.
- Several recommendations carry a level-of-evidence-C rating because of a lack of precise data.

The first implantable pacemaker was developed about 50 years ago. Since that time, cardiac implantable electronic device therapy (CIED) has undergone dramatic changes. Two of the most significant advances are the development of implantable defibrillators (ICDs) to treat ventricular tachyarrhythmias and prevent sudden death and left ventricular–based pacing to achieve cardiac resynchronization therapy (CRT). Along with the rapid advance in technology, clinical trials have helped to establish the appropriate populations that benefit most from these devices.

As our understanding of the pathophysiology and treatment options of sudden cardiac death (SCD) and heart failure (HF) have progressed, the role of devices has changed. This change requires periodic updates and modifications of guidelines. In this article, the authors review the current indications for ICDs and CRT, with a particular emphasis on recent updates in the guidelines. Of note, many countries and regions of the world now have guidelines for CIED use. In this article, the authors only focus on US guidelines.

ICD THERAPY

Early clinical trials established a mortality benefit of defibrillator therapy compared with medical therapy in populations with ventricular tachycardia, prior cardiac arrest, or syncope with inducible arrhythmias (ie, secondary prevention).[1] Because of a continued high incidence of out-of-hospital sudden death among patient populations with no prior symptomatic arrhythmias, such as patients with HF or ischemic cardiomyopathy, indications for defibrillator therapy as the primary prevention progressed to include larger groups of patients with systolic dysfunction and other risk factors.[2,3]

Secondary Prevention

The initial indications for ICD therapy were for patients with documented, life-threatening ventricular arrhythmias. These secondary prevention trials showed the benefits of ICD implantation primarily in patients with reduced systolic dysfunction. The Antiarrhythmics versus Implantable Defibrillators (AVID) trial demonstrated a 38%

Medical University of South Carolina, Charleston, SC 29425, USA
* Corresponding author. Division of Cardiology, Medical University of South Carolina, 25 Courtenay Drive, Room 7031 ART, MSC 592, Charleston, SC 29425.
E-mail address: goldmr@musc.edu

Cardiol Clin 32 (2014) 181–190
http://dx.doi.org/10.1016/j.ccl.2013.12.004
0733-8651/14/$ – see front matter © 2014 Elsevier Inc. All rights reserved.

relative reduction of death in patients with ICDs compared with class III antiarrhythmic drug therapy (AAD) therapy. Inclusion criteria for the trial were resuscitated ventricular fibrillation, sustained ventricular tachycardia (VT) with syncope, and sustained VT with hemodynamic compromise. Patients were randomized to ICD or medical therapy. Enrollment criteria also consisted of left ventricular ejection fraction (LVEF) less than 40% among patients with VT.[4]

The Canadian Implantable Defibrillator Study (CIDS) was a randomized, multicenter, clinical trial that compared (ICD) therapy versus amiodarone among patients with prior cardiac arrest or hemodynamically unstable VT. Although the trial demonstrated that a 33% reduction occurred in arrhythmic mortality with the ICD therapy group, this reduction did not reach statistical significance. However, subgroup analysis of the CIDS study did show a benefit in ICD therapy by age, functional status, and poor left ventricular systolic function. Specifically, the benefit was greatest among patients with LVEF less than 35% and advanced New York Heart Association (NYHA) functional status.

The CASH (Cardiac Arrest Study Hamburg) trial evaluated ICD therapy compared with AAD in survivors of SCD.[5] Patients were randomized to ICD therapy versus amiodarone, propafenone, or metoprolol. ICD therapy provided a significant reduction in mortality compared with drug therapy alone. A meta-analysis of the AVID, CIDS, and CASH trials showed a 28% relative risk reduction in mortality with ICD therapy compared with amiodarone therapy; the mortality benefit was attributed to a 50% reduction to arrhythmic deaths in the ICD group.[6] Additionally, there was a 34% reduction in mortality with ICD therapy in patients with LVEF less than 35%.

Secondary prevention of SCD trials established the clear benefits of ICD therapies in patients with aborted SCD and ventricular arrhythmias compared with AAD. Additionally, the secondary prevention trials provided the basis for primary prevention therapy by suggesting that patients with poor left ventricular systolic function had the potential for significant mortality reduction from ICD implantation.

Primary Prevention

Subsequent guidelines addressed the risk of SCD in several patient populations at risk for ventricular fibrillation and VT. Multiple trials have evaluated the risks and benefits of the ICD in the prevention of sudden death and have improved survival in a variety of patient populations, including those with prior coronary artery disease, myocardial infarction, and reduced left ventricular systolic function secondary to both ischemic and nonischemic causes.

The MADIT (Multicenter Automatic Defibrillator Implantation Trial) was the first to demonstrate a mortality benefit for ICD versus medical therapy for primary prevention. The patients included in the trial had ischemic heart disease with prior myocardial infarction demonstrated with either Q waves on the electrocardiogram or a history of positive biomarkers for myocardial infarction. The LVEF was required to be 35% or less and nonsustained VT (NSVT) documented; NYHA class IV functional status was excluded. All patients underwent an electrophysiology study. If VT or ventricular fibrillation was inducible, the patients were then randomized to implantable defibrillator or conventional medical therapy. The primary outcome was 5-year mortality, which was 16% in the ICD group compared with 39% in the control group.[7] The MUSTT (Multicenter Unsustained Tachycardia Trial) was performed concomitantly with MADIT. It evaluated the prognostic value of electrophysiology testing and efficacy of AADs in reducing the risk of sudden death among patients with coronary artery disease, left ventricular dysfunction, and asymptomatic, NSVT. Patients with inducible sustained VT were randomized to medical therapy alone or a strategy of programmed ventricular stimulation to guided antiarrhythmic drug therapy. If patients remained inducible on AADs, then an ICD was implanted. Patients who received ICD therapy showed marked mortality reduction. Additionally, the nonrandomized patients with no inducible sustained arrhythmias still had a significant mortality risk.[8]

The results of MADIT and MUSTT established the role of ICDs for primary prevention. MADIT II simplified the risk stratification by eliminating the requirement for NSVT as well as electrophysiology studies. Patients with myocardial infarction 1 month or more before enrollment and LVEF of 30% or less were randomized to ICD or medical therapy. There were 105 of 742 (14.2%) and 97 of 490 (17.9%) deaths in the ICD and conventional groups, respectively (hazard ratio [HR] 0.69, $P = .016$). Thus, the ICD arm showed a 31% reduction in mortality despite no qualifying electrophysiology study for inclusion.[9] The Sudden Cardiac Death Heart Failure Trial (SCD-HeFT) was the first large randomized trial to evaluate the efficacy of ICD therapy in patients with systolic HF with reduced left ventricular systolic dysfunction in patients with both ischemic and nonischemic cardiomyopathies. Patients were randomized to placebo, amiodarone, or ICD therapy. The enrollment criteria included patients with class II or III HF with LVEF less than 35%.

Single-chamber ICD implantation resulted in a 23% relative risk reduction of all-cause mortality compared with placebo, and no benefit of amiodarone therapy was demonstrated. SCD-HeFT showed that regardless of cause, patients with reduced systolic HF and a markedly reduced LVEF benefited from ICD implantation.[10]

These landmark mortality studies led to the early guidelines for ICD use. They also led to policy decisions regarding reimbursement for this therapy. The 2005 Centers for Medicare and Medicaid Service National Coverage Determination document was based on the results of these early ICD primary prevention trials. The updated document allows ICD implantation 40 days after myocardial infarction. However, following revascularization by either percutaneous coronary intervention (PCI) or coronary artery bypass graft (CABG), device implantation must be delayed for 3 months on medical therapy. It is important to note that the 3-month PCI and CABG restrictions are not included in the current guidelines of the American College of Cardiology (ACC)/American Heart Association (AHA)/Heart Rhythm Society (HRS).[11] The coverage decisions also require a waiting period of at least 3 months following the initial diagnosis of HF, although such a delay in treatment was not part of the primary prevention trials. These differences highlight that coverage and reimbursement rules do not always align with the guidelines or inclusion criteria of clinical studies.

The current guidelines (2008) also provide recommendations for less common conditions, such as cardiac sarcoidosis, arrhythmogenic right ventricular dysplasia, Brugada syndrome, and hypertrophic cardiomyopathy. However, because of the rarity of these diseases, there is a paucity of prospective data to guide recommendations.[12]

Patients with cardiac sarcoidosis have areas of scar and granuloma that are substrate for VT, increasing their risk for SCD. Studies showed that about one-third of the patients implanted for secondary prevention received appropriate ICD therapies in the follow-up. About one-quarter of the patients implanted for primary prevention received appropriate ICD therapies.[13,14] Although these ICD therapies tend to overestimate the risk of sudden death, this frequency of appropriate shocks and antitachycardia pacing supports the implantation of ICDs in high-risk patients with cardiac sarcoidosis.

Patients with arrhythmogenic right ventricular dysplasia (ARVD) also have an increased risk of SCD but without clear criteria for prophylactic devices. In a multicenter study that enrolled 106 patients, patients with ARVD and no history of ventricular fibrillation or VT underwent ICD implantation for primary prevention because they had at least one risk factor for SCD. Appropriate ICD therapies were observed in 24% of patients in the follow-up. Of the patients with syncope as a risk factor for SCD, 43% had appropriate device therapies. Of the asymptomatic patients with NSVT, 17.5% had appropriate therapies, whereas no patients with only a family history of SCD received therapies.[15] Another study of 84 patients with ARVD that underwent prophylactic ICD placement found that 48% of the patients received appropriate therapies.[16]

Patients with symptomatic Brugada syndrome (BrS) as evidenced by a history of ventricular arrhythmias or syncope maintain a class IIa indication for ICD implantation in current guidelines. Indications for ICD implantation in asymptomatic patients are less clear as perceived risk factors, such as inducibility of ventricular tachyarrhythmias and family history of SCD, are not reliable predictors of cardiac events.[17] Because asymptomatic patients have a low but not immeasurable risk of SCD, a recent large study evaluated patients with structurally normal hearts with type I Brugada syndrome.[18] Of the 378 patients enrolled, 166 patients were asymptomatic before ICD implantation. Although the patients with BrS or spontaneous type I on electrocardiogram (ECG) had a higher incidence of appropriate ICD shock compared with asymptomatic patients, a substantial portion (12%) of asymptomatic patients did receive appropriate ICD therapy. The rate of inappropriate shocks was twice that of appropriate shocks in asymptomatic patients. Although inappropriate therapy was mitigated by less aggressive programing, a concerning rate of lead failure as well as other complications were present in all groups. The investigators of the study emphasized the importance of risk stratification and careful patient assessment before implantation in asymptomatic patients. In general, a spontaneous type I Brugada ECG pattern, rather than ECG abnormalities provoked by diagnostic pharmacotherapy, is considered a high risk.

Hypertrophic cardiomyopathy (HCM) is a well-recognized cause of SCD, particularly among young patients. Thus, there has been a need to identify high-risk patients that would benefit from prophylactic ICDs. The indications for ICD placement for HCM fall under 3 different categories: patients with diminished LVEF, patients with previous SCD or ventricular arrhythmias, and patients with multiple risk factors for SCD. The 2011 ACCF/AHA Guideline for the Diagnosis and Treatment of Hypertrophic Cardiomyopathy outlines the risk factors for SCD in this population: history of sustained VT or SCD events, a family history for SCD, unexplained syncope, documented NSVT, a failure to augment blood pressure with exercise, and left ventricular septal wall thickness of 30 mm or more.[19] The benefit of prophylactic ICD therapy has been demonstrated in patients with one or more of these risk factors.[20] In a large, international, multicenter cohort, 383 patients with HCM who have received ICD were judged to be at high risk based on the risk factors noted earlier. Although 51 patients (13%) experienced an appropriate ICD discharge, the number of risk factors did not correlate with the rate of subsequent appropriate ICD discharges. In light of these findings as well as the low incidence of SCD in patients with HCM[21] and a lack of large amounts of clinical data, the writing committee emphasized that the clinical decision for implantation for primary prevention should be made on an individual basis and account for multiple patient variables.

ICD Guideline Changes

The previous guidelines for device-based therapy separated ICD recommendations based on the indications for primary prevention and secondary prevention separately. The updated 2008 ICD recommendations are combined into a single list because of the overlap between primary and secondary indications (**Box 1**). The 2006 guidelines of the ACC/AHA/European Society of Cardiology used an LVEF of less than 40% as a critical cutoff to justify ICD implantation for primary prevention of SCD.[12] The LVEF used in clinical trials assessing the ICD for primary prevention of SCD ranged from 30% to 40%.[8,9] Two trials, MADIT I and SCD-HeFT, used LVEFs of 35% or less as the entry criterion. The writing committee stated the desire to include "patients with clinical profiles as similar to those included in the trials as possible."[12] Thus, the primary prevention ICD indications for both ischemic and nonischemic cardiomyopathy are clarified using data from SCD-HeFT. ICD therapy is indicated in patients with nonischemic dilated cardiomyopathy who have an LVEF of 35% or less and who have NYHA functional class II or III symptoms.

The MADIT II enrollment criteria (ie, ischemic cardiomyopathy and LVEF ≤30%, NYHA I) are now class I indications, elevated from class IIa. The guidelines also emphasize that primary prevention ICD recommendations apply only to patients receiving optimal medical therapy and a reasonable expectation of survival, with good functional capacity for more than 1 year. Independent risk assessment preceding ICD implantation is emphasized, including the consideration of patient preferences, which is underscored by the recurring indications for candidacy for device-based therapy in patients with greater than 1-year survival. Importantly, the updated guidelines now include a discussion of ICD and pacemaker programming at the end of life, such as ethical considerations for clinicians and device deactivation at the end of life.

The 2012 ACCF/AHA/HRS Focused Update of the 2008 Guidelines for Device-Based Therapy of Cardiac Rhythm Abnormalities was released in September 2012. These new guidelines mentioned that, although there has been new data in the interim, there is not sufficient new information to change the recommendations from the 2008 guidelines. However, the 2012 focused update addressed new data and changes to the recommendations for CRT.

CRT

Notable changes in the 2012 ACCF/AHA/HRS Focused Update for CRT are based on HF severity, QRS morphology, QRS duration, and atrial fibrillation. Patients with left ventricular systolic dysfunction and electrocardiographic evidence of conduction disease, based solely on QRS duration, were the focus of early CRT studies. It was originally hypothesized that electrical conduction abnormalities contribute to worsened left ventricular systolic dysfunction by multiple mechanisms. The development of biventricular pacing improves cardiac hemodynamics in part by reducing ventricular dyssynchrony.[22] Effects of multisite biventricular pacing in patients with heart failure and intraventricular conduction delay (MUSTIC) was an early trial that evaluated the efficacy of CRT in patients with electrocardiographic evidence of intraventricular conduction delay.[23] Patients with NYHA class III symptoms, LVEF less than 35%, and a QRS duration of more than 150 ms were included. MUSTIC demonstrated improvements in the 6-minute walk distance with active CRT therapy. Larger, subsequent studies demonstrated other benefits of CRT therapy. However, patient selection has remained a controversial issue (**Box 2**).

QRS duration had been specifically addressed in the 2008 guidelines. Although the greatest benefits were observed among patient populations with a QRS duration of more than 150 ms, the 2008 guidelines did not make separate recommendations based on the QRS duration or morphology because most of the clinical trials of resynchronization therapy at that time focused on patients with left bundle branch block (LBBB). Furthermore, no single large trial demonstrated a clinical benefit among patients without QRS prolongation, even when they have been selected for echocardiographic evidence of dyssynchrony.[24] The

Box 1
ICD guidelines

Class I

1. ICD therapy is indicated in patients who are survivors of cardiac arrest caused by ventricular fibrillation or hemodynamically unstable sustained VT after evaluation to define the cause of the event and to exclude any completely reversible causes (level of evidence: A).

2. ICD therapy is indicated in patients with structural heart disease and spontaneous sustained VT, whether hemodynamically stable or unstable (level of evidence: B).

3. ICD therapy is indicated in patients with syncope of undetermined origin with clinically relevant, hemodynamically significant sustained VT or ventricular fibrillation induced at electrophysiologic study (level of evidence: B).

4. ICD therapy is indicated in patients with an LVEF of 35% or less caused by prior myocardial infarction, at least 40 days after myocardial infarction, and in NYHA functional class II or III (level of evidence: A).

5. ICD therapy is indicated in patients with nonischemic dilated cardiomyopathy who have an LVEF of 35% or less and are in NYHA functional class II or III (level of evidence: B).

6. ICD therapy is indicated in patients with LV dysfunction caused by prior myocardial infarction who are at least 40 days after myocardial infarction, have an LVEF of 30% or less, and are in NYHA functional class I (level of evidence: A).

7. ICD therapy is indicated in patients with NSVT caused by prior myocardial infarction, LVEF of 40% or less, and inducible ventricular fibrillation or sustained VT at electrophysiologic study (level of evidence: B).

Class IIa

1. ICD implantation is reasonable for patients with unexplained syncope, significant LV dysfunction, and nonischemic dilated cardiomyopathy (level of evidence: C).

2. ICD implantation is reasonable for patients with sustained VT and normal or near-normal ventricular function (level of evidence: C).

3. ICD implantation is reasonable for patients with HCM who have 1 or more major risk factors for SCD (level of evidence: C).

4. ICD implantation is reasonable for the prevention of SCD in patients with arrhythmogenic right ventricular dysplasia/cardiomyopathy who have 1 or more risk factors for SCD (level of evidence: C).

5. ICD implantation is reasonable to reduce SCD in patients with long-QT syndrome who are experiencing syncope and/or VT while receiving beta-blockers (level of evidence: B).

6. ICD implantation is reasonable for nonhospitalized patients awaiting transplantation (level of evidence: C).

7. ICD implantation is reasonable for patients with Brugada syndrome who have had syncope (level of evidence: C).

8. ICD implantation is reasonable for patients with Brugada syndrome who have documented VT that has not resulted in cardiac arrest (level of evidence: C).

9. ICD implantation is reasonable for patients with catecholaminergic polymorphic VT who have syncope and/or documented sustained VT while receiving beta-blockers (level of evidence: C).

10. ICD implantation is reasonable for patients with cardiac sarcoidosis, giant cell myocarditis, or Chagas disease (level of evidence: C).

Class IIb

1. ICD therapy may be considered in patients with nonischemic heart disease who have an LVEF of 35% or less and who are in NYHA functional class I (level of evidence: C).

2. ICD therapy may be considered for patients with long-QT syndrome and risk factors for SCD (level of evidence: B).

3. ICD therapy may be considered in patients with syncope and advanced structural heart disease in whom thorough invasive and noninvasive investigations have failed to define a cause (level of evidence: C).

4. ICD therapy may be considered in patients with a familial cardiomyopathy associated with sudden death (level of evidence: C).

5. ICD therapy may be considered in patients with LV noncompaction (level of evidence: C).

Class III

1. ICD therapy is not indicated for patients who do not have a reasonable expectation of survival with an acceptable functional status for at least 1 year, even if they meet ICD implantation criteria specified in the class I, IIa, and IIb recommendations described earlier (level of evidence: C).

2. ICD therapy is not indicated for patients with incessant VT or ventricular fibrillation (level of evidence: C).

3. ICD therapy is not indicated in patients with significant psychiatric illnesses that may be aggravated by device implantation or that may preclude systematic follow-up (level of evidence: C).

4. ICD therapy is not indicated for NYHA class IV patients with drug-refractory congestive HF who are not candidates for cardiac transplantation or implantation of a CRT device that incorporates both pacing and defibrillation capabilities (level of evidence: C).

5. ICD therapy is not indicated for syncope of undetermined cause in patients without inducible ventricular tachyarrhythmias and without structural heart disease (level of evidence: C).

6. ICD therapy is not indicated when ventricular fibrillation or VT is amenable to surgical or catheter ablation (eg, atrial arrhythmias associated with Wolff-Parkinson-White syndrome, right ventricular or LV outflow tract VT, idiopathic VT, or fascicular VT in the absence of structural heart disease) (level of evidence: C).

7. ICD therapy is not indicated for patients with ventricular tachyarrhythmias caused by a completely reversible disorder in the absence of structural heart disease (eg, electrolyte imbalance, drugs, or trauma) (level of evidence: B).

From Epstein AE, Dimarco JP, Ellenbogen KA, et al. ACC/AHA/HRS 2008 guidelines for device-based therapy of cardiac rhythm abnormalities: executive summary a report of the American College of Cardiology/American Heart Association Task Force on Practice Guidelines (Writing Committee to Revise the ACC/AHA/NASPE 2002 Guideline Update for Implantation of Cardiac Pacemakers and Antiarrhythmia Devices): developed in collaboration with the American Association for Thoracic Surgery and Society of Thoracic Surgeons. J Am Coll Cardiol 2008;21(51):2085–105; with permission.

guidelines are reinforced in that there may be harm of CRT in this group as evidenced by the recent Echocardiography Guided Cardiac Resynchronization Therapy (EchoCRT) study.[25]

Previous trials, including Resynchronization for Ambulatory Heart Failure Trial (RAFT), Multicenter Automatic Defibrillator Implantation Trial-Cardiac Resynchronization Therapy (MADIT-CRT), Resynchronization Reverses Remodeling in Systolic Left Ventricular Dysfunction (REVERSE), Cardiac Resynchronization in Heart Failure Study (CARE-HF), and Comparison of Medical Therapy, Pacing, and Defibrillation in Heart Failure (COMPANION), were not powered to detect whether the benefit from CRT is consistent across all degrees of QRS widening, although a greater benefit was noted consistently in the wider QRS subgroups. Therefore, a meta-analysis of those trials addressed the effect of CRT as a function of the baseline QRS duration (**Fig. 1**).[26] CRT significantly decreased the primary end point of death or hospitalization for HF in patients with a QRS of 150 ms or more (HR 0.58, 95% confidence interval [CI] 0.50–0.68; $P<.0001$) but not in patients with a QRS less than 150 ms (HR 0.95, 95% CI 0.83–1.10; $P = .51$). These results were consistent across all degrees of HF severity. Despite these

analyses, the dichotomization of a continuous variable (eg, grouping QRS duration as >150 ms or <150 ms) is potentially problematic. This point has been shown recently in an individual patient meta-analysis, which demonstrated the strong impact of QRS duration on outcomes but no clear threshold at 150 ms (**Fig. 2**).[27] Rather, the curves seem to show no effect or adverse effect at less than 120 to 130 ms, consistent with studies of narrow QRS cohorts.[25]

Early CRT trials investigated patients with more advanced HF symptoms (NYHA functional class III and IV), whereas 3 subsequent trials investigated the benefit of CRT in asymptomatic or mildly symptomatic HF (NYHA functional class I and II). In the REVERSE trial, patients with an LVEF of 40% or less, a QRS duration of more than 120 ms, and NYHA class I or II functional status were randomized to CRT therapy (CRT ON) or no CRT therapy (CRT OFF) for 12 months, with a primary end point of HF clinical response and a secondary end point of change in left ventricular end systolic volume index (LVESVI). Although there was no difference in quality-of-life scores, the CRT ON group had a significant delay in the time to first HF hospitalization (HR 0.47, $P = .03$). Importantly, there was a significant decrease in the

Box 2
Indications for CRT[a]

Class I

- Left ventricular ejection fraction (EF) less than 35%, sinus rhythm, QRS duration more than 150 ms, NYHA class II, III, or ambulatory IV

Class IIa

- EF less than 35%, sinus rhythm, left bundle branch block (LBBB) with QRS duration 120 to 149 ms, NYHA class II, III, ambulatory class IV

- EF less than 35%, sinus rhythm, non-LBBB with QRS duration more than 150 ms, NYHA III, or ambulatory class IV

- EF less than 35%, undergoing device replacement and anticipated significant (>40%) ventricular pacing

- EF less than 35%, AF, if

  1. Requires ventricular pacing or otherwise meets CRT criteria

  2. Atrioventricular nodal ablation or rate control will allow near 100% biventricular pacing

Abbreviation: AF, atrial fibrillation.
[a] Patients must be on guide line–directed medical therapy, including beta-blocker and angiotensin-converting enzyme inhibitor or angiotensin receptor blocker.[34]

asymptomatic patients.[28] In addition, a post hoc subanalysis of the trial results investigated the significance of QRS morphology and duration on reverse remodeling. This subanalysis showed a marked reduction in LVESVI in the patients with LBBB with CRT ON versus CRT OFF (-25.3 ± 28.5 mL/m^2 vs -1.7 ± 25.8 mL/m^2, $P \leq .001$). In the patients with non-LBBB morphology, there was less reverse remodeling effects (6.7 ± 25.8 mL/m^2) and no difference between the study groups ($P = .18$). In addition, as the QRS duration prolonged, the LVESVI decreased in almost a linear fashion.[29]

In the RAFT trial, patients with an LVEF of 30% or less, a QRS duration of more than 120 ms, NYHA class II or III symptoms, and sinus rhythm or permanent atrial fibrillation with a controlled rate were randomized to ICD or cardiac resynchronization therapy with implantable cardioverter-defibrillator (CRT-D); the composite primary outcome was all-cause death or HF hospitalization. Approximately 80% of patients in each group had NYHA class II symptoms. CRT-D performed significantly better than ICD for preventing the primary outcome (33.2% CRT-D vs 40.3% ICD alone, HR 0.75, $P \leq .001$). The CRT-D group also showed a reduction of all-cause mortality (HR 0.75, $P = .003$), death from cardiovascular cause (HR 0.76, $P = .02$), and HF hospitalizations (HR 0.68, $P \leq .001$) as the preplanned secondary end points. In the analysis of patient subgroups, only those in sinus rhythm with a QRS duration of more than 150 ms in an LBBB pattern showed a benefit of CRT-D over ICD. There was no difference between the two groups for the composite primary end point in

LVESVI in the CRT ON group (-18.4 ± 29.5 mL/m^2) versus CRT OFF (-1.3 ± 23.4 mL/m^2; $P = .0001$). This trial was the first trial to show a reverse remodeling effect of CRT in mildly symptomatic or

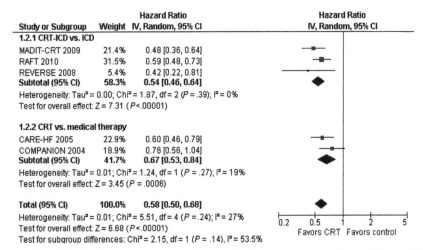

Fig. 1. Patients with QRS of 150 ms or more assigned to CRT versus control. CI, confidence interval. (*From* Stavrakis S, Lazzara R, Thadani U, et al. The benefit of cardiac resynchronization therapy and QRS duration: a meta-analysis. J Cardiovasc Electrophysiol 2012;23(2):163–8; with permission.)

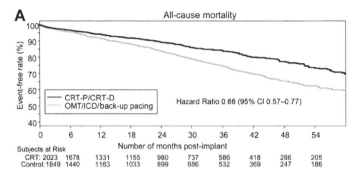

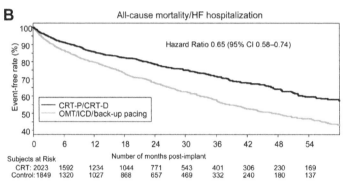

Fig. 2. Overall effect of CRT versus control on all-cause mortality (*A*) and on death or HF hospitalization (*B*). CI, confidence interval. CRT-D, cardiac resynchronization therapy with implantable cardioverter-defibrillator; CRT-P, cardiac resynchronization therapy; OMT, optimal medical therapy. (*From* Cleland JG, Abraham WT, Linde C, et al. An individual patient meta-analysis of five randomized trials assessing the effects of cardiac resynchronization therapy on morbidity and mortality in patients with symptomatic heart failure. Eur Heart J 2013;34(46): 3547–56; with permission.)

patients with an intrinsic QRS duration of less than 150 ms or non-LBBB QRS morphology.[30] In a subanalysis of the trial data looking only at patients with permanent atrial fibrillation, there was no difference in the composite primary outcome between the two study groups,[31] although the ventricular pacing group was disappointingly low for the CRT-D cohort confounding the analysis.

In the MADIT-CRT trial, patients were enrolled if they had ischemic cardiomyopathy and NYHA class I and II symptoms or nonischemic cardiomyopathy and NYHA class II symptoms, an LVEF less than 30%, and a QRS duration of more than 130 ms. Patients then underwent implantation of CRT-D or ICD alone and were followed until the trial ended with a primary end point of death from any cause or nonfatal HF events. The primary end point occurred less in the CRT-D group than the ICD group (17.2% vs 25.3%, P = .001). This difference was caused by a decrease in HF events in the CRT-D group (13.9% vs 22.8%, P≤.001), with no difference in all-cause mortality between groups (6.8% CRT-D vs 7.3% ICD, P = .99). Also, only patients with a QRS duration of more than 150 ms experienced a benefit from CRT-D. Echocardiographic indices of reverse remodeling (left ventricular end-diastolic volume, LVESV, and LVEF) were all significantly greater with CRT-D compared

with ICD only.[32] A subanalysis of the MADIT-CRT data investigated whether specific QRS morphologies identified patients that improved with CRT. Patients were identified as having an LBBB, right bundle branch block (RBBB), or intraventricular conduction delay (IVCD) at baseline. In the ICD arm, there was no difference in primary end point or in death alone between the different QRS morphologies. In the CRT-D arm, the LBBB group had significant improvement in the primary end point and in death from any cause compared with patients with either RBBB or IVCD. Only patients with LBBB had improvement in the primary end point with CRT-D compared with ICD only, whereas patients with either RBBB or IVCD had similar outcomes regardless of CRT-D or ICD only.[33]

Based on the results of these recent trials, CRT is no longer recommended for non-LBBB patients and mild HF (NYHA I or II). For more severe HF, the recommendation is strongest for LBBB; but in the presence of non-LBBB, there are still class II recommendations. In addition, a QRS duration more than 150 ms is a class I recommendation, whereas a QRS duration of 120 to 149 ms is now a class II recommendations. Furthermore, the 2012 focused update emphasizes class I recommendations for CRT in patients in sinus rhythm, whereas patients with atrial fibrillation have a class II indication.

SUMMARY

Device-based therapy has progressed greatly since the days of the first pacemakers. With the advent of the ICD, SCD can now be aborted successfully. With CRT, HF symptoms and mortality are improved; in addition, LV remodeling can actually be reversed. However, patient selection continues to be an imperfect science for many reasons, including a lack of data or a lack of complete understanding of the underlying mechanisms. Accordingly, several recommendations carry a level-of-evidence-C rating because of a lack of precise data. As more data are collected and the pathophysiology of certain diseases is better understood, guidelines will continue to be updated to hone patient selection.

REFERENCES

1. Connolly SJ, Gent M, Roberts RS, et al. Canadian Implantable Defibrillator Study (CIDS): a randomized trial of the implantable cardioverter defibrillator against amiodarone. Circulation 2000;101(11): 1297–302.
2. Kadish A, Dyer A, Daubert JP, et al. Prophylactic defibrillator implantation in patients with nonischemic dilated cardiomyopathy. N Engl J Med 2004; 350(21):2151–8.
3. Huikuri HV, Castellanos A, Myerburg RJ. Sudden death due to cardiac arrhythmias. N Engl J Med 2001;345(20):1473–82.
4. A comparison of antiarrhythmic-drug therapy with implantable defibrillators in patients resuscitated from near-fatal ventricular arrhythmias. The Antiarrhythmics versus Implantable Defibrillators (AVID) Investigators. N Engl J Med 1997;337(22):1576–83.
5. Kuck KH, Cappato R, Siebels J, et al. Randomized comparison of antiarrhythmic drug therapy with implantable defibrillators in patients resuscitated from cardiac arrest. Circulation 2000;102(7):748–54.
6. Connolly SJ, Gent M, Roberts RS, et al. Meta-analysis of the implantable cardioverter defibrillator secondary prevention trials. AVID, CASH and CIDS studies. Antiarrhythmics vs Implantable Defibrillator study. Cardiac Arrest Study Hamburg. Canadian Implantable Defibrillator Study. Eur Heart J 2000; 21(24):2071–8.
7. Moss AJ, Hall WJ, Cannom DS, et al. Improved survival with an implanted defibrillator in patients with coronary disease at high risk for ventricular arrhythmia. Multicenter Automatic Defibrillator Implantation Trial Investigators. N Engl J Med 1996; 335(26):1933–40.
8. Buxton AE, Lee KL, DiCarlo L, et al. Electrophysiologic testing to identify patients with coronary artery disease who are at risk for sudden death.

Multicenter Unsustained Tachycardia Trial Investigators. N Engl J Med 2000;342(26):1937–45.
9. Moss AJ, Zareba W, Hall WJ, et al. Prophylactic implantation of a defibrillator in patients with myocardial infarction and reduced ejection fraction. N Engl J Med 2002;346(12):877–83.
10. Bardy GH, Lee KL, Mark DB, et al. Amiodarone or an implantable cardioverter-defibrillator for congestive heart failure. N Engl J Med 2005;352(3):225–37.
11. Available at: http://www.cms.gov/medicare-coverage-database/details/ncd-details.aspx?NCDId=110 &ncdver=3&IsPopup=y&NCAId=102&NcaName= Implantable+Defibrillators+-+Clinical+Trials&bc= AAAAAAAAIAAA&. Accessed January 20, 2014.
12. Epstein AE, Dimarco JP, Ellenbogen KA, et al. ACC/AHA/HRS 2008 Guidelines for device-based therapy of cardiac rhythm abnormalities: executive summary a report of the American College of Cardiology/American Heart Association Task Force on Practice Guidelines (Writing Committee to Revise the ACC/AHA/NASPE 2002 Guideline Update for Implantation of Cardiac Pacemakers and Antiarrhythmia Devices): developed in collaboration with the American Association for Thoracic Surgery and Society of Thoracic Surgeons. J Am Coll Cardiol 2008;21(51): 2085–105.
13. Betensky BP, Tschabrunn CM, Zado ES, et al. Long-term follow-up of patients with cardiac sarcoidosis and implantable cardioverter-defibrillators. Heart Rhythm 2012;9(6):884–91.
14. Schuller JL, Zipse M, Crawford T, et al. Implantable cardioverter defibrillator therapy in patients with cardiac sarcoidosis. J Cardiovasc Electrophysiol 2012; 23(9):925–9.
15. Corrado D, Calkins H, Link MS, et al. Prophylactic implantable defibrillator in patients with arrhythmogenic right ventricular cardiomyopathy/dysplasia and no prior ventricular fibrillation or sustained ventricular tachycardia. Circulation 2010;12(122):1144–52.
16. Bhonsale A, James CA, Tichnell C, et al. Incidence and predictors of implantable cardioverter-defibrillator therapy in patients with arrhythmogenic right ventricular dysplasia/cardiomyopathy undergoing implantable cardioverter-defibrillator implantation for primary prevention. J Am Coll Cardiol 2011;58(14):1485–96.
17. Sacher F, Probst V, Maury P, et al. Long-term prognosis of patients diagnosed with Brugada syndrome: results from the FINGER Brugada Syndrome Registry. Circulation 2010;121(5):635–43.
18. Probst V, Veltmann C, Eckardt L. Outcome after implantation of a cardioverter-defibrillator in patients with Brugada syndrome: a multicenter study-part 2. Circulation 2013;128(16):1739–47.
19. Gersh BJ, Maron BJ, Bonow RO, et al. 2011 ACCF/AHA guideline for the diagnosis and treatment of hypertrophic cardiomyopathy: a report of

the American College of Cardiology Foundation/ American Heart Association Task Force on Practice Guidelines Developed in Collaboration With the American Association for Thoracic Surgery, American Society of Echocardiography, American Society of Nuclear Cardiology, Heart Failure Society of America, Heart Rhythm Society, Society for Cardiovascular Angiography and Interventions, and Society of Thoracic Surgeons. J Am Coll Cardiol 2011;25(58):212–60.

20. Maron BJ, Spirito P, Shen WK, et al. Implantable cardioverter defibrillators and prevention of sudden cardiac death in hypertrophic cardiomyopathy. JAMA 2007;298(4):405–12.

21. Maron BJ, Shen WK, Link MS, et al. Contemporary insights and strategies for risk stratification and prevention of sudden death in hypertrophic cardiomyopathy. Circulation 2010;121(3):445–6.

22. Burkhardt JD, Wilkoff BL. Interventional electrophysiology and cardiac resynchronization therapy: delivering electrical therapies for heart failure. Circulation 2007;115(16):2208–20.

23. Cazeau S, Leclercq C, Lavergne T, et al. Effects of multisite biventricular pacing in patients with heart failure and intraventricular conduction delay. N Engl J Med 2001;344(12):873–80.

24. Beshai JF, Grimm RA, Nagueh SF, et al. Cardiac-resynchronization therapy in heart failure with narrow QRS complexes. N Engl J Med 2007;357(24):2461–71.

25. Ruschitzka F, Abraham WT, Singh JP, et al. Cardiac-resynchronization therapy in heart failure with a narrow QRS complex. N Engl J Med 2013;369(15):1395–405.

26. Stavrakis S, Lazzara R, Thadani U, et al. The benefit of cardiac resynchronization therapy and QRS duration: a meta-analysis. J Cardiovasc Electrophysiol 2012;23(2):163–8.

27. Cleland JG, Abraham WT, Linde C, et al. An individual patient meta-analysis of five randomized trials assessing the effects of cardiac resynchronization therapy on morbidity and mortality in patients with symptomatic heart failure. Eur Heart J 2013;34(46):3547–56.

28. Linde C, Abraham WT, Gold MR, et al. Randomized trial of cardiac resynchronization in mildly symptomatic heart failure patients and in asymptomatic patients with left ventricular dysfunction and previous heart failure symptoms (REVERSE trial). J Am Coll Cardiol 2008;23(52):1834–43.

29. Gold MR, Thebault C, Linde C, et al. Effect of QRS duration and morphology on cardiac resynchronization therapy outcomes in mild heart failure: results from the Resynchronization Reverses Remodeling in Systolic Left Ventricular Dysfunction (REVERSE) study. Circulation 2012;126(7):822–9.

30. Tang AS, Wells GA, Talajic M, et al. Cardiac-resynchronization therapy for mild-to-moderate heart failure. N Engl J Med 2010;363(25):2385–95.

31. Healey JS, Hohnloser SH, Exner DV, et al. Cardiac resynchronization therapy in patients with permanent atrial fibrillation: results from the Resynchronization for Ambulatory Heart Failure Trial (RAFT). Circ Heart Fail 2012;5(5):566–70.

32. Moss AJ, Hall WJ, Cannom DS. Cardiac-resynchronization therapy for the prevention of heart-failure events. N Engl J Med 2009;361(14):1329–38.

33. Zareba W, Klein H, Cygankiewicz I, et al. Effectiveness of cardiac resynchronization therapy by QRS morphology in the Multicenter Automatic Defibrillator Implantation Trial-Cardiac Resynchronization Therapy (MADIT-CRT). Circulation 2011;123(10):1061–72.

34. Tracy CM, Epstein AE, Darbar D, et al. American College of Cardiology Foundation; American Heart Association Task Force on Practice Guidelines; Heart Rhythm Society: 2012 ACCF/AHA/HRS focused update of the 2008 guidelines for device-based therapy of cardiac rhythm abnormalities: a report of the American College of Cardiology Foundation/American Heart Association Task Force on Practice Guidelines. Circulation 2012;126:1784–818.

Shock Avoidance and the Newer Tachycardia Therapy Algorithms

Kushwin Rajamani, MD, Adam S. Goldberg, MD,
Bruce L. Wilkoff, MD*

KEYWORDS

- Inappropriate shocks • Avoidable shocks • Antitachycardia pacing (ATP) • ICD programming

KEY POINTS

- Patients who receive shock therapy have an associated reduction in the mortality benefit from implantable cardioverter defibrillators (ICDs).
- Prolonging the time to therapy and restricting therapy to faster tachycardias can significantly reduce shocks overall, with an associated mortality benefit.
- The decision on single-chamber versus dual-chamber defibrillator implantation needs to be individualized.
- Remote monitoring facilitates earlier recognition of patient-related and device-related issues, reducing the risk of inappropriate therapy.
- Medical therapy and catheter ablation are effective adjunctive strategies in patients with ICD shocks to reduce or eliminate future events.

INTRODUCTION

Implantable cardioverter defibrillator (ICD) therapy has been proven in several large-scale clinical trials to reduce mortality in patients with primary and secondary indications.[1–4] There is evidence to suggest that receiving shocks may reduce the mortality benefit; however, more recent study has suggested that this maybe due to the arrhythmia or comorbidities rather than the shock itself.[5,6] Shock therapy, despite the benefits, is also associated with significant psychological issues, including anxiety, depression, and posttraumatic stress.[7–9] Therefore, reducing both appropriate and inappropriate shocks, without compromising patient safety, is desirable. This can be achieved with a multifaceted approach with medical therapy, improved device-based programming, and ablation strategies. This article discusses these strategies.

BACKGROUND

The first ICD was implanted in 1980, and was revolutionary in the approach to cardiac arrhythmias and sudden cardiac death.[10] It is now well established that ICD therapy improves mortality and is generally considered to be cost-effective.[2,3,11] Over many years, large randomized trials have identified patients with greatest potential benefit

Drs K. Rajamani and A.S. Goldberg have no disclosures.
Dr B.L. Wilkoff is on the Medical Advisory Board for Medtronic, St. Jude Medical, and Spectranetics. He has received speaker honoraria from Boston Scientific and royalties from Medtronic.
Section of Cardiac Pacing and Electrophysiology, Robert and Suzanne Tomsich Department of Cardiovascular Medicine, Sydell and Arnold Miller Family Heart and Vascular Institute, Cleveland Clinic Foundation, 9500 Euclid Avenue, Cleveland, OH 44195, USA
* Corresponding author.
E-mail address: wilkofb@ccf.org

Cardiol Clin 32 (2014) 191–200
http://dx.doi.org/10.1016/j.ccl.2014.01.002

from ICD placement and therapy, and this is reflected in current guidelines.[12]

ICD implantation has become a cornerstone of therapy for many patient groups, including those with inherited or acquired cardiomyopathies and channelopathies. Although sudden cardiac death (SCD) is a leading cause of death in the United States and Europe, identification of those at higher risk of death than the general population has been critical in reducing mortality in select groups. Although there are inherent risks associated with ICD implantation (infection or lung, vascular, or cardiac injury), in these populations the benefits of prophylaxis outweigh the risks.

Despite these benefits, ICD shocks can have a profound effect on patients when a shock is delivered, such as physical and psychological trauma, as well as impairment of their quality of life and general health.[7–9,13–15] As a result, reduction in shock exposure is an ideal strategy, and various methods have been developed to avoid both appropriate and inappropriate shocks. In this pursuit, it is important to understand the types of shocks that patients are exposed to (**Box 1**).

It has been reported that among patients with an ICD who have received a shock from the device, about one-third were inappropriate.[3] There are conflicting data regarding the effect of ICD shocks on survival. Some studies have indicated that mortality is increased among patients with an ICD who receive shock for any reason compared with receiving no shock.[5,16] An analysis of 2135 patients from 4 trials of antitachycardia pacing (ATP) therapy to reduce shock therapy revealed that shocked ventricular arrhythmic events were associated with increased mortality risk compared with ATP-terminated tachycardia.[17] This was attributed to the substantially higher ventricular arrhythmia burden among these patients and a poorer survival compared with ATP-only treated patients. A recent study supported this finding

that the increased mortality is due to the underlying arrhythmia, and not the physical effect of the shock itself, as those who receive shock for inappropriate reasons did not have increased mortality compared with those without any shock.[6]

In the United States, more than 250,000 ICD implantations occurred in 2011, with most (>70%) for primary prevention indications.[18] Inevitably, clinicians will be faced with increasingly complex management issues pertaining to shock therapy, both appropriate and inappropriate. Knowledge in strategies to reduce shock therapy is vital, as it is associated with significant beneficial implications to the patient, as well as the health care system (**Box 2**).

Management Options to Minimize Shock Therapy

1. Medical therapy
2. Catheter ablation
3. Advanced device programming

General measures, such as electrolyte replacement and avoidance of aggravating factors like sleep deprivation, caffeine, alcohol, over-the-counter medications, herbal remedies (eg, gingko, ephedra, ginseng, guarana, and yohimbine), and cardiac stimulants (eg, theophylline, cocaine, and amphetamines), should be used. Patients with underlying heart disease should be on optimal medical therapy (eg, aspirin, angiotensin-converting enzyme inhibitor/angiotensin receptor blocker, beta-blockers, aldosterone antagonists, statins). Treatment of other underlying structural or ischemic heart disease should be considered, as these are associated with proarrhythmia.

MEDICAL THERAPY

Beta-blocker therapy can be beneficial in reducing shocks of any type, as they can suppress supraventricular tachycardias, as well as ventricular ectopy and arrhythmias. Recently, analysis of the

---

Box 1
Classifications of shock therapy

1. Appropriate shocks: triggered by life-threatening ventricular arrhythmias, which can be further classified as follows:

    a. Necessary shocks: shock delivered due to failure of antitachycardia pacing (ATP) therapy/other means

    b. Avoidable shocks: as a result of underutilization of other termination methods

2. Inappropriate shocks: shocks triggered from incorrect detection

---

Box 2
Benefits of shock-avoidance techniques

1. Improved survival
2. Better quality of life
3. Reduced hospitalizations
4. Increased ICD battery life
5. Lower health care expenditure
6. Less need for post-shock care
7. Greater acceptance of ICD therapy

Multicenter Automatic Defibrillator Implantation With Cardiac Resynchronization Therapy (MADIT-CRT) trial found that there were even intraclass differences in the rates of inappropriate ICD therapy (ATP or shock without the presence of ventricular arrhythmia) among beta-blockers. Carvedilol was associated with a 36% lower rate of inappropriate ICD therapies compared with metoprolol, and a 50% reduction in inappropriate therapies due to atrial fibrillation.[19]

Amiodarone is a commonly utilized antiarrhythmic but has serious long-term adverse effects. In the Sudden Cardiac Death in Heart Failure (SCD-HeFT) trial, although amiodarone was not associated with increased mortality overall, among patients with New York Heart Association Class III heart failure, increased deaths were observed.[3] A recent meta-analysis found that amiodarone was associated with a 29% reduction of sudden cardiac death and 18% reduction of cardiovascular mortality.[20] The Optimal Pharmacologic Therapy in Cardioverter Defibrillator Patients (OPTIC) study was a randomized trial that compared amiodarone plus beta-blocker with sotalol alone or beta-blocker alone in 412 patients who had received a dual-chamber ICD for inducible or spontaneous ventricular tachycardia (VT) or ventricular fibrillation (VF) and left ventricular ejection fraction lower than 40% or syncope. During 1 year of follow-up, shocks occurred in 41 patients (38.5%) assigned to beta-blocker alone, in 26 (24.3%) assigned to sotalol alone, and in 12 (10.3%) assigned to amiodarone plus beta-blocker, a difference that was statistically significant.[21]

Despite the lack of clinical data applicable to current defibrillation systems, it has been noted that chronic amiodarone administration causes a significant increase in defibrillation threshold (DFT). In addition, clinicians need to be aware that antiarrhythmic drugs can influence antitachycardia pacing and tachycardia detection.[22,23]

CATHETER ABLATION

Although medications are often the first line of adjunctive therapy in patients with repeated episodes of shock for ventricular arrhythmia, they are associated with considerable side effects and inherent risks. Further, medical therapy is not universally successful in preventing further ventricular arrhythmia, and in some patients a more invasive approach must be taken with catheter ablation. Determining the effectiveness of catheter ablation in clinical studies has been somewhat challenging as a result of maintenance of antiarrhythmic therapy pre and post ablation.

More recent studies have shown that in patients with recurrent VT and subsequent ICD therapies, catheter ablation significantly decreases the frequency of subsequent VT events. In one trial using THERMOCOOL catheters (Biosense Webster, CA), patients had a median of 11.5 episodes of VT in the 6 months preceding ablation, compared with a median of 0 episodes in the 6 months following, and frequency of VT was reduced by more than 75% in two-thirds of patients.[24] VT recurrence after ablation was associated with the presence of increased patient comorbidities, age, and higher number of inducible VTs at time of ablation.

Initial attempts at catheter ablation were complicated by the need for hemodynamic stability while in the arrhythmia, allowing mapping to be performed. However, with improved technology, specifically electroanatomic mapping, targets and foci of arrhythmia could be identified and tagged as areas of low voltage or scar.[25] This allowed for mapping and successful ablation of targets while in sinus or with pace mapping, rather than the need for induction of ventricular arrhythmia, with an associated reduction in VT recurrence and subsequent need for ICD therapies.[25,26]

Despite advancements in catheter ablation techniques and technology, it remains an invasive procedure with relatively high procedural mortality. Furthermore, the previously mentioned ablation trials have shown that there is still a high post procedure follow-up mortality, with one-third attributable to arrhythmic death, and another third to heart failure mortality.

Perhaps most importantly, few data remain regarding ablation in nonischemic disease, and this substrate differs in that there is diffuse scar, often with more epicardial origin than the endocardial scar seen with prior infarction.[27]

In electrical storm and in incessant VT presentations, catheter ablation has been shown to improve outcomes by altering the substrate or by targeting triggers of arrhythmia (premature ventricular contractions). Studies have shown the ability to eliminate electrical storm, and to reduce ICD therapies in patients who underwent ablation.[28,29]

Finally, studies have also evaluated the utility of catheter ablation before ICD implantation. These have shown that ablation significantly decreases the rate of ICD shocks and increases the time to first ventricular arrhythmic event.[30,31]

DEVICE PROGRAMMING

There are many different adjustable parameters in ICDs that allow for the reduction of shocks, both avoidable and inappropriate, and thus improve patient satisfaction and outcomes.

Lowest Detected Rate

Patients who receive defibrillators for primary prevention tend to have spontaneous VT rates that are significantly faster in comparison with patients implanted for secondary prevention indications. Among 829 patients with an ICD in a primary prevention study, 269 patients (33.2%) received a shock, of which 128 patients received only appropriate shocks, based on a slowest detection rate of 188 beats per minute (bpm) (<320 ms).[16] In the primary prevention MADIT Reduce Inappropriate Therapy (MADIT-RIT) trial, patients were randomized to conventional tachycardia detection choices, high tachycardia rate detection (200 bpm), or prolonged tachycardia detection at slower detection time (60 seconds) with slow detection rate (170 bpm). This pivotal randomized study demonstrated that by restricting the delivery of initial therapy only to rates that exceed 200 bpm or delaying tachycardia detection at conventional detection rates resulted in a 50% relative risk reduction in any inappropriate shocks and a 55% risk reduction in mortality in comparison with conventional programming.[32] Of interest, although not the focus of the publication, these programming choices also reduced appropriate therapies and appropriate shocks in a differential manner, suggesting that there is value to both delaying detection and raising the detection rate in patients receiving primary prevention.

Patients on antiarrhythmic drug therapy and patients with secondary prevention indications because of sustained monomorphic VT tend to experience slower tachycardias. Therefore, for patients with secondary prevention indications, a safety margin of 40 ms between the slowest spontaneous or induced VT cycle length and the cutoff rate cycle length is recommended.[33]

By comparison, clinical supraventricular tachycardias (SVT) usually range between 160 and 180 bpm. In the Primary Prevention Parameters Evaluation (PREPARE) study there was a 3.6% event rate with SVT discrimination limit rate set at less than 200 bpm.[34] Volosin and colleagues[35] proposed an even greater SVT discrimination limit of 230 bpm, as most patients have SVT rates up to this rate. Increasing the SVT discrimination rate limit is increasingly important, as the slowest tachycardia rate is increased and as ATP is programmed in the 230 to 250 bpm range.

Detection Duration

Early clinical trials with ICD therapy had aggressive protocols to detect and deliver therapy. However, it has been increasingly recognized that many VTs terminate without the need for ICD therapy. The PREPARE trial found that with increased detection durations to declare VT (30 of 40 consecutive beats had to be in the therapy zone) and deliver therapy, with ATP and SVT discriminators programmed, there was a reduction in all ICD shocks compared with standard programming (8.5% vs 16.9%), and there was no change in the rates of untreated VT or arrhythmic syncope.[34] Further, mortality was reduced with delayed detection (4.9% vs 8.7%).

In the MADIT-RIT trial, patients in the duration delay arm had therapy delayed for 60 seconds for rates greater than 170 bpm, 12 seconds for rates greater than 200 bpm, and 2.5 seconds for rates greater than 250 bpm. As many arrhythmias would terminate without therapy, this programming strategy resulted in a 50% reduction in inappropriate ICD therapies.[32]

Antitachycardia Pacing (ATP)

ATP, the process by which a defibrillator delivers a burst of pacing at a cycle length slightly shorter than the VT cycle length to terminate the arrhythmia, has been proven in multiple studies to significantly diminish the number of shocks delivered by the device.[15,34,36,37] When first developed, ATP was used primarily for slow VT, but these same studies showed that ATP also could be used to terminate faster VT.

There are different types of ATP programming available, namely burst (at a set fraction of the VT cycle length) or ramp (pacing starts at a fraction of the VT cycle length with each subsequent pulse coming with incrementally shorter coupling intervals); however, the purpose is the same: to enter the arrhythmia circuit and create bidirectional block that terminates the reentry. The number of stimuli to enter the circuit and block may vary, and in some cases require an extra stimulus at the end of a pacing burst to achieve block. Further, location of the VT circuit relative to the pacing stimulus (lead location) may lead to difficulty in entering the circuit and creating block, and in some instances left ventricular or simultaneous right and left ventricular stimuli may improve efficacy.[38] Slower VTs usually will require more aggressive ATP (shorter cycle length relative to tachycardia cycle length) to terminate the arrhythmia, but the faster the cycle becomes the greater the risk of accelerating the cycle length of the arrhythmia.

The delay between ATP therapy and shock, in cases in which ATP is unsuccessful in terminating VT, may be lessened by the ability to charge while delivering ATP therapy. Although this has the benefit of decreasing the time to shock therapy, it does increase the risk of an avoidable shock for rhythms that were successfully terminated with ATP, due to the differences in confirmation of rhythm when charged versus redetection post-ATP by the device.[39]

Ultimately, ATP is a key feature of ICDs, which can prevent shocks by either delaying the time to shock therapy and, more importantly, by terminating the ventricular arrhythmia before shock is necessary.

SVT Discrimination

The most common causes of inappropriate shocks in the MADIT-II trial were atrial fibrillation (44%) followed by SVT (36%).[40] This finding, replicated in several studies, has culminated in many device algorithms being developed to distinguish these arrhythmias from VT. Among the various algorithms, morphology criteria and AV relationship add importantly to discrimination accuracy.

However, detection rate and duration, discussed previously, are fundamental to SVT and VT discrimination, which not only distinguishes nonsustained from sustained arrhythmias, but also between SVT and atrial fibrillation versus VT. The primary importance of detection rate and duration was emphatically documented in the PREPARE and MADIT-RIT trials. These additional discrimination techniques differ according to the type of device: single-chamber versus dual-chamber defibrillators. The primary modes available in single-chamber defibrillators to discriminate SVT from VT include sudden onset, stability, and morphology. Each of these programmable features enhances accurate rhythm identification and work optimally in certain situations.

Sudden Onset

The quickness of onset of tachycardia can be used to distinguish sinus tachycardia from VT, as sinus tachycardia has a gradual onset. Once a tachycardia has been detected, the device measures the difference between the shortest RR interval before the onset of the tachycardia and that at the beginning of the tachycardia. VT is declared if this difference is greater than the programmed value. This feature may inappropriately identify SVTs that are also of sudden onset as ventricular arrhythmias. Conversely, slow VT may go unrecognized as "nonsudden."[41–43] In the case of exercise-induced VT, in which there is a gradual onset, appropriate therapy could be potentially withheld. Ultimately, while used initially in earlier-model ICDs, the significance placed on sudden onset criteria for SVT discrimination is waning.

Stability

Analysis of cycle length beat-to-beat stability was developed to differentiate VT from the variable ventricular rate seen in atrial fibrillation. Each device manufacturer uses different methods of discrimination. Medtronic devices (Medtronic, Minneapolis, MN, USA) compare the current RR interval with the 3 previous RR intervals since the VT episode was declared. If this value is greater than the programmed stability value, it is considered irregular. It also incorporates "PR logic," where it calculates the percentage of how often the 2 most frequent intervals occur and are labeled as atrial fibrillation if less than 50%.

St Jude devices (St. Jude Medical Inc, St. Paul, MN, USA) classify the rhythm as atrial fibrillation based on "sinus interval history" and if the difference between the second longest and second shortest RR intervals is beyond the programmed stability interval. There is constant re-analysis of the rhythm; therefore, if the tachycardia became subsequently stable, or the sustained rate duration period is satisfied, therapy may well be initiated if the rate persisted above the programmed cutoff rate.

In general, there is a trade-off between increasing the programmed stability interval, which increases sensitivity but reduces specificity.[44] The combination of sudden-onset and stability criteria performs well at ventricular rates less than 190 bpm, and accuracy deteriorates with faster heart rates.[41] False-positive detections could occur in the setting of fast atrial fibrillation with a pseudo-regular ventricular response. Underdetection of VT is of concern if the patient has polymorphic VT, and in the setting of ischemic VT with a varying reentrant circuit.[41] Overall, application of sudden-onset and stability criteria with a time-related override has a sensitivity of 100% and specificity of 83% for ventricular arrhythmia detection.[41] Interestingly, in the EMPIRIC and PREPARE trials, in which additional safety features such as high-rate time-out and sustained rate duration were switched off, there was no difference in adverse events.[34,36] The value of cycle length stability is also reduced with greater insights into programming, detection rate, duration, AV relationship, and morphology.

Morphology

The introduction of morphology criteria enhanced the appropriate classification of SVT, particularly sudden-onset arrhythmia with regular RR intervals (eg, atrial flutter and atrial tachycardia) from VT. This algorithm is based on the creation of a template in sinus rhythm, SVT, and VT with subsequent quantification of the percentage match (programmable). The differences in the algorithm are based primarily on filtering and alignment methods, plus the waveform characteristics used to differentiate the tachycardia versus the stored electrogram template. Inaccuracies of the baseline template can lead to inappropriate classification of normal rhythms. Furthermore, inaccurate classifications can occur when the morphology of the VT is similar to the intrinsic. Changes in electrogram (EGM) morphology due to truncation of high-voltage signals, acute ischemic EGM changes, EGM maturation, and myopotential interference are potential situations that are prone to inaccurate categorization.[45]

Among device manufacturers, where morphology criteria were used as the sole discriminator, trials involving Medtronic (Wavelet) quote a sensitivity of 98.6% (accurate identification of VT/VF) and a specificity of 78.2% (proportion of SVT accurately identified).[46] Sensitivity and specificity ranges for a St. Jude device vary between 77% and 94%, and 71% and 95%, respectively.[47–49] Preliminary trials with Boston Scientific's Rhythm ID algorithm (Boston Scientific, Natick, MA, USA) using vector timing and correlation algorithm have demonstrated both a high sensitivity (99%) and specificity (97%).[50] Among the 3 discrimination modalities, morphology criterion is perhaps the most effective tool to discriminate SVT from VT in a single-chamber device.

AV Relationship and Choosing Single-Chamber or Dual-Chamber ICDs

Choosing between single-chamber or dual-chamber defibrillators to improve ICD discrimination has been a topic of substantial controversy. The presence of an atrial lead enables the timing and pattern of atrial activity and determines the association with ventricular signals, in addition to using single-chamber ICD discrimination algorithms. PR Logic (Medtronic), PARAD+ (Sorin, Arvada, CO, USA), SMART (Biotronik, Lake Oswego, OR, USA), Rhythm ID (Guidant/Boston Scientific), and the St. Jude dual-chamber algorithm are various dual-chamber discrimination algorithms that are based on the premise that the ventricular rate exceeds the atrial rate in vast majority of ventricular arrhythmias. Although the various manufacturers quote different specificities for their dual-chamber discrimination algorithm, determining superiority requires head-to-head trials; some of which are under way.

The critical question is whether dual-chamber defibrillators add value to ICD discrimination in a patient without pacing. Although several trials have attempted to address this important question, because of the small size of these studies, a

definite recommendation cannot be made.[43,51,52] A meta-analysis of 5 prospective trials showed that there was a 36% reduction in inappropriately treated episodes per patient with dual-chamber discrimination algorithms compared with single-chamber devices.[53] There was no reduction in the total number of individuals receiving inappropriate therapy. The reason behind this finding has been attributed to undersensing atrial activity and functional undersensing due to atrial blanking. Attempts at correcting the latter has unfortunately led to increased far-field R-wave sensing. Recently, Biotronik introduced Linox^{SMART}S DX, which is a single ventricular lead with ring electrodes located at the junction of the atrium and superior vena cava and the other free-floating in the atrium.[54] Presently, there is a need for further trials to demonstrate morbidity, mortality, and financial implications of newer-generation single-chamber versus dual-chamber ICDs to assist with this decision-making process. More significant outcome improvements have been made with programming prolonged tachycardia detection durations and increased tachycardia detection rates than by adding an atrial lead.

Ventricular Oversensing

Ventricular oversensed events broadly encompass the inappropriate recognition of non-QRS complexes of the electrogram waveform, as well as electrical artifacts originating from both internal and external sources. The ALTITUDE study evaluated 1570 inappropriate shocks, of which 134 (8.5%) were attributed to noise, artifact, and oversensing. Of these 134 events, 76 (57%) were attributed to external noise, 37 (28%) had lead connector–related problems, muscle noise present in 11 (8%), oversensing of atrial events in 7 (5%), T-wave oversensing in 2 (2%), and other noise in 1 (1%).[55]

Breakdown in lead integrity, such as the widely publicized Riata and Fidelis leads, culminated in the development of lead-monitoring systems. Medtronic's lead integrity alert system continuously monitors for changes in impedance, sensing integrity counter episodes, and very fast nonsustained VTs. Subsequently, the patient and clinician are alerted of this, while the VF number of intervals for detection is extended to 30/40. This setup has shown to provide at least a 3-day advanced warning for 75% of patients with lead fractures.[56] Presently all major device manufacturers have developed lead-monitoring systems with some functional differences.

Any apparatus that emits radiofrequency waves between 0 and 10^9 Hz can generate electromagnetic interference (EMI) and therefore prevent proper device function. The incidence of EMI has been significantly reduced with the modern-generation ICDs that routinely use bipolar leads, minimizing the physical zone of electrical reception. There is no significant difference in oversensing between true bipolar leads and integrated bipolar leads.[55] Improved lead-shielding material (eg, titanium), advanced filtration methods, and proprietary noise detection and rejection algorithms have dramatically reduced shocks due to EMI.

T-wave oversensing has been reported in some studies to be the commonest cause of ventricular oversensing, leading to inappropriate shocks as a result of double-counting.[57] Various solutions have been proposed to reduce this problem without undersensing VT or VF. Medtronic's T-wave discrimination algorithm uses stored information differentiating R waves from T waves based on amplitude, frequency content, and pattern in contrast to R and T patterns from VT/VF.[58] Some algorithms automatically increase the sensitivity threshold after a sensed ventricular event followed by a smooth decay to minimize detection of the T wave. The percentage change in sensitivity threshold and the decay time interval are programmable. Certain clinical situations require particular attention, including prominent T waves (hypertrophic cardiomyopathy, hyperkalemia, and short QT syndrome) and prolonged QT interval (long QT syndrome). St. Jude and Biotronik's "decay-delay" algorithm was designed to manage this issue by commencing the delay after a programmable time interval.

Remote Interrogation and Monitoring

The Lumos-T Safely RedUceS RouTine Office Device Follow-Up (TRUST) trial investigated Biotronik's home monitoring system which does not require a land telephone connection and has the capability of transmitting information from any location worldwide. This technology facilitated time-sensitive review of patients with specific device-related issues (eg, impedance changes) and provided an opportunity for early detection/therapy of asymptomatic SVT/atrial fibrillation, which could potentially lead to inappropriate shock therapy.[59] It also demonstrated that more consistent follow-up is possible in comparison with the conventional in-hospital device checks. Importantly, this setup has reduced both appropriate and inappropriate shock delivery with a significant reduction in the need for hospitalization.[60] Remote monitoring capabilities are now provided by most of the major device manufacturers.

In addition, remote interrogation data registries of more than 100,000 patients from both Medtronic (Carelink) and Boston Scientific (Lattitude) have documented a huge variance in the programming of tachycardia-detection parameters from the standards discussed previously. Use of ATP, detection duration, detection rate, and SVT discrimination algorithms was remarkably low in clinical practice. Use of remote monitoring to detect atrial fibrillation, rapid ventricular response, suboptimal programming choices, lead integrity issues that could lead to noise and inappropriate therapies, and frequent nonsustained arrhythmias are examples of the substantial value to remote interrogation and monitoring.

SUMMARY

ICDs have indisputable benefit in the reduction in mortality in select patient populations, and are proven in both primary and secondary prevention of sudden cardiac death. Despite this benefit, ICD shocks carry a tremendous burden to patients, including physical and emotional stress, and have been associated with depression, anxiety, and trauma like experiences; these effects lead some to live in fear of further shocks, or disarm the therapies entirely. Recent evidence suggests that shocks may reduce the mortality benefit, as well as affect patient satisfaction and quality-of-life substantially, and therefore shock avoidance is desirable.

Improvements in medication and catheter ablation techniques and technologies have allowed for alteration in the cardiac milieu and reductions in sustained ventricular arrhythmias, which in turn leads to a reduction in the need for shock.

ICD technology has been most dynamic with regard to shock avoidance. Through improved programming, application of advanced algorithms for arrhythmia detection, mechanisms to minimize ventricular oversensing, and remote monitoring, ICD shocks can be significantly reduced without compromising patient safety. The evidence that prolongation of time to therapy and restriction of therapy to faster tachycardias has shifted conventional thinking, and has profoundly reduced patient exposure to therapy.

REFERENCES

1. Moss AJ, Hall WJ, Cannom DS, et al. Improved survival with an implanted defibrillator in patients with coronary disease at high risk for ventricular arrhythmia. Multicenter Automatic Defibrillator Implantation Trial Investigators. N Engl J Med 1996; 335(26):1933–40.
2. Moss AJ, Zareba W, Hall WJ, et al. Prophylactic implantation of a defibrillator in patients with

myocardial infarction and reduced ejection fraction. N Engl J Med 2002;346(12):877–83.

3. Bardy GH, Lee KL, Mark DB, et al. Amiodarone or an implantable cardioverter-defibrillator for congestive heart failure. N Engl J Med 2005;352(3):225–37.

4. Buxton AE, Lee KL, Fisher JD, et al. A randomized study of the prevention of sudden death in patients with coronary artery disease. Multicenter Unsustained Tachycardia Trial Investigators. N Engl J Med 1999;341(25):1882–90.

5. Larsen GK, Evans J, Lambert WE, et al. Shocks burden and increased mortality in implantable cardioverter-defibrillator patients. Heart Rhythm 2011;8(12):1881–6.

6. Powell BD, Saxon LA, Boehmer JP, et al. Survival after shock therapy in implantable cardioverter-defibrillator and cardiac resynchronization therapy-defibrillator recipients according to rhythm shocked: the ALTITUDE survival by rhythm study. J Am Coll Cardiol 2013;62(18):1674–9.

7. Pelletier D, Gallagher R, Mitten-Lewis S, et al. Australian implantable cardiac defibrillator recipients: quality-of-life issues. Int J Nurs Pract 2002;8(2):68–74.

8. Ahmad M, Bloomstein L, Roelke M, et al. Patients' attitudes toward implanted defibrillator shocks. Pacing Clin Electrophysiol 2000;23(6):934–8.

9. Heller SS, Ormont MA, Lidagoster L, et al. Psychosocial outcome after ICD implantation: a current perspective. Pacing Clin Electrophysiol 1998;21(6):1207–15.

10. Mirowski M, Mower MM, Staewen WS, et al. Standby automatic defibrillator. An approach to prevention of sudden coronary death. Arch Intern Med 1970;126(1):158–61.

11. Kuck KH, Cappato R, Siebels J, et al. Randomized comparison of antiarrhythmic drug therapy with implantable defibrillators in patients resuscitated from cardiac arrest: the Cardiac Arrest Study Hamburg (CASH). Circulation 2000;102(7):748–54.

12. Epstein AE, DiMarco JP, Ellenbogen KA, et al. ACC/AHA/HRS 2008 guidelines for device-based therapy of cardiac rhythm Abnormalities: a report of the American College of Cardiology/American Heart Association Task Force on Practice Guidelines (Writing Committee to Revise the ACC/AHA/NASPE 2002 Guideline Update for Implantation of Cardiac Pacemakers and Antiarrhythmia Devices): developed in collaboration with the American Association for Thoracic Surgery and Society of Thoracic Surgeons. Circulation 2008;117(21):e350–408.

13. Irvine J, Dorian P, Baker B, et al. Quality of life in the Canadian Implantable Defibrillator Study (CIDS). Am Heart J 2002;144(2):282–9.

14. Sears SE Jr, Conti JB. Understanding implantable cardioverter defibrillator shocks and storms: medical and psychosocial considerations for research and clinical care. Clin Cardiol 2003;26(3):107–11.

15. Wathen MS, DeGroot PJ, Sweeney MO, et al. Prospective randomized multicenter trial of empirical antitachycardia pacing versus shocks for spontaneous rapid ventricular tachycardia in patients with implantable cardioverter-defibrillators: pacing fast ventricular tachycardia reduces shock therapies (PainFREE Rx II) trial results. Circulation 2004;110(17):2591–6.

16. Poole JE, Johnson GW, Hellkamp AS, et al. Prognostic importance of defibrillator shocks in patients with heart failure. N Engl J Med 2008;359(10):1009–17.

17. Sweeney MO, Sherfesee L, DeGroot PJ, et al. Differences in effects of electrical therapy type for ventricular arrhythmias on mortality in implantable cardioverter-defibrillator patients. Heart Rhythm 2010;7(3):353–60.

18. Kremers MS, Hammill SC, Berul CI, et al. The National ICD Registry Report: version 2.1 including leads and pediatrics for years 2010 and 2011. Heart Rhythm 2013;10(4):e59–65.

19. Ruwald MH, Abu-Zeitone A, Jons C, et al. Impact of carvedilol and metoprolol on inappropriate implantable cardioverter-defibrillator therapy: the MADIT-CRT trial (Multicenter Automatic Defibrillator Implantation With Cardiac Resynchronization Therapy). J Am Coll Cardiol 2013;62(15):1343–50.

20. Piccini JP, Berger JS, O'Connor CM. Amiodarone for the prevention of sudden cardiac death: a meta-analysis of randomized controlled trials. Eur Heart J 2009;30(10):1245–53.

21. Connolly SJ, Dorian P, Roberts RS, et al. Comparison of beta-blockers, amiodarone plus beta-blockers, or sotalol for prevention of shocks from implantable cardioverter defibrillators: the OPTIC Study: a randomized trial. JAMA 2006;295(2):165–71.

22. Jung W, Manz M, Luderitz B. Effects of antiarrhythmic drugs on defibrillation threshold in patients with the implantable cardioverter defibrillator. Pacing Clin Electrophysiol 1992;15(4 Pt 3):645–8.

23. Bollmann A, Husser D, Cannom DS. Antiarrhythmic drugs in patients with implantable cardioverter-defibrillators. Am J Cardiovasc Drugs 2005;5(6):371–8.

24. Stevenson WG, Wilber DJ, Natale A, et al. Irrigated radiofrequency catheter ablation guided by electroanatomic mapping for recurrent ventricular tachycardia after myocardial infarction: the multicenter thermocool ventricular tachycardia ablation trial. Circulation 2008;118(25):2773–82.

25. Marchlinski FE, Callans DJ, Gottlieb CD, et al. Linear ablation lesions for control of unmappable ventricular tachycardia in patients with ischemic

and nonischemic cardiomyopathy. Circulation 2000;101(11):1288–96.

26. Soejima K, Suzuki M, Maisel WH, et al. Catheter ablation in patients with multiple and unstable ventricular tachycardias after myocardial infarction: short ablation lines guided by reentry circuit isthmuses and sinus rhythm mapping. Circulation 2001;104(6):664–9.

27. Soejima K, Stevenson WG, Sapp JL, et al. Endocardial and epicardial radiofrequency ablation of ventricular tachycardia associated with dilated cardiomyopathy: the importance of low-voltage scars. J Am Coll Cardiol 2004;43(10):1834–42.

28. Della Bella P, Riva S, Fassini G, et al. Incidence and significance of pleomorphism in patients with post-myocardial infarction ventricular tachycardia. Acute and long-term outcome of radiofrequency catheter ablation. Eur Heart J 2004;25(13):1127–38.

29. Carbucicchio C, Santamaria M, Trevisi N, et al. Catheter ablation for the treatment of electrical storm in patients with implantable cardioverter-defibrillators: short- and long-term outcomes in a prospective single-center study. Circulation 2008; 117(4):462–9.

30. Kuck KH, Schaumann A, Eckardt L, et al. Catheter ablation of stable ventricular tachycardia before defibrillator implantation in patients with coronary heart disease (VTACH): a multicentre randomised controlled trial. Lancet 2010;375(9708):31–40.

31. Reddy VY, Reynolds MR, Neuzil P, et al. Prophylactic catheter ablation for the prevention of defibrillator therapy. N Engl J Med 2007;357(26): 2657–65.

32. Moss AJ, Schuger C, Beck CA, et al. Reduction in inappropriate therapy and mortality through ICD programming. N Engl J Med 2012;367(24): 2275–83.

33. Kuhlkamp V, Wilkoff BL, Brown AB, et al. Experience with a dual chamber implantable defibrillator. Pacing Clin Electrophysiol 2002;25(7):1041–8.

34. Wilkoff BL, Williamson BD, Stern RS, et al. Strategic programming of detection and therapy parameters in implantable cardioverter-defibrillators reduces shocks in primary prevention patients: results from the PREPARE (Primary Prevention Parameters Evaluation) study. J Am Coll Cardiol 2008;52(7): 541–50.

35. Volosin KJ, Exner DV, Wathen MS, et al. Combining shock reduction strategies to enhance ICD therapy: a role for computer modeling. J Cardiovasc Electrophysiol 2011;22(3):280–9.

36. Wilkoff BL, Ousdigian KT, Sterns LD, et al. A comparison of empiric to physician-tailored programming of implantable cardioverter-defibrillators: results from the prospective randomized multicenter EMPIRIC trial. J Am Coll Cardiol 2006; 48(2):330–9.

37. Wathen MS, Sweeney MO, DeGroot PJ, et al. Shock reduction using antitachycardia pacing for spontaneous rapid ventricular tachycardia in patients with coronary artery disease. Circulation 2001;104(7):796–801.

38. Yee R, Birgersdotter-Green U, Belk P, et al. The relationship between pacing site and induction or termination of sustained monomorphic ventricular tachycardia by antitachycardia pacing. Pacing Clin Electrophysiol 2010;33(1):27–32.

39. Schoels W, Steinhaus D, Johnson WB, et al. Optimizing implantable cardioverter-defibrillator treatment of rapid ventricular tachycardia: antitachycardia pacing therapy during charging. Heart Rhythm 2007;4(7):879–85.

40. Daubert JP, Zareba W, Cannom DS, et al. Inappropriate implantable cardioverter-defibrillator shocks in MADIT II: frequency, mechanisms, predictors, and survival impact. J Am Coll Cardiol 2008; 51(14):1357–65.

41. Brugada J, Mont L, Figueiredo M, et al. Enhanced detection criteria in implantable defibrillators. J Cardiovasc Electrophysiol 1998;9(3):261–8.

42. Swerdlow CD, Ahern T, Chen PS, et al. Underdetection of ventricular tachycardia by algorithms to enhance specificity in a tiered-therapy cardioverter-defibrillator. J Am Coll Cardiol 1994;24(2): 416–24.

43. Bansch D, Steffgen F, Gronefeld G, et al. The 1+1 trial: a prospective trial of a dual- versus a single-chamber implantable defibrillator in patients with slow ventricular tachycardias. Circulation 2004; 110(9):1022–9.

44. Nanthakumar K, Paquette M, Newman D, et al. Inappropriate therapy from atrial fibrillation and sinus tachycardia in automated implantable cardioverter defibrillators. Am Heart J 2000;139(5): 797–803.

45. Tzeis S, Andrikopoulos G, Kolb C, et al. Tools and strategies for the reduction of inappropriate implantable cardioverter defibrillator shocks. Europace 2008;10(11):1256–65.

46. Klein GJ, Gillberg JM, Tang A, et al. Improving SVT discrimination in single-chamber ICDs: a new electrogram morphology-based algorithm. J Cardiovasc Electrophysiol 2006;17(12):1310–9.

47. Boriani G, Occhetta E, Pistis G, et al. Combined use of morphology discrimination, sudden onset, and stability as discriminating algorithms in single chamber cardioverter defibrillators. Pacing Clin Electrophysiol 2002;25(9):1357–66.

48. Theuns DA, Rivero-Ayerza M, Goedhart DM, et al. Evaluation of morphology discrimination for ventricular tachycardia diagnosis in implantable cardioverter-defibrillators. Heart Rhythm 2006;3(11):1332–8.

49. Gronefeld GC, Schulte B, Hohnloser SH, et al. Morphology discrimination: a beat-to-beat algorithm

for the discrimination of ventricular from supraventricular tachycardia by implantable cardioverter defibrillators. Pacing Clin Electrophysiol 2001;24(10): 1519–24.

50. Gold MR, Shorofsky SR, Thompson JA, et al. Advanced rhythm discrimination for implantable cardioverter defibrillators using electrogram vector timing and correlation. J Cardiovasc Electrophysiol 2002;13(11):1092–7.

51. Theuns DA, Klootwijk AP, Goedhart DM, et al. Prevention of inappropriate therapy in implantable cardioverter-defibrillators: results of a prospective, randomized study of tachyarrhythmia detection algorithms. J Am Coll Cardiol 2004;44(12): 2362–7.

52. Friedman PA, McClelland RL, Bamlet WR, et al. Dual-chamber versus single-chamber detection enhancements for implantable defibrillator rhythm diagnosis: the detect supraventricular tachycardia study. Circulation 2006;113(25):2871–9.

53. Theuns DA, Rivero-Ayerza M, Boersma E, et al. Prevention of inappropriate therapy in implantable defibrillators: a meta-analysis of clinical trials comparing single-chamber and dual-chamber arrhythmia discrimination algorithms. Int J Cardiol 2008;125(3):352–7.

54. Bansch D, Schneider R, Akin I, et al. A new single chamber implantable defibrillator with atrial sensing: a practical demonstration of sensing and ease of implantation. J Vis Exp 2012;(60). pii: 3750.

55. Saxon LA, Hayes DL, Gilliam FR, et al. Long-term outcome after ICD and CRT implantation and influence of remote device follow-up: the ALTITUDE survival study. Circulation 2010;122(23):2359–67.

56. Swerdlow CD, Gunderson BD, Ousdigian KT, et al. Downloadable algorithm to reduce inappropriate shocks caused by fractures of implantable cardioverter-defibrillator leads. Circulation 2008; 118(21):2122–9.

57. Gilliam FR 3rd. T-wave oversensing in implantable cardiac defibrillators is due to technical failure of device sensing. J Cardiovasc Electrophysiol 2006;17(5):553–6.

58. Cao J, Gillberg JM, Swerdlow CD. A fully automatic, implantable cardioverter-defibrillator algorithm to prevent inappropriate detection of ventricular tachycardia or fibrillation due to T-wave oversensing in spontaneous rhythm. Heart Rhythm 2012;9(4): 522–30.

59. Varma N, Michalski J, Epstein AE, et al. Automatic remote monitoring of implantable cardioverter-defibrillator lead and generator performance: the Lumos-T Safely RedUceS RouTine Office Device Follow-Up (TRUST) trial. Circ Arrhythm Electrophysiol 2010;3(5):428–36.

60. Guedon-Moreau L, Lacroix D, Sadoul N, et al. A randomized study of remote follow-up of implantable cardioverter defibrillators: safety and efficacy report of the ECOST trial. Eur Heart J 2013;34(8): 605–14.

Lead Extractions
Indications, Procedural Aspects, and Outcomes

Ulrika M. Birgersdotter-Green, MD[a],*,
Victor G. Pretorius, MBChB[b]

KEYWORDS

- Lead extraction • Lead extraction indications • Lead recall • Lead extraction tools
- Device infections

KEY POINTS

- The number of implantable cardiac devices (cardiac implantable electronic devices [CIEDs]) is increasing.
- There is a trend toward increasing CIED infections.
- Lead malfunction and recalls require careful and potentially difficult lead management issues.
- There is an increased demand for lead extraction skills and comprehensive lead management programs.

INTRODUCTION

An estimated 10,000 to 15,000 pacemaker and implantable cardioverter defibrillator (ICD) leads are extracted annually worldwide.[1] New indications for device therapy and with that an increasing number of CIEDs placed contribute to the need for lead extractions. A higher lead prevalence due to an increased life expectancy as well as implantation of cardiac resynchronization therapy (CRT) devices requiring more leads per patient also play a role. CIED infections are a common indication for system extraction. Therefore, infection rates have increased as the number and complexity of devices increase.[2] Most recently, the complex question of lead recalls and lead malfunctions have added to the increasing number of lead extractions.

INDICATIONS FOR LEAD EXTRACTION

The Heart Rhythm consensus statement from 2009 contains the current recommendations for lead extraction.[3] The recommendations are summarized in **Table 1**. Overall, the most common indication for an extraction is infection, but the indications will vary somewhat depending on the referral base, volume, and expertise of the extraction center. **Fig. 1** shows the lead extraction indications at the University of California, San Diego.

CIED Infection

The indications for lead extraction as a result of CIED infection are outlined in **Table 2**. The patient vignette (**Box 1**) demonstrates a *Class I* indication for lead extraction. His ICD system was extracted, and a new ICD system was placed only after an appropriate antibiotic course as per Infectious Disease recommendations.

Device infection rates reportedly range from 1% to 7%. ICDs have a higher rate of infection compared with pacemakers. Factors that increase the risk of device infection include diabetes mellitus,

Disclosures: U.M. Birgersdotter-Green research grants, honorarium—Medtronic, Boston Scientific, St Jude, Biotronik; V.G. Pretorius honorarium—Spectranetics.
[a] Division of Cardiology, UCSD Health System, 9444 Medical Center Drive, La Jolla, San Diego, CA 92037, USA;
[b] Division of Cardiothoracic Surgery, UCSD Health System, 9444 Medical Center Drive, La Jolla, San Diego, CA 92037, USA
* Corresponding author. 9444 Medical Center Drive, MC 7411, La Jolla, CA 92037.
E-mail address: ubgreen@ucsd.edu

Table 1
Indications overview

	Class I	Class IIa	Class IIb	Class III
Infection	X	X		X
Chronic pain		X		
Thrombosis or venous stenosis	X	X		
Functional leads	X		X	X
Nonfunctional leads	X	X	X	X

Adapted from Wilkoff BL, Love CJ, Byrd CL, et al. Transvenous lead extraction: heart rhythm society expert consensus on facilities, training, indications, and patient management. Heart Rhythm 2009;6(7):1085–104; with permission.

previous glucocorticoid therapy, underlying malignancy, operator inexperience, multiple lead placement, advanced patient age, oral anticoagulant use, frequent generator replacement, heart failure, fever before device implantation, use of temporary pacing catheters[4] nonpectoral (abdominal or thoracoscopic) implantations, and renal dysfunction.[3] CIED infections are associated with substantial morbidity and mortality, but it has also been shown that early and complete removal of CIED infected systems is associated with better outcomes.[5] Therefore, awareness of best management for infected CIED systems is imperative as is system-wide measurements to prevent infections.

Chronic Pain Indication

Severe chronic pain at the device or lead insertion site that failed medical management and had no alternative is a *Class IIa* indication. It would be appropriate to refer this patient for a discussion of the risks and benefits of an extraction procedure (**Box 2**).

Thrombosis or Venous Stenosis Indications

Ipsilateral venous occlusion if there is a contraindication for contralateral lead placement (arteriovenous [AV] fistula, mastectomy) is a *Class I* indication for extraction. This patient underwent a successful extraction of her left-sided right ventricular (RV) pacemaker lead and was upgraded to a biventricular ICD (CRT-D) device (**Box 3**). Other *Class I* indications include significant thromboembolic events originating from leads, bilateral subclavian or superior vena cava (SVC) occlusion precluding implantation of needed leads, SVC stenosis or occlusion with limiting symptoms, and also planned venous stent deployment to avoid lead entrapment. In the case of an ipsilateral occlusion at the time of placement of an additional lead, the current recommendation calls this a *Class IIa* indication.

Functional Lead Indications

There are several *Class I* indications for removal of functional leads, including when leads interfere

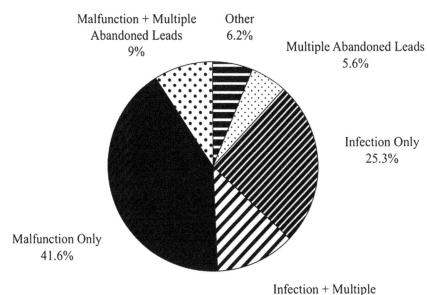

Fig. 1. University of California, San Diego, data from August 2010 to October 2013.

Table 2
Indications for transvenous extraction as a result of CIED infection

Definite CIED infection with
  Lead endocarditis
  Valvular endocarditis
Pocket infection with abscess formation
Superficial erosion
Chronic draining sinus
Occult gram-positive bacteremia
Persistent occult gram-negative bacteremia
Valvular endocarditis without evidence of
  device infection

Box 2
Patient vignette

- A 43-year-old woman status after pacemaker placement in 2003
- Has never used the pacemaker as per device interrogations
- Persistent pain at the PM site. Feels that it is firing and gives her a metallic taste in her mouth. Extensive negative workup
- Patient referred for lead extraction

with treatment of a malignancy such as radiation or reconstructive surgery (**Box 4**). Perhaps, the classic functional lead extraction indication is seen in leads that may pose an immediate threat to a patient because of design or failure, which is seen in the problematic Accufix "J" lead (Telectronics Pacing Systems, Englewood, CO, USA), with wire fracture and protrusion. This lead was recalled after 2 deaths and 2 nonfatal injuries related to protrusion of an electrically inactive "J" retention wire, resulting in laceration of the right atrium.[6] Other *Class I* indications include life-threatening arrhythmias due to retained leads and leads interfering with the operation of implanted cardiac devices. These clinical scenarios are generally less common, and one should keep in mind that although a *Class I* indication may exist for removal of a functional lead, an acceptable risk-to-benefit ratio needs to be in place.

Management of recalled leads typically falls under the Functional Lead indication for extraction, and although there is no consensus statement directly addressing the ongoing issues with the Sprint Fidelis ICD (Medtronic, Minneapolis, MN, USA) lead or the Riata ICD lead (St. Jude Medical, Inc, St. Paul, MN, USA), the HRS consensus statement[7] has classified a lead with potential future threat due to design as a *Class IIb* indication for

extraction. This classification indicates that the usefulness/efficacy of an extraction is less established by evidence/opinion and appropriately reflects the difficult clinical decision making in managing patients with these leads. Recommendations for clinicians managing lead advisory notices were included in a task force paper by Heart Rhythm Society on lead performance policies and guidelines,[8] and these recommendations are listed in **Table 3**.

The patient whose vignette is given in **Box 5** will clearly need a new ICD lead and would likely be better served by an extraction and new lead rather than with an additional lead. This is, however, a discussion between patient/family and physicians based on the extraction center's volume, expertise, and outcomes. In this case, the patient underwent an extraction with replacement of a single-coil ICD lead.

Other *Class IIb* indications include leads no longer used (RV lead in ICD upgrade), patients requiring specific imaging techniques with no alternative, and removal in consideration of upgrade to a magnetic resonance imaging (MRI)-conditional device.

There are also circumstances when there is no indication for extraction of functional leads, *Class III* indications. These circumstances include a functional but redundant lead if the life

Box 1
Patient vignette

- A 69-year-old man with history of coronary artery disease s/p coronary artery bypass graft in 1991 and VT s/p ICD in 2006. Battery at elective replacement indicator (ERI)
- Presents with fevers/chills, dry cough, and shortness of breath for 10 days
- Blood cultures growing *Staphylococcus aureus*, on IV antibiotics
- Patient referred for ICD generator replacement

Box 3
Patient vignette

- A 65-year-old woman with history of breast cancer, s/p right mastectomy
- Pacemaker placed on the left side for complete heart block 6 years ago
- Diagnosed with dilated cardiomyopathy with an indication for upgrade to a CRT-D device
- An occluded left subclavial vein is found
- The patient is referred for extraction and upgrade

Box 4
Patient vignette

- A 56-year-old woman with history of dual chamber pacemaker for sick sinus syndrome (SSS) in May 2010
- Recent left upper lobe nodule c/w lung cancer and need for irradiation of left side of chest
- Patient referred for pacemaker lead extraction and reimplantation of device to right side

---

Box 5
Patient vignette

- A 14-year-old boy with history of tetralogy of fallot (ToF), status postsurgical ventricular septal defect (VSD) repair at the age of 1 year followed by the RV conduit to pulmonary artery repair at the age of 7 years
- At age of 9 years, he had ventricular tachycardia causing syncope, s/p placement of a single-chamber Medtronic ICD with Sprint Fidelis lead
- Has had several episodes of VT requiring appropriate shocks
- Documentation of ICD lead fracture on remote monitoring
- Patient referred for lead extraction

---

expectancy is less than 1 year and known anomalous placement of a lead (subclavian artery, aorta, pleura, atrial or ventricular wall, or mediastinum) or through a systemic venous atrium or systemic ventricle. An anomalous lead may need to be removed but will likely need additional techniques including surgical consultation.

Table 3
Recommendations for clinicians managing lead advisory notices

1. Conservative noninvasive management with periodic device monitoring (remote or inperson, as appropriate) should be strongly considered particularly for:
   Patients who are not pacemaker dependent
   Patients with an ICD for primary prevention of sudden cardiac death who have not required device therapy for a ventricular arrhythmia
   Patients whose operative risk is high or patients who have other significant competing morbidities even when the risk of lead malfunction or patient harm is substantial
2. Lead revision or replacement should be considered if in the clinician's judgment:
   The risk of malfunction is likely to lead to patient's death or serious harm
   The risk of revision or replacement is believed to be less than the risk of patient harm from the lead malfunction
3. Reprogramming of the pacemaker or ICD should be performed when this can mitigate the risk of an adverse event from a lead malfunction

Adapted from Maisel WH, Hauser RG, Hammill SC, et al. Recommendations from the Heart Rhythm Society Task Force on Lead Performance Policies and Guidelines: developed in collaboration with the American College of Cardiology (ACC) and the American Heart Association (AHA). Heart Rhythm 2009;6(6):869–85; with permission.

Nonfunctional Lead Indications

The same *Class I* indications for extraction apply for nonfunctioning leads as well as for functioning leads. The patient described in **Box 6** has a *Class IIa* indication; more than 4 leads from one side or more than 5 leads through the SVC. He underwent an extraction of the right-sided RV lead with placement of a new ICD lead and left ventricular (LV) lead.

PROCEDURAL ASPECTS
Facilities and Training Requirements

Lead extraction procedures are often technically challenging with a risk of life-threatening complications in complex patients. Therefore, these procedures should only be done in hospitals where the environment provides full support of a lead management program, which includes a team-based approach involving the electrophysiologist,

---

Box 6
Patient vignette

- A 44-year-old man with history of congenital CHB, s/p transvenous pacemaker from left side at the age of 14 years
- At the age of 29 years, he had evidence of atrial and RV lead fractures and underwent placement of new right-sided dual chamber pacemaker
- Requires upgrade to CRT-D because of heart failure with low ejection fraction (EF) and pacemaker dependence
- Patient referred for lead extraction

cardiothoracic surgeon, anesthesia support, as well as operating room staff and electrophysiology laboratory staff. Available equipment should include all tools needed for extraction, including laser, mechanical rotational sheaths, and femoral extraction kit, as well as surgical instruments needed for an open extraction or emergency surgery.[9] The primary operator needs to both be properly trained and maintain a continued procedural volume. The current recommendations from the Heart Rhythm Society expert consensus[7] are as follows:

1. A physician being trained in lead extractions should extract a minimum of 40 leads as the primary operator under the direct supervision of a qualified training physician.
2. An operator should perform a minimum of 20 lead extractions per year to maintain competency.

Preprocedural Considerations

Considering the complexity of lead extraction and the potential for life-threatening complications, a written informed consent should be obtained, which should include an explanation of the critical elements of the planned procedure as well as the hospital's and physician's extraction volume and outcomes.

A thorough history and physical examination should be performed to identify not only the indication and need for lead extraction but also the presence of comorbidities that could affect the procedure or postoperative recovery.

Consultation with an infectious disease specialist to guide antibiotic therapy should be undertaken for infected device cases.

Preprocedural investigations could include the following:

- Chest radiograph to identify the number, location, and type of leads, as well as the lead's fixation mechanism. Superior vena cava defibrillator coils make the procedure more complex and riskier.[10]
- Chest computed tomographic (CT) scanning with three-dimensional reconstruction can be helpful if lead perforation of the vasculature or heart is expected.
- Venous Doppler or venography should be performed to determine patency of upper limb veins to plan extraction and device upgrade or replacement procedure.
- Echocardiography can identify the presence of lead vegetations and concomitant valvular and ventricular function that might aid procedural and anesthesia planning.

- Essential CIED interrogation to determine if the patient is pacer dependent and will require temporary pacing during extraction. Preprocedural settings and parameters should be recorded. Tachycardia therapies should be disabled to prevent inappropriate device shocks during electrocautery use.

Procedure Considerations

Older leads may not be removed with simple traction and might require complex extraction techniques. These techniques as well as simple traction have been associated with vascular injury or perforation that can lead to cardiac tamponade, hemothorax, AV fistula, tricuspid valve disruption or pulmonary embolism. To prevent these complications from resulting in mortality or severe morbidity, the following guiding principles should be followed:

- Extractions should be performed in an operating room with adequate fluoroscopy. Modern hybrid operating rooms are ideally suited for lead extractions.
- General anesthesia with endotracheal intubation allows for airway safety even in emergent situations and is routinely used.
- Intraoperative transesophageal echocardiography allows real-time monitoring of fluid status and cardiac function and can identify the development of pericardial or pleural effusions.
- Hemodynamic monitoring with an arterial line and large-bore central vascular access should be available for anesthesia for resuscitation in an emergency. Preferably, a low-placed right internal jugular Cordis can be used at the end of the procedure for access to place a temporary permanent external pacemaker system in patients with device infection who are pacer dependent.[11]
- Sterile preparation and exposure of the entire anterior chest and both groin areas should be performed to allow conversion to an open procedure.
- On-site cardiothoracic surgery involvement can help with planning of procedure and management of vascular or cardiac injuries.
- Four units of packed red blood cells should be available in the operating room.
- Femoral arterial and venous sheaths are placed for emergency establishment of cardiopulmonary bypass. Femoral venous access can also be used for temporary pacing purposes or for femoral extraction purposes.
- Antibiotic prophylaxis is administered 30 minutes before skin incision.

Device Pocket Preparation

Good surgical technique and strict hemostasis should be adhered to at all times. Complete capsulectomy should be performed for device infection cases with removal of all vascular and foreign material. Infected pockets can be treated with iodoform packing after extraction until healing by secondary intent or by negative-pressure wound therapy through application of a vacuum pump (**Fig. 2**) that promotes faster healing by inducing rapid granulation tissue formation.[12]

Findings of very dense adhesions or calcifications should alert the extractor to the potential of similar intravascular reactions around the leads. Calcifications are commonly seen in patients with renal failure. Avoidance of blood entrainment into the lead inner channel will improve the likelihood of passing the locking stylet all the way to the lead tip. If existing leads are to be left in place, avoidance of injury to the lead insulation is essential and plasma blade cautery should be used for lead dissection in these instances.

Lead Extraction Procedure

- The active fixation helix is retracted, and the lead is transected distal to the lead connector.
- A locking stylet (Liberator Universal Locking Stylet [Cook Medical Inc, Bloomington, IN, USA] or LLD EZ locking stylet [Spectranetics Corporation, Colorado Springs, CO, USA]) is inserted through the inner lead coil all the way to the tip of the lead for fixation. Correct location of the lead is enhanced by the radiopaque tip of these stylets making them visible on fluoroscopy. Lead fractures often occur at the costoclavicular junction, and extraction of these leads can be challenging because of inability to advance a locking stylet all the way to the tip.
- Insulation and conductor materials are secured to the locking stylet with a non-stretchable suture (Supramid S Jackson, Inc, Alexandria, VA, USA) to provide support and to form a rail to hold countertraction on multiple sites along the lead.
- A variety of specialized sheaths can then be advanced over the prepared lead to dissect the fibrous tissue and free the lead within the vasculature. Polypropylene, Teflon, and stainless-steel sheaths were initially used but have now been replaced by next-generation laser sheaths (CV-300 Eximer Laser and laser SLS II sheaths, Spectranetics Corporation) and rotating mechanical sheaths (Evolution, Cook Medical Inc), which yield higher success rates and are easier and safer to use. The laser sheath lyses adhesions via photochemolysis and photothermal ablation, whereas the mechanical sheath has a rotating treaded barrel tip that can separate binding sites mechanically. Often, densely calcified adhesions cannot be dissolved with laser, and the rotating mechanical sheath might be superior to break up the adhesions. The techniques for lead preparation, countertraction, and dissection

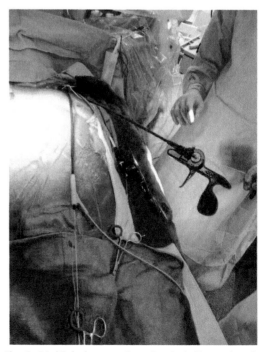

Fig. 3. Multiple laser and mechanical dilator sheaths working simultaneously.

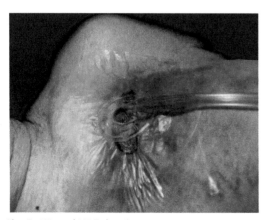

Fig. 2. Wound VAC dressing.

remain the same regardless of the instruments used or indications for extraction. Sheaths are lubricated with sterile light mineral oil to reduce friction and allow improved control of the sheath-lead interface. The sheath tip has to remain coaxial to the lead to reduce the likelihood of vascular injury. Sheath advancement forces and lead retraction forces should be balanced allowing the laser or rotating mechanical tip to free the adhesions up. Occasionally, it might be necessary to use a variety of sheaths on different leads simultaneously to break through very dense bindings (**Fig. 3**). Initially, it was thought that laser or mechanical rotation should not be used inside the coronary sinus when extracting an LV lead, but recently, such cases have been performed with good success and no complications. Due to its design with 3 expandable

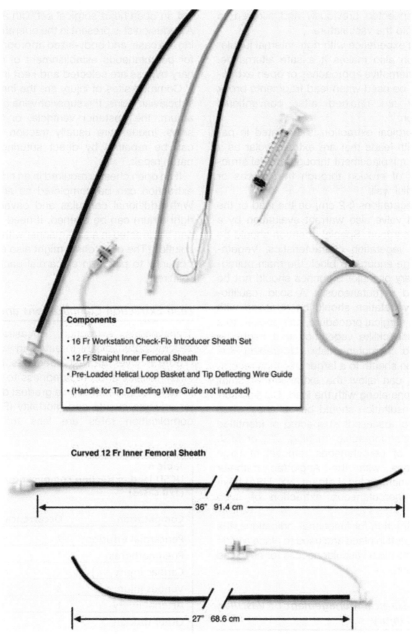

Components

- 16 Fr Workstation Check-Flo Introducer Sheath Set
- 12 Fr Straight Inner Femoral Sheath
- Pre-Loaded Helical Loop Basket and Tip Deflecting Wire Guide
- (Handle for Tip Deflecting Wire Guide not included)

Curved 12 Fr Inner Femoral Sheath

— 36" 91.4 cm —

— 27" 68.6 cm —

Fig. 4. Byrd workstation femoral intravascular retrieval set. (Permission for use granted by Cook Medical Incorporated, Bloomington, Indiana.)

polyurethane lobes, the Attain StarFix lead, Medtronic, can pose significant challenge in coronary sinus extraction.[13]

- Occasionally, when the superior approach fails, alternative routes of extraction should be considered. A variety of femoral extraction tools and snares have been developed for lead extraction including the Byrd Workstation Femoral Intravascular Retrieval Set (**Fig. 4**) and the Needle's Eye Snare (Cook Vascular, Inc, Leechburg, PA, USA). Femoral extraction is the preferred method in leads that have been transected previously and allowed to retract into the vasculature.
- Growing experience with right internal jugular extraction also makes it a safe alternative. These alternative approaches or open extraction can be used when lead fragments break off and are retained after conventional extraction.[14]
- Open surgical extraction is indicated in patients with leads that are extravascular as a result of misplacement through arterial structures or of erosion through the venous or myocardial wall.
- Large vegetations (>2 cm) on the lead or the tricuspid valve also warrant evaluation by a cardiac surgeon. Special attention should be paid to vegetation characteristics. Vegetations large enough to block the main pulmonary artery or major branches should not be extracted percutaneously. A solid, cauliflowerlike vegetation should be removed with an open surgical procedure, as opposed to a thin windsocklike vegetation that might be extracted percutaneously. Upgrading the extraction sheath to a larger size than recommended can allow the extraction of small vegetations along with the lead. Cardiac surgical consultation should be obtained when a cardiac abscess is suspected or identified on echocardiographic imaging, CT, or MRI. Reports of percutaneous removal of large vegetations with the AngioVac catheter (AngioDynamics Inc, Latham, NY, USA) have allowed percutaneous extraction of such cases.[4]
- After extraction for functional indications, the sheath is left in place and used to place a glide wire to maintain vascular access for new lead placement.

Emergency Surgical Management of Vascular and Cardiac Injury

Considering the frail state of many patients who require lead extraction, it is not unexpected that despite diligent technique, cardiac and vascular injuries can occur. These injuries can range from minor hematomas to catastrophic bleeding and even cardiac tamponade and death. Emergency preparedness can avoid these mortalities. A significant number of patients requiring lead extraction have had prior open heart surgery. In an emergency, surgical access can be achieved via an anterior thoracotomy or redo sternotomy. Circulatory support with blood transfusion and administration of inotropic and/or presser agents is required. Cardiac scrub technicians routinely lay out an open heart surgical set with a sternal saw. A perfusionist is present in the operating room during the case, and body-sized appropriate cannulas for percutaneous establishment of cardiopulmonary bypass are selected and kept in the room.

Common sites of injury are the innominate and subclavian veins, the superior vena cava, the right atrium, the posterior ventricle, or the coronary sinus. Injuries are usually traction induced and can be repaired by direct suturing or biologic patch repair.

If an open chest is required in an emergency, the extraction can be completed as an open case. With additional cannulas and caval snares, the right atrium can be opened. If need be, the heart can be arrested in a safe manner with cardioplegia solution. The open chest might also afford the opportunity to place an epicardial pacing system if required.

Lead Extraction Complications and Outcomes

Transvenous extraction is associated with several potential life-threatening complications (**Table 4**). Over the past 3 decades, improvement in techniques and preparedness to handle complications has resulted in a gradual decline in major adverse events and mortality (**Fig. 5**). Major complication rates are less than 2%, and

Table 4 UCSD lead extraction complication rate (170 cases)		
Complication	**Occurrence**	**Percent**
Pericardial effusion	2	1.2
Pneumothorax	1	0.6
Cardiac injury	1	0.6
Venous injury	3	1.7
Arterial injury	1	0.6
Other (pocket hematoma)	1	0.6

Abbreviation: UCSD, University of California, San Diego.

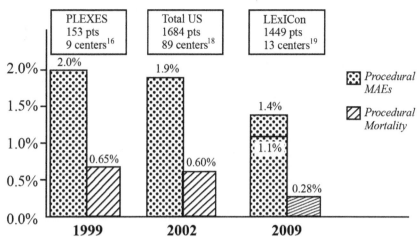

Fig. 5. Procedural outcome of laser-assisted lead extraction demonstrating major adverse events (MAEs) and procedural mortality. PLEXES, Pacemaker lead extraction with the laser sheath: results of the pacing lead extraction with the excimer sheath.

in-hospital mortality is less than 1% in experienced centers.[15–17] Older leads, extraction of ICD leads, female sex, renal failure, and low body mass index are independent predictors of major complications.[18] Extraction of infected leads, especially when lead vegetations are present, poses the potential risk of septic emboli to the lung, which can result in acute pulmonary hypertension and hypoxemia from large pulmonary emboli, acute septic shock, respiratory failure, or lung abscess formation.

Over a 3-year span at the University of California, San Diego, the lead management team has extracted 309 leads during 170 cases. No hospital mortality occurred. Although complications were infrequent (**Table 5**), 2 cases required emergent sternotomy for vascular injuries. Complete removal of all leads was achieved in 97.7% of lead extraction attempts. These results compare favorably to the *Lead Extraction Device Evaluation and Results Database (LEADER database)*[18,19] or the *LExICon Study* results.

Table 5
Potential lead extraction complications

Major Complications	Minor Complications
Death	Pericardial effusion not requiring intervention
Cardiac avulsion requiring intervention (percutaneous or surgical)	Hemothorax not requiring intervention
Vascular injury requiring intervention (percutaneous or surgical)	Pocket hematoma requiring reoperation
Pulmonary embolism requiring surgical intervention	Upper extremity thrombosis resulting in medical treatment
Respiratory arrest/anesthesia-related complication prolonging hospitalization	Vascular repair near implant site or venous entry site
Stroke	Hemodynamically significant air embolism
CIED infection at previously noninfected site	Migrated lead fragment without sequelae Blood transfusion as a result of intraoperative blood loss Pneumothorax requiring a chest tube Pulmonary embolism not requiring surgical intervention

From Maytin M, Epstein LM. Arrhythmias: the challenges of transvenous lead extraction. Heart 2011;97:425–34; with permission.

SUMMARY

As a result of more CIEDs being placed, there is a trend toward increasing device infections and increased concerns regarding lead malfunction. There is a greater need for lead extraction skills and comprehensive lead management programs. The current indications for lead extractions as per the 2009 Heart Rhythm consensus statement provide a systematic approach to different clinical scenarios where an extraction may be considered. Recent ICD lead recalls have added to the complexity of appropriate lead management and underscore the need for a comprehensive approach. A successful lead management program should offer trained operators collaborating together in a facility that provides full professional and technical support. Under these circumstances, lead extractions can be performed safely and can be an important addition to patient care.

REFERENCES

1. Hauser RG, Katsiyiannis WT, Gornick CC, et al. Deaths and cardiovascular injuries due to device-assisted implantable cardioverter-defibrillator and pacemaker lead extraction. Europace 2010;12(3): 395–401.

2. Greenspon AJ, Patel JD, Lau E, et al. 16-year trends in the infection burden for pacemakers and implantable cardioverter-defibrillators in the United States 1993 to 2008. J Am Coll Cardiol 2011;58(10):1001–6.

3. Mulpuru SK, Pretorius VG, Birgersdotter-Green UM. Device infections: management and indications for lead extraction. Circulation 2013;128(9):1031–8.

4. Patel N, Azemi T, Zaeem F, et al. Vacuum assisted vegetation extraction for the management of large lead vegetations. J Cardiovasc Surg 2013;28(3): 321–4. http://dx.doi.org/10.1111/jocs.12087 Source Henry Low Heart Center, Hartford Hospital, Hartford, Connecticut 06102, USA.

5. Le KY, Sohail MR, Friedman PA, et al. Impact of timing of device removal on mortality in patients with cardiovascular implantable electronic device infections. Heart Rhythm 2011;8(11):1678–85.

6. Lloyd MA, Hayes DL, Holmes DR Jr. Atrial "J" pacing lead retention wire fracture: radiographic assessment, incidence of fracture, and clinical management. Pacing Clin Electrophysiol 1995;18(5 Pt 1): 958–64.

7. Wilkoff BL, Love CJ, Byrd CL, et al. Transvenous lead extraction: heart rhythm society expert consensus on facilities, training, indications, and patient management: this document was endorsed by the American Heart Association (AHA). Heart Rhythm 2009;6(7):1085–104.

8. Maisel WH, Hauser RG, Hammill SC, et al. Recommendations from the heart rhythm society task force on lead performance policies and guidelines: developed in collaboration with the American College of Cardiology (ACC) and the American heart Association (AHA). Heart Rhythm 2009;6(6):869–85.

9. Love CJ, Wilkoff BL, Byrd CL, et al. Recommendations for extraction of chronically implanted transvenous pacing and defibrillator leads: indications, facilities, training. North American Society of Pacing and Electrophysiology Lead Extraction Conference Faculty. Pacing Clin Electrophysiol 2000;23(4 Pt 1): 544–51.

10. Epstein LM, Love CJ, Wilkoff BL, et al. Superior vena cava defibrillator coils make transvenous lead extraction more challenging and riskier. J Am Coll Cardiol 2013;61(9):987–9.

11. Kawata H, Pretorius V, Phan H, et al. Utility and safety of temporary pacing using active fixation leads and externalized re-usable permanent pacemakers after lead extraction. Europace 2013;15(9): 1287–91.

12. McGarry TJ, Joshi R, Kawata H, et al. Pocket infections of cardiac implantable electronic devices treated by negative pressure wound therapy. Europace 2013. http://dx.doi.org/10.1093/europace/eut305. [Epub ahead of print].

13. Maytin M, Carrillo RG, Baltodano P, et al. Multicenter experience with transvenous lead extraction of active fixation coronary sinus leads. Pacing Clin Electrophysiol 2012;35(6):641–7.

14. Bongiorni MG, Soldati E, Zucchelli G, et al. Transvenous removal of pacing and implantable cardiac defibrillating leads using single sheath mechanical dilatation and multiple venous approaches: high success rate and safety in more than 2000 leads. Eur Heart J 2008;29(23):2886–93.

15. Wilkoff BL, Byrd CL, Love CJ, et al. Pacemaker lead extraction with the laser sheath: results of the pacing lead extraction with the excimer sheath (PLEXES) trial. J Am Coll Cardiol 1999;33(6):1671–6.

16. Byrd CL, Wilkoff BL, Love CJ, et al. Clinical study of the laser sheath for lead extraction: the total experience in the United States. Pacing Clin Electrophysiol 2002;25(5):804–8.

17. Kennergren C, Schaerf RH, Sellers TD, et al. Cardiac lead extraction with a novel locking stylet. J Interv Card Electrophysiol 2000;4(4):591–3.

18. Wazni O, Epstein LM, Carrillo RG, et al. Lead extraction in the contemporary setting: the LExICon study: an observational retrospective study of consecutive laser lead extractions. J Am Coll Cardiol 2010;55(6): 579–86.

19. Love CJ, Kutalek SP, Starck C, et al. Results of the Lead Extration Device Evaluation and Results (LEADER) Datebase. Journal of Heart Disease 2012;9(1):78.

Is Defibrillation Testing Necessary?

Andrea M. Russo, MD[a],*, Mina K. Chung, MD[b]

KEYWORDS

• Defibrillation testing • Implantable cardioverter defibrillator • Sudden cardiac death

KEY POINTS

- Whether or not defibrillation testing is necessary at the time of implantable cardioverter defibrillator (ICD) implantation is one of the most frequently debated topics in electrophysiology.
- With advancements in ICD technology, an inadequate safety margin for defibrillation at the time of implantation now occurs infrequently.
- Testing of ICDs seems safe in most patients, and modifications of the system are often easily performed at the time of the implantation procedure.
- Clinical trials demonstrating the efficacy of ICD therapy for the primary and secondary prevention of sudden cardiac death (SCD) all used some form of defibrillation testing at the time of implantation.
- The authors recommend that defibrillation testing be considered a standard part of initial ICD implantation in the absence of contraindications.

INTRODUCTION

ICDs are effective for the primary and secondary prevention of SCD in high-risk populations.[1–7] At the time of implantation, ventricular fibrillation (VF) is typically induced to demonstrate effective arrhythmia termination. Instructions for use of ICDs approved by the Food and Drug Administration (FDA) in the United States include recommendations for defibrillation testing at the time of implantation. Defibrillation testing, in the absence of contraindications, still seems to be the standard of care at most centers in the United States, with testing performed in 71% of patients, according to National Cardiovascular Data Registry (NCDR) data.[8]

With advanced technology, the practice of performing defibrillation threshold (DFT) testing has been questioned due to potential risks of testing

as well as doubts about its ability to improve clinical shock efficacy or survival. Current technology includes biphasic waveform shocks, pectoral active can systems, and higher-output devices that result in higher defibrillation efficacy.[9–16]

In the absence of results of prospective randomized data, the topic of defibrillation testing continues to spark much debate. This article describes reasons to perform testing as well as reasons to avoid defibrillation testing at the time of initial ICD implantation.

DEFINITION OF DEFIBRILLATION THRESHOLD

The term, DFT, refers to the minimum shock strength that defibrillates.[17] This has been used as a patient-specific measure of defibrillation efficacy, and a threshold below a specific value has been used as a criterion for successful device

Disclosures: A.M. Russo: Honoraria/Consulting (Medtronic, Boston Scientific, St. Jude, Biotronik); Research trials (Medtronic, Boston Scientific, Biotronik); Fellowship support (Medtronic, Boston Scientific); M.K. Chung: Honoraria/Consulting $0 (Medtronic, Boston Scientific, St. Jude, Biotronik); Research trials (Medtronic, Boston Scientific, St. Jude, Biotronik).

[a] Electrophysiology and Arrhythmia Services, Cooper University Hospital, Cooper Medical School of Rowan University, 426 Dorrance Building, 1 Cooper Plaza, Camden, NJ 08103, USA; [b] Cleveland Clinic Foundation, Cleveland Clinic Lerner College of Medicine of Case Western Reserve University, 9500 Euclid Avenue, Cleveland, OH 44195, USA
* Corresponding author.
E-mail address: russo-andrea@cooperhealth.edu

Cardiol Clin 32 (2014) 211–224
http://dx.doi.org/10.1016/j.ccl.2014.01.003
0733-8651/14/$ – see front matter © 2014 Elsevier Inc. All rights reserved.

implantation.[18,19] A detailed review of ICD implantation testing has been published.[20] Given the probabilistic nature of defibrillation, clinical measurement of DFT has only fair reproducibility and represents an estimate of a point on a patient's defibrillation probability-of-success curve.

A variety of methods have been used to determine DFT, including step-down, step-up, and binary search approaches. These methods often involved multiple VF inductions, however. With advancements in defibrillator technology, most centers now limit defibrillation testing and use safety margin testing. With this method, an adequate safety margin for defibrillation may be defined as successful shock therapy at 10 J below the maximum output of the device. Many implanting physicians may elect to induce VF only once or twice and, for example, accept successful defibrillation at 25 J with an ICD capable of delivering 35 J. In this article, the term DFT is used interchangeably with defibrillation safety margin testing, despite the differences in meaning.

REASONS TO SUPPORT DEFIBRILLATION TESTING

Assessment of System Integrity and Reliable Sensing

DFT testing can confirm the electrical integrity of connections between the leads and pulse generator, reliable sensing, and appropriate detection and redetection of VF.[21] Opponents of DFT testing, however, note that connection integrity can usually be evaluated without defibrillation testing by assessing low-voltage pulses introduced during sinus rhythm, pacing thresholds and impedances, and recorded electrograms. R wave amplitude in the native rhythm correlates well with reliable sensing during VF.[22,23] With modern ICDs, undersensing of spontaneous VF is rare if the native rhythm R wave is adequate ($\geq$5–7 mV). Some inner insulation failures may be detected, however, only by postshock oversensing, and some lead failures may pass with normal shock impedance values at low-voltage but fail with high-voltage testing. Postshock redetection issues are more important with older integrated bipolar leads with short tip-to-coil spacing.[24]

Discovery of High DFTs Needing System Modification

The primary goal of DFT testing is to increase the likelihood that the ICD will effectively terminate spontaneous ventricular tachycardia (VT) or VF and to identify patients who require system revision if implant testing demonstrates a high DFT.[21] The yield by defibrillation testing of discovering high DFTs needing system modification ranges from 2.2% to 12% of implants (**Table 1**). One study examining high DFTs at implantation suggests that an inadequate safety margin is more likely to occur with a single-coil compared with a dual-coil transvenous system (4.6% vs 2.6%, $P<.0001$).[25]

Although the sickest patients are likely at highest risk for hemodynamic complications of DFT testing, these patients are also at highest risk for DFT failure and thus have the highest yield of testing. In 138 patients undergoing cardiac resynchronization therapy (CRT) defibrillator implantation, 12% had a less than 10-J safety margin.[26] A less than 10-J safety margin requiring system revision was seen in 28% of patients with New York Heart Association (NYHA) class IV compared with only 3% to 4% of patients with NYHA class I-III heart failure ($P<.0001$).[27]

If a high DFT is identified, system revisions can be performed and an adequate DFT can almost always be obtained at the time of implantation. After system modification, 67% to 100% of patients who did not initially meet implant criteria achieved an adequate safety margin for defibrillation.[24,26–34] System revisions may include moving the right ventricular coil, capping off the superior vena cava (SVC) coil (in a dual-coil system), changing to a higher-output device, reversing polarity, optimizing the biphasic waveform, or adding an extra lead (such as a subcutaneous, transvenous SVC, or azygous lead). In addition, discontinuing drugs that may increase the DFT, such as amiodarone, may help. The REPLACE study demonstrated major complications occurring in 15.3% of patients undergoing ICD replacement with planned lead revisions[35]; therefore, such revisions might be best performed at the time of initial implantation.

Poor Predictive Value of Clinical Factors in Identifying High DFTs

Unfortunately, there is a poor predictive value of clinical factors in identifying patients who are likely to have ineffective defibrillation at implantation testing.[21] Factors that may influence defibrillation success include (1) patient characteristics (2) ICD system features (leads, shock waveform, and defibrillation pathway) (3) drug effects, in particular, chronic amiodarone, which has increased DFT in several studies[28,36–44]; and (4) implant-related factors or complications (such as pneumothorax, which may increase the DFT).

Common patient-specific factors that are associated with higher DFTs identified in multiple studies include lower left ventricular ejection fraction (LVEF),[28,32,36,45–48] larger left ventricular (LV) size[37,49] or mass,[50–53] worse clinical heart

Table 1
Yield of defibrillation testing

Study	N	Implant Criteria	Age, y (Mean ± SD or Median)	Gender (% Female)	LVEF, % (Mean ± SD)	# Patients Not Meeting Implant Criteria	Percentage Implants with High DFT
Russo, Heart Rhythm 2005	1139	10-J safety margin	66 ± 13	25	32 ± 14	71	6.2
Bardy, NEJM 2005; Blatt, JACC 2008	717	30-J (max 2 inductions)	60.1	23	24	0	0 (2.2 <10-J safety margin)
Leong-Sit, AHJ 2006	168	10-J safety margin	61.6 ± 12.7	23	27 ± 13	16	9.5
Mainigi, Heart Rhythm 2006	121	10-J safety margin	67 ± 11	15	21 ± 8	14	12.0
Day, Europace 2008	1530	10-J safety margin	63.6 ± 11	21	—	59	3.9
Healey, JCE 2010	1268	10-J safety margin	62.9 ± 12.8	22	30.0 ± 12.0	44	3.5
Sauer, PACE 2011	853	10-J safety margin (follow-up test)	—	—	—	21	2.4
Healey, JCE 2012	71	≤25 J	65.9 ± 9.3	20	24.7 ± 4.6	3	4.2
Keyser, Inter CV Surg 2013	716	≤21 J	60.0 ± 14.2	20	27.4 ± 11.8	28	3.9
Vischer, JCE 2013	309	10-J safety margin	63 ± 14	18	33 ± 13	7	2.3
Lin, PACE 2013	240	10-J safety margin	58.5 ± 16.1	27	28.3 ± 14.5	48	2.2
Havel, Heart Rhythm 2010	3335[a]	10-J safety margin	—	—	—	155	4.6
	100,804[b]	10-J safety margin	—	—	—	2579	2.6

[a] Single coil.
[b] Dual coil.
Data from Refs.[7,24–34,64]

failure,[28,36,37,47–49,51,54] QRS duration greater than or equal to 200 ms in CRT defibrillator implants,[26] nonischemic cardiomyopathy,[28] male gender,[37,46,49,51,55] greater body surface area,[37,49,51] right-sided pectoral implantation,[56,57] and the presence of hypertrophic cardiomyopathy.[58–60] The strengths of these associations are not consistent, however, between studies. Other studies have demonstrated that no clinical variables were strong predictors of a high DFT.[38,61]

Increased Assurance that Defibrillation of VF Will Be Successful During Clinical Events

There are few data to predict if implant defibrillation testing predicts effective defibrillation during follow-up.[21] First-shock success for spontaneous VT/VF in VF zone for patients who passed implant criteria is only 83% to 92%,[62–65] not 100%. Success rates might be even lower, however, if defibrillation testing were not performed. Although ICDs can deliver up to 5 to 6 shocks for VT/VF, so subsequent shocks may be successful even if the first shock fails, there is still benefit from achieving successful conversion after the first shock. Shocks are painful, and prolonged VT/VF can cause syncope or other adverse effects related to prolonged hypotension.

A post hoc analysis of the Sudden Cardiac Death in Heart Failure Trial (SCD-HeFT) is frequently used to justify not performing DFT testing at implantation.[64] First-shock efficacy in SCD-HeFT was 83.0% and did not differ when the cohort was subdivided by baseline DFT. The investigators chose an arbitrary cutoff of greater than 10 J to define a high DFT and less than or equal to 10 J to define a low DFT. Most patients with a high DFT still had a greater than or equal to 10-J safety margin for defibrillation, which is a common criterion used for determining an adequate safety margin at implantation testing. Only 16 patients had a less than 10-J safety margin in this study and all patients had a DFT less than or equal to 30 J. CRT patients were not included in SCD-HeFT; patients in clinical trials might not be representative of sicker patients seen in "contemporary" clinical practice. Therefore, results of this post hoc analysis should not be used as sole justification to omit testing.

Discovery of Low DFTs that May Allow Programming of Lower First-Shock Energies

Identifying lower DFTs at implant might permit lower programmed first-shock energies that result in faster charge times.[21] Although considered an issue with longer charge times in some earlier-generation devices, there are few clinical data to support such a benefit. Lower-shock strengths may result in a reduction in postshock ventricular dysfunction that may result in electromechanical dissociation (EMD).[66–69] Animal models demonstrate myocardial dysfunction and damage with high shock magnitudes, although these magnitudes are generally higher than those used clinically.[67–69] Nevertheless, in a study of sudden deaths in patients with ICDs, postshock EMD was noted in 29% of sudden deaths, suggesting that some deaths may have occurred from overly large or frequent shocks.[66]

Assurance of a Safety Margin for Testing After Addition of Antiarrhythmic Drugs, such as Amiodarone, that May Raise DFTs

Dynamic clinical factors can have an impact on defibrillation efficacy, including changes in underlying substrate, ischemia, or addition of drugs (such as amiodarone) that may increase the DFT. Demonstration of an adequate safety margin at the time of initial implantation may help offset these adverse changes in DFT during follow-up.[21]

Assurance that the Device Is Not a Lemon

Once detection of VT/VF occurs, it is unlikely that a device fails to deliver the programmed energy. A search of the Manufacturer and User Facility Device Experience database from 01/01/2000 through 06/28/2013 of non-CRT ICDs revealed 5 devices that failed to deliver energy and 1 device with failure to power up and difficulty programming.[21] These rare problems should be detectable at the time of the implant procedure.

Assessment of Lead Problems that May Only Be Identified with High-Voltage Testing

A case report identified a concealed lead fracture demonstrating normal shock impedances measured with subthreshold test pulses, whereas abnormal shock impedances (>200 Ω) were noted after DFT testing.[70] Case reports of electrical abnormalities detected by defibrillation testing, but not by high-voltage lead integrity testing, have also been published for Riata leads (St. Jude Medical, St. Paul, MN, USA).[71,72]

Assessment for Device-Device Interaction in Patients with More than One Cardiac Implantable Electrical Device

Some patients with single-chamber ICDs may have a separate permanent pacemaker in place for concomitant bradyarrhythmias. In addition, the recently approved totally subcutaneous ICD (S-ICD) does not have standard bradycardia pacing (with the exception of postshock pacing). If a separately implanted pacemaker is present, additional testing is required to exclude adverse pacemaker-ICD interactions.[21] In addition to potential oversensing of pacemaker spikes resulting in inappropriate device therapy, the most serious and potentially life-threatening problem is related to undersensing of VF. If the separately implanted pacemaker undersenses VF, pacemaker-delivered pacing stimuli can be sensed by the ICD (and misinterpreted as QRS complexes), whereas the smaller VF signals remain undetected, resulting in failure of the ICD to deliver potentially life-saving therapy. During defibrillation testing to exclude significant device interactions, VF can be induced with the pacemaker programmed to worst-case scenario parameters that minimize sensitivity and maximize output. With availability of the S-ICD, this two-device combination may be seen more frequently in upcoming years.

Evidence-Based Medicine, Clinical Trials, and Standard of Care

All clinical trials demonstrating a mortality benefit of ICD therapy have included some form of DFT testing at the time of implantation. Up to this point, DFT testing has been the standard of care and the FDA instructions for use in device company manuals have included labeling with defibrillation testing.[21] There may be medical-legal implications of implanting devices without DFT testing, in the absence of contraindications, particularly in the event that appropriate shocks from a nontested device fail to terminate clinical VT/VF.

It was DFT-tested ICDs, not nontested ICDs, that were demonstrated to reduce mortality in primary and secondary prevention trials.[21] The Multicenter Automatic Defibrillator Implantation Trial (MADIT) I and MADIT II made every effort made to achieve a 10-J safety margin.[3,4] Although SCD-HeFT specified a maximum of 2 DFT inductions, few patients had a high DFT and defibrillation was always successful at less than or equal to 30 J.[7] In MADIT-CRT, testing details were not specified.[73] In the Multicenter Unsustained Tachycardia Trial, intraoperative testing of VF energy requirements was mandated and confirmation of adequate defibrillation was repeated prior to hospital discharge if DFT was greater than 20 J.[74] In the Antiarrhythmics Versus Implantable Defibrillators trial, virtually all patients (99%) achieved an adequate DFT.[1]

REASONS TO AVOID DEFIBRILLATION TESTING
Low Probability of High DFTs

With modern technology, mean DFT was reported to be 8.5 ± 4.2 J with dual-coil and 11.2 ± 6.6 J with single-coil systems.[75] Because most devices now deliver a maximum output of 35 to 40 J, a large safety margin for defibrillation is often present. Low thresholds (<15 J) were seen in 96% of patients with dual-coil and in 81% of patients with single-coil configurations. As described previously, the yield of discovering high DFTs needing system modification ranges from 2.2% to 12% of implants (see **Table 1**). If a high-output device were used upfront, one study reported that the percentage of patients requiring system modification would be reduced in half, from 6% to 3%.[28]

Even if a high DFT is noted, maximum shock energies may be effective. With the capacity to deliver multiple shocks, subsequent shocks may be effective, even if a first shock is unsuccessful.

Majority of Treated Events Are VT, Effectively Treated with Antitachycardia Pacing

Most patients currently receive ICDs for primary prevention indications and may never require shock therapy, particularly due to the availability of antitachycardia pacing (ATP) and contemporary device programming based on recent studies demonstrating reduction of unnecessary ICD therapy with high rate cutoffs and prolonged detection times.[76,77] The annual incidence of appropriate shocks seems to be only 5% to 10% per year.[28,78–80] Shocks are still required, however, in many of these patients for potentially life-threatening arrhythmias, and efficacy should be assured when this therapy is necessary.

Even If a First Shock Fails, Subsequent Shocks Likely Are Successful

Contemporary ICDs can deliver up to 5 to 6 shocks per episode. If the first shock fails, subsequent shocks may be successful in terminating VT/VF. Because shocks are painful, however, and may lead to syncope or other adverse effects related to prolonged periods of hypotension, there seem to be advantages to successful first-shock therapy.

DFT Testing Requires Heavier Sedation and Additional Personnel

Intravenous conscious sedation is used for most patients undergoing DFT testing. Risks of anesthetic agents include adverse hemodynamic effects, respiratory depression, and aspiration. Most contemporary agents used for this purpose are, however, short-lived or can be easily reversed. Some centers require support from the anesthesia department to administer agents used for deep conscious sedation, and these additional personnel may not always be readily available.

Complications Related to Defibrillation Testing Can Lead to Morbidity or Even Mortality

One of the most common reasons cited to avoid DFT testing is related to the presumed increased risk of complications related to testing. Risks include those related to VF itself, which may lead to prolonged hypotension, hypoperfusion and circulatory arrest, the shocks themselves, or the anesthetic drugs required for shock testing.

During defibrillation testing, transient central nervous system hypoperfusion can be demonstrated during intraoperative electroencephalographic monitoring.[81–83] This does not, however, seem clinically relevant. One study demonstrated that DFT testing did not cause cognitive dysfunction 24 to 48 hours after ICD implantation.[84,85] Hypotension due to prolonged episodes of VF could result in myocardial ischemia in patients with coronary artery disease, although true intraoperative myocardial infarction seems rare, even in patients who underwent extensive DFT testing.[86–89] One study showed no evidence for significant tissue injury, without change in biomarkers (creatine kinase [CK], CK-MB, myoglobin, and N-terminal pro b-type natriuretic peptide) before and after DFT testing.[90] DFT slightly increased troponin T in the group with preserved LVEF and troponin I in the group with reduced LVEF, but the values did not exceed normal ranges.[90] Both shocks alone and VF may transiently depress contractile function[90] although fatal pulseless electrical activity is also rare at the time of ICD implantation.[91–94]

Refractory VF has been reported to occur during defibrillation testing. One study published in 2005 reported that all tested ICD shocks failed and greater than or equal to 3 external rescue shocks were required in 0.5% of patients.[95] Multiple failed shocks are now extremely rare, however, with the availability of biphasic ICD and external defibrillator waveforms. A Canadian study (with implants from 2000 to 2006) reported 27 of 19,067 (0.14%) prolonged resuscitations during DFT testing.[96]

Thromboembolic complications may occur in the presence of intracardiac thrombus, although these adverse events should be preventable by appropriate screening. A Canadian study reported 5 of 19,067 (0.026%) strokes or transient ischemic attacks (TIAs) occurring within 24 hours of DFT testing.[96] In patients with atrial fibrillation, preprocedure tranesophageal echocardiography can be performed to exclude left atrial appendage thrombus, and atrial fibrillation can be reinduced, if converted by shocks off anticoagulation. Alternatively, DFT testing can be deferred for several weeks until an appropriate duration of therapeutic anticoagulation is maintained. LV thrombus may be a less likely source of thromboembolism in patients undergoing defibrillation testing, although this should also be excluded by transthoracic echocardiography.

Anesthetic agents may contribute to complications related to a primary depressant effect on myocardial contractility or secondary effect leading to respiratory depression. This may lead to hypoxia or hypercapnea, which is more likely in patients with underlying obstructive pulmonary disease or sleep apnea. This may also occur in patients, however, who do not undergo DFT testing; therefore, special attention to avoid respiratory depression is necessary for all patients undergoing ICD implantation.

Improved ICD technology has led to the need for fewer inductions of VF at the time of implantation testing. With transvenous systems and biphasic waveforms, the procedure-related mortality rate within 30 days of implantation is 0.2% to 0.4%.[28,65,92,95] In-hospital mortality was less than 0.5% in the NCDR ICD Registry,[97] and data from 21 Canadian centers estimated a mortality rate of 0.016% related to DFT testing.[96]

In the absence of randomized trial data, it is often difficult to identify which complications are directly (or indirectly) related to DFT testing itself. Based on presumed risks of DFT testing, **Table 2** lists possible implantation complications that might be directly or indirectly related to testing. For example, risks that may be directly related to DFT testing include stroke or TIA, because intracardiac thrombus may dislodge during conversion of atrial fibrillation in the absence of therapeutic anticoagulation, or hypotension could result in reduced cerebral perfusion. In contrast, DFT testing may indirectly increase the risk for pneumothorax or infection because more leads may be placed and the procedure may be prolonged due to system revisions aimed at improving defibrillation efficacy. All these complications may also occur, however, in the absence of DFT testing. Adverse events are driven primarily by mechanical complications or infection, most of which are not related to defibrillation testing itself.

A small randomized study and a larger prospective observational study demonstrated no significant difference in perioperative complications,

Table 2
Implant-related complications that may be directly or indirectly related to DFT testing

Implant Complications	Complication Rates	Potentially Directly or Indirectly Related to DFT
Pneumothorax	0.4%–0.8%	Indirect
Lead dislodgement	1%–6%	Indirect
Perforation or tamponade	0.1%	Indirect
Hemodynamic complications	1%	Direct
Multiple external defibrillations	0.5%	Direct
Pulseless electrical activity	0.1%–0.3%	Direct
Stroke/TIA	0.03%–0.09%	Direct
Respiratory depression	0.5%	Direct
Infection	0.8%–2.0%	Indirect
Death	0.2%–0.5%	Direct
All complications	~8%–10%	

Data from Refs.[1,28,35,65,92–94,96,97]

regardless of whether DFT testing was performed.[33,98] The absence of randomization and confounding differences in baseline characteristics using observational data, however, does not provide conclusive evidence related to DFT testing. In the randomized pilot study, the number of patients reaching the primary endpoint was small, and the study was underpowered to detect a difference between the two groups. Other nonrandomized studies demonstrated worse outcomes of patients who did not undergo DFT testing compared with those who did. These include a large analysis of DFT testing from the NCDR ICD Registry in which patients who did not undergo defibrillation testing had a higher in-hospital mortality (0.61% vs 0.24%, $P<.001$), even after multivariate analysis.[8] Although this supports an overall absence of harm from DFT testing, selection bias cannot be excluded, because sicker patients are more likely excluded from DFT testing.[8,65]

There are some patients who should be excluded from DFT testing at implantation because risks clearly outweigh any potential benefits. Absolute and relative contraindications are listed in **Box 1**. In some cases, testing may be reconsidered several weeks or months after initial implantation, such as a situation where left atrial (LA) thrombus resolves. In other cases, such as unrevascularized severe 3-vessel disease or left main disease, this is not appropriate.

Shocks May Increase Mortality

Data suggest that patients receiving ICD shocks for clinical events, whether shocks are appropriate

Box 1
Absolute and relative contraindications to DFT testing

- Thromboembolic risks
  - Presence of LA thrombus
  - Presence of LV thrombus
  - Atrial fibrillation in the absence of adequate (therapeutic) anticoagulation
- Hemodynamic risks or structural heart disease
  - Hemodynamic instability during implantation procedure
  - Ongoing inotropic support (eg, class IV heart failure)
  - Severe aortic stenosis
- Ischemic risks
  - Unrevascularized severe proximal 3 vessel coronary artery disease or significant left main disease
  - Unstable angina
  - Recent percutaneous coronary intervention*
- Cerebrovascular disease
  - Recent stroke or TIA
- Pulmonary disease
  - Severe COPD*
  - Respiratory issues that preclude adequate sedation
- Others
  - Known inadequate external defibrillation
  - Inadequate anesthesia support

* Denotes relative contraindications.

or inappropriate, are at increased risk for adverse outcomes, including increased risk for mortality.[99–102] Because ATP did not seem to increase mortality risk, it has been suggested that shocks may themselves be detrimental.[99]

Outcomes after shocks for clinical events do not extrapolate, however, to outcomes after defibrillation testing. ICD shocks delivered during induced ventricular arrhythmias do not seem to increase the risk of death.[103,104] A post hoc analysis of MADIT-CRT revealed that an increasing number of ICD shocks delivered during DFT testing was not associated with an increased risk for heart failure or death (primary endpoint), heart failure alone, VT/VF, or death.[103] In addition, shock energy level (defined as high, >20 J, or low, ≤20 J) was not associated with adverse clinical outcomes. This suggests that the ICD shocks themselves may not be responsible for the increased risk of adverse outcomes. Instead, the occurrence of spontaneous arrhythmias more likely explains the increased mortality risk of patients who receive shocks for clinical arrhythmias during follow-up.

Defibrillation Testing Limits Expansion of Device Implantation

Although recent reports suggest potential overuse of ICDs in clinical practice,[105] data from a prospective cohort study (Registry to Improve the Use of Evidence-Based Heart Failure Therapies in the Outpatient Setting [IMPROVE HF]) suggest potential underuse.[106] This outpatient cardiology registry demonstrated that only 50.7% of patients with chronic HF and LVEF less than or equal to 35% who were eligible for ICDs based on guidelines actually received ICDs with or without CRT.[106] Although nonelectrophysiologists may implant devices at some centers, they are typically not trained to perform DFT testing. Increased adherence to ICD usage was associated with electrophysiologists on staff in one study, even after multivariate analysis.[106] Opponents of DFT testing suggest that requirements for testing may limit expansion of devices to areas without electrophysiologists. This is purely speculative, however.

Defibrillation Testing Increases Costs

Costs related to DFT testing include (1) additional time to perform testing, (2) additional personnel, (3) additional charges for testing itself, and (4) any costs related to additional complications related of testing. **Table 3** estimates these costs. Anesthesia personnel used for the procedure lead to additional professional charges. Additional time spent testing may add to laboratory staff time to perform the procedure (and perhaps not

Table 3
Estimated costs related to DFT testing

Procedure	Reimbursement
Electrophysiologic testing of ICD (with DFT testing) 93641	$358
Anesthesia (professional) 33249	$1002
Laboratory staff × 3 @$51/h for extra 1 h	$153
Total[a]	$1512

[a] Does not include the extra laboratory time/hospital costs, medications, or any increased costs related to complications and prolonged hospital stay (150,000 ICDs in US each year × $1512 = $226,800 unnecessary expenses, with approximately 2/3 medicare).

performing another procedure). There are also professional fees for the implanting physician based on electrophysiologic testing of the device during the procedure. These do not include additional overhead for the hospital, cost of medications required for heavier sedation, increased recovery time, or any increased costs related to complications or a prolonged hospital stay. If it is estimated that 150,000 ICDs are implanted each year in the United States, and it may cost an extra $2151 to perform testing, this equals $324,150,000 in unnecessary expenses, and approximately two-thirds of these may be performed in Medicare patients. These costs may vary by region.

DFT IMPACT ON MORTALITY AND ARRHYTHMIC DEATH

Early investigation demonstrated that a high DFT was associated with worse outcome and arrhythmic death; thus, defibrillation testing was considered mandatory. With monophasic devices implanted through a thoracotomy approach, a high DFT of greater than or equal to 25 J resulted in an actuarial rate of sudden arrhythmic death in 16% of patients over 5 years.[55]

The most common mechanism of sudden death in patients with an ICD is VT/VF treated with an appropriate shock. Postmortem interrogation of ICDs revealed that 25% of sudden deaths in ICD patients were caused by failure to defibrillate VF.[66] Multiple shocks may be required to defibrillate VF, and postdefibrillation EMD accounted for 29% of deaths in one study.[107] It is feasible, however, that failed shocks during follow-up and mortality might be higher if DFT testing (and subsequent system revisions) were not performed at implantation. Devices are typically implanted when patients are in a stable or best possible state. Factors that may not be present at the time of implantation, such as ischemia, progressive heart failure, metabolic abnormalities, or drug effects, may subsequently lead to increased DFTs, failed shocks, or even sudden death. System modifications to allow a safety margin at implantation testing may help ameliorate subsequent increases in DFT, still allowing effective defibrillation at follow-up.

Some retrospective studies and a prospective observational study suggest no difference in mortality in patients who underwent DFT testing versus those who did not.[28,98,108,109] These studies were often limited by size and short follow-up with few treated arrhythmic events. Large variations in the practice between centers and selection bias also cannot be excluded. In contrast, one small retrospective study revealed a lower total survival in the no-DFT group (69.1% vs 91.2%, $P = .004$), although after adjusting for differences in baseline characteristics, multivariate analysis revealed only a trend toward increased risk of death in the no-DFT group (hazard ratio 3.18; 95% CI, 0.82–12.41; $P = .095$).[110] A much larger study (64,227 initial ICD implantation procedures performed at 1261 facilities from the NCDR ICD Registry), reported by Russo and colleagues,[8] demonstrated higher in-hospital mortality in patients who did not undergo defibrillation testing compared with those who did undergo testing (0.61% vs 0.24%, $P<.001$), even after multivariate analysis. Similarly, in a retrospective study by Pires and colleagues,[65] overall long-term survival was significantly lower in the no-testing (58%) compared with the DFT (74%) and safety margin testing (69%) groups ($P<.0005$); lack of ICD testing was an independent predictor of mortality in multivariate analysis.

Worse outcomes in patients who do not undergo DFT testing are most likely related to exclusion of testing in the sickest patients. Fortunately, most patients undergoing DFT testing are able to achieve adequate safety margins with system modification or drug changes. With this strategy, elevated DFTs seem to have no impact on mortality.[26,28] Russo and colleagues reported that long-term survival was not significantly different in patients requiring system modification compared with those who did not require modification.[28] Although this survival outcome could be interpreted to support lack of a need for DFT testing, another interpretation is that the strategy of DFT testing and system revision for those with high DFTs allowed achievement of similar survival to those patients with lower DFTs. A recent study demonstrated that a high-implant DFT predicts

an adverse prognosis, even when an adequate safety margin is present, suggesting that a high DFT may just be one marker of a sicker patient.[111] Therefore, whether or not a mortality difference exists between patients who undergo DFT testing versus those who do not is best answered by a prospective randomized trial.

CURRENT PRACTICE TRENDS

There is a trend toward ICD implantation without DFT testing.[21,112,113] A decrease in defibrillation testing has been noted over time, with devices implanted without testing in 10.4% of patients in 2000–2002, 18.6% in 2003–2005, and 29.6% in 2006–2008 at a US university center.[112] Only 25% of patients who did not have defibrillation testing at implant underwent testing within 6 months postimplant. In Italy, 30% to 67% of devices were implanted without DFT testing.[113–115] Two Canadian studies reported that 20% to 35% of devices were implanted without DFT testing.[29,96] In the NCDR, DFT testing was not performed in 29% of 64,227 initial ICD implant procedures.[8] The use of DFT testing in clinical practice seems to vary by geographic region, hospital, year of implant, physician training, and country.[8,111,113,114]

PAUCITY OF RANDOMIZED TRIAL DATA

Based on ongoing controversy and paucity of prospective data, randomized trial data are needed to support or refute the need for DFT testing.[21] A randomized controlled pilot study comparing ICD implantation with and without intraoperative defibrillation testing in 145 patients with heart failure and severe LV dysfunction, a substudy of the Resynchronization for Ambulatory Heart Failure Trial, revealed no significant differences in perioperative complications, failed appropriate shocks, or arrhythmic death, regardless of whether or not DFT testing was performed.[33] This was a small study, however, with few events and was underpowered.

Additional prospective randomized trials are currently underway. These include the following: (1) Shockless Implant Evaluation trial, which is being performed at centers in Canada, Europe, Israel, and Asia Pacific, sponsored by Boston Scientific (NCT00800384)[116]; (2) NORDIC ICD, which is being performed in Europe, sponsored by Biotronik (NCT01282918); and (3) Test-No Test ICD, which is being performed at two centers in the United States (NCT01905007). Depending on clinical trial results, it may become apparent that a much larger study with longer follow-up is needed.

Because the benefit of ICD therapy was demonstrated in primary and secondary clinical trials that examined total mortality, the primary endpoint for trials evaluating the benefit of ICD therapy without DFT testing ideally would use mortality as a primary endpoint. This would require, however, a very large study with long follow-up.

SUMMARY

Whether or not defibrillation testing is necessary at the time of ICD implantation is one of the most frequently debated topics in electrophysiology. With advancements in ICD technology, including biphasic waveforms, active cans, and high-output devices, an inadequate safety margin for defibrillation at the time of implantation now occurs infrequently. On the other hand, testing of ICDs seems safe in most patients, and modifications of the system are often easily performed at the time of the implantation procedure. The paucity of prospective randomized data is responsible for the wide differences in opinion related to this topic. Although data are not currently available to demonstrate that testing translates into improved mortality or increased efficacy of therapy for clinical VT/VF, available studies do not show demonstrable harm, and clinical trials demonstrating the efficacy of ICD therapy for the primary and secondary prevention of SCD all used some form of defibrillation testing at the time of implantation. If systems were not tested and revised based on the results of DFT testing, it is currently unknown whether or these trials would have demonstrated the same benefit from ICD therapy.

Once additional prospective data become available, it is anticipated that future guidelines or consensus documents will address recommendations related to defibrillation testing. Although ongoing trials may not answer the mortality question, they will help address first-shock efficacy and frequency of adverse events related to DFT testing. Until then, the authors recommend that defibrillation testing should be considered a standard part of initial ICD implantation in the absence of contraindications.

REFERENCES

1. Antiarrhythmics versus Implantable Defibrillator (AVID) Investigators. A comparison of antiarrhythmic drug therapy with implantable defibrillators in patients resuscitated from near fatal ventricular arrhythmias. N Engl J Med 1997;337:1576–83.
2. Connolly SJ, Hallstrom AP, Cappato R, et al. Meta-analysis of the implantable cardioverter defibrillator secondary prevention trials. AVID, CASH and CIDS studies. Antiarrhythmics vs Implantable Defibrillator study. Cardiac Arrest Study Hamburg. Canadian Implantable Defibrillator Study. Eur Heart J 2000;21:2071–8.
3. Moss AJ, Hall WJ, Cannom DS, et al. Improved survival with an implanted defibrillator in patients with coronary disease at high risk for ventricular arrhythmia. N Engl J Med 1996;335:1933–40.
4. Moss AJ, Zareba W, Hall J, et al, Multi-center Automatic Defibrillator Implantation II Trial Investigators. Prophylactic implantation of a defibrillator in patients with myocardial infarction and reduced ejection fraction. N Engl J Med 2002;346:877–83.
5. Buxton AE, Lee KL, Fisher JD, et al, Multicenter Unsustained Tachycardia Trial Investigators. A randomized study of the prevention of sudden death in patients with coronary artery disease. N Engl J Med 1999;341:1882–90.
6. Kadish A, Dyer A, Daubert JP, et al, for the Defibrillators in Non-Ischemic Cardiomyopathy Treatment Evaluation (DEFINITE) Investigators. Prophylactic defirillator implantation in patients with nonischemic dilated cardiomyopathy. N Engl J Med 2004; 350:2151–8.
7. Bardy GH, Lee KL, Mark DB, et al, Ip JH for the Sudden Cardiac Death in Heart Failure Trial (SCD-HeFT) Investigators. Amiodarone or an implantable cardioverter-defibrillator for congestive heart failure. N Engl J Med 2005;352:225–37.
8. Russo A, Wang Y, Curtis J, et al. Patient, physician, and procedural factors influencing the use of defibrillation testing during initial implantable cardioverter insertion: findings of the NCDR®. Pacing Clin Electrophysiol 2013;36:1522–31.
9. Wyse DG, Kavanagh KM, Gillis AM, et al. Comparison of biphasic and monophasic shocks for defibrillation using a nonthoracotomy system. Am J Cardiol 1993;71:197–202.
10. Neuzner J, Pitschner HF, Huth C, et al. Effect of biphasic waveform pulse on endocardial defibrillation efficacy in humans. Pacing Clin Electrophysiol 1994;17:207–12.
11. Natale A, Sra J, Krum D, et al. Comparison of biphasic and monophasic pulses: does the advantage of biphasic shocks depend on the waveshape? Pacing Clin Electrophysiol 1995;18:1354–61.
12. Olsovsky MR, Hodgson DM, Shorofsky SR, et al. Effect of biphasic waveforms on transvenous defibrillation thresholds in patients with coronary artery disease. Am J Cardiol 1997;80(8):1098–100.
13. Gold MR, Foster AH, Shorofsky SR. Effects of an active pectoral-pulse generator shell on defibrillation efficacy with a transvenous lead system. Am J Cardiol 1996;78:540–3.
14. Bardy GH, Yee R, Jung W. Multicenter experience with a pectoral unipolar implantable

cardioverter-defibrillator. Active Can Investigators. J Am Coll Cardiol 1996 Aug;28(2):400–10.

15. Bardy GH, Johnson G, Poole JE, et al. A simplified, single-lead unipolar transvenous cardioversion-defibrillation system. Circulation 1993; 88(2):543–7.

16. Natale A, Sra J, Axtell K, et al. Preliminary experience with a hybrid nonthoracotomy defibrillating system that includes a biphasic device: comparison with a standard monophasic device using the same lead system. J Am Coll Cardiol 1994;24: 406–12.

17. Rattes MF, Jones DL, Sharma AD, et al. Defibrillation threshold: a simple and quantitative estimate of the ability to defibrillate. Pacing Clin Electrophysiol 1987;10:70–7.

18. Singer I, Lang D. Defibrillation threshold: clinical utility and therapeutic implications. Pacing Clin Electrophysiol 1992;15:932–9.

19. Marchlinski FE, Flores B, Miller JM, et al. Relation of the intraoperative defibrillation threshold to successful postoperative defibrillation with an automatic implantable cardioverter defibrillator. Am J Cardiol 1988;62:393–8.

20. Swerdlow CD, Russo AM, Degroot PJ. The dilemma of ICD implant testing. Pacing Clin Electrophysiol 2007;30:675–700.

21. Russo AM, Chung MK. Defibrillation testing is necessary at the time of implantable cardioverter defibrillator implantation. Circ Arrhythm Electrophysiol 2014, in press.

22. Ellenbogen KA, Wood MA, Stambler BS, et al. Measurement of ventricular electrogram amplitude during intraoperative induction of ventriclar tachyarrhythmias. Am J Cardiol 1992;70:1017–22.

23. Swerdlow CD. Implantation of cardioverter defibrillators without induction of ventricular fibrillation. Circulation 2001;103:2159–64.

24. Sauer WH, Lowery CM, Bargas RL, et al. Utility of postoperative testing of implantable cardioverter-defibrillators. Pacing Clin Electrophysiol 2011;34: 186–92.

25. Havel WJ, Johnson J. Effect of number of shock coils on defibrillation testing outcome: analysis from the Medtronic Discovery™ Hub database. Heart Rhythm 2010;7(Suppl):S75.

26. Mainigi SK, Cooper JM, Russo AM, et al. Elevated defibrillation thresholds in patients undergoing biventricular defibrillator implantation: incidence and predictors. Heart Rhythm 2006;3:1010–6.

27. Day JD, Olshansky B, Moore S, et al, INTRINSIC RV Study Investigators. High defibrillation energy requirements are encountered rarely with modern dual-chamber implantable cardioverter-defibrillator systems. Europace 2008;10:347–50.

28. Russo AM, Sauer W, Gerstenfeld EP, et al. Defibrillation threshold testing: is it really necessary at the time of implantable cardioverter-defibrillator insertion? Heart Rhythm 2005;2:456–61.

29. Healey JS, Birnie DH, Lee DS, et al, Ontario ICD Database Investigators. Defibrillation testing at the time of ICD insertion: an analysis from the Ontario ICD Registry. J Cardiovasc Electrophysiol 2010;21:1344–8.

30. Keyser A, Hilker MK, Schmidt S, et al. Shock or no shock - a question of philosophy or should intraoperative implantable cardioverter defibrillator testing be recommended? Interact Cardiovasc Thorac Surg 2013;16:321–5.

31. Vischer AS, Sticherling C, Kühne MS, et al. Role of defibrillation threshold testing in the contemporary defibrillator patient population. J Cardiovasc Electrophysiol 2013;24:437–41.

32. Lin EF, Dalal D, Cheng A, et al. Predictors of high defibrillation threshold in the modern era. Pacing Clin Electrophysiol 2013;36:231–7.

33. Healey JS, Gula LJ, Birnie DH, et al. A randomized-controlled pilot study comparing ICD implantation with and without intraoperative defibrillation testing in patients with heart failure and severe left ventricular dysfunction: a substudy of the RAFT trial. J Cardiovasc Electrophysiol 2012;23:1313–6.

34. Leong-Sit P, Gula LJ, Diamantouros P, et al. Effect of defibrillation testing on management during implantable cardioverter-defibrillator implantation. Am Heart J 2006;152:1104–8.

35. Poole JE, Gleva MJ, Mela T, et al, REPLACE Registry Investigators. Complication rates associated with pacemaker or implantable cardioverter-defibrillator generator replacements and upgrade procedures: results from the REPLACE registry. Circulation 2010;122:1553–61.

36. Shukla HH, Flaker GC, Jayam V, et al. High defibrillation thresholds in transvenous biphasic implantable defibrillators: clinical predictors and prognostic implications. Pacing Clin Electrophysiol 2003;26(Pt I): 44–8.

37. Khalighi K, Daly B, Leino V, et al. Clinical predictors of transvenous defibrillation energy requirements. Am J Cardiol 1997;79:150–3.

38. Hohnloser SH, Dorian P, Roberts R, et al. Effect of amiodarone and sotalol on ventricular defibrillation threshold: the optimal pharmacological therapy in cardioverter defibrillator patients (OPTIC) trial. Circulation 2006;114:104–9.

39. Zhou L, Chen BP, Kluger J, et al. Effects of amiodarone and its active metabolite desethylamiodarone on the ventricular defibrillatoin threshold. J Am Coll Cardiol 1998;31:1672–8.

40. Troup PJ, Chapman PD, Olinger GN, et al. The implanted defibrillator: relation of defibrillating lead configuration and clinical variables to defibrillation threshold. J Am Coll Cardiol 1985;6:1315–21.

41. Pelosi F, Oral H, Kim MH, et al. Effect of chronic amiodarone therapy on defibrillation energy

requirements in humans. J Cardiovasc Electrophysiol 2000;11:736–40.

42. Dorian P. Amiodarone and defibrillation thresholds: a clinical conundrum. J Cardiovasc Electrophysiol 2000;11:741–3.

43. Jung W, Manz M, Pizzulli L, et al. Effects of chronic amiodarone therapy on defibrillation threshold. Am J Cardiol 1992;70:1023–7.

44. Verma A, Kaplan AJ, Sarak B, et al. Incidence of very high defibrillation thresholds (DFT) and efficacy of subcutaneous (SQ) array insertion during implantable cardioverter defibrillator (ICD) implantation. J Interv Card Electrophysiol 2010;29:127–33.

45. Pinski SL, Vanerio G, Castle LW, et al. Patients with a high defibrillation threshold: clinical characteristics, management, and outcome. Am Heart J 1991;122:89–95.

46. Leitch JW, Yee R. Predictors of defibrillation efficacy in patients undergoing epicardial defibrillator implantation. The Multicenter Pacemaker Cardioverter-Defibrillator (PCD) Investigators Group. J Am Coll Cardiol 1993;21:1632–7.

47. Horton RP, Canby RC, Roman CA, et al. Determinants of nonthoractotomy biphasic defibrillation. Pacing Clin Electrophysiol 1997;20:60–4.

48. Lubinski A, Lewicka-Nowak E, Zienciuk A, et al. Clinical predictors of defibrillation threshold in patients with implantable cardioverter defibrillators. Kardiol Pol 2005;62:317.

49. Brooks R, Garaan H, Torchiana D, et al. Determinants of successful nonthoracotomy cardioverter-defibrillator implantation: experience in 101 patients using two different lead systems. J Am Coll Cardiol 1993;22:1835–42.

50. Chapman PD, Sagar KB, Wetherbee JN, et al. Relationship of left ventricular mass to defibrillation threshold for the implantable defibrillator: acombined clinical and animal study. Am Heart J 1987;114:274–8.

51. Schwartzman D, Concato J, Ren JF, et al. Factors associated with successful implantation of nonthoracotomy defibrillation lead systems. Am Heart J 1996;131:1127–36.

52. Jain SK, Ghanbari H, Hourani R, et al. Echocardiographic parameters to predict inadequate defibrillation safety margin in patients receiving implantable cardioverter defibrillators for primary prevention. J Interv Card Electrophysiol 2013;37:79–85.

53. Raitt MH, Johnson G, Dolack GL, et al. Clinical predictors of the defibrillation threshold with the unipolar implantable defibrillation system. J Am Coll Cardiol 1995;25:1576–83.

54. Russo AM, Al-Khatib SM, Wang Y, et al. Predictors of high defibrillation energy requirements: results from the NCDR ICD registry. Circulation 2012;126(Suppl):A9039.

55. Epstein AE, Ellenbogen KA, Kirk KA, et al. Clinical characteristics and outcome of patients with high defibrillation thresholds. A multicenter study. Circulation 1992;86:1206–16.

56. Flaker GC, Tummala R, Wilson J. Comparison of right and left-sided pectoral implantation parameters with the Jewel active can cardiodefibrillator. The World Wide Jewel Investigators. Pacing Clin Electrophysiol 1998;21:447–51.

57. Roberts PR, Allen S, Betts T, et al. Increased defibrillation threshold with right-sided active pectoral can. J Interv Card Electrophysiol 2000;4:245–9.

58. Jastrzebski M, Czarnecka D, Bacior B, et al. Massive myocardial hypertrophy in hypertrophic cardiomyopathy: a risk factor for sudden death and high defibrillation threshold during cardioverter-defibrillator implantation. Kardiol Pol 2005;63:191–5 [in Polish].

59. Almquist AK, Montgomery JV, Haas TS, et al. Cardioverter-defibrillator implantation in high risk patients with hypertrophic cardiomyopathy. Heart Rhythm 2005;2:814–9.

60. Roberts BD, Hood RE, Saba MM, et al. Defibrillation threshold testing in patients with hypertrophic cardiomyopathy. Pacing Clin Electrophysiol 2010;33:1342–6.

61. Hodgson DM, Olsovsky MR, Shorofsky SR, et al. Clinical predictors of defibrillation thresholds with an active pectoral puse generator lead system. Pacing Clin Electrophysiol 2002;25:408–13.

62. Gold MR, Higgins S, Klein R, et al. Efficacy and temporal stability of reduced safety margins for ventricular defibrillation: primary results from the Low Energy Safety Study (LESS). Circulation 2002;105:2043–8.

63. Sweeney M, DeGroot P, Stark A, et al, Investigators PRI. Relationship between defibrillation threshold, programmed energy and first shock efficacy for fast ventricular tachycardia and ventricular fibrillation in PainFREE Rx II. Circulation 2004;110:503A.

64. Blatt JA, Poole JE, Johnson GW, et al, SCD-HeFT Investigators. No benefit from defibrillation threshold testing in the SCD-HeFT (Sudden Cardiac Death in Heart Failure Trial). J Am Coll Cardiol 2008;52:551–6.

65. Pires LA, Johnson KM. Intraoperative testing of the implantable cardioverter defibrillator: how much is enough? J Cardiovasc Electrophysiol 2006;17:140–5.

66. Mitchell LB, Pineda EA, Titus JL, et al. Sudden death in patients with implantable cardioverter defibrillators: the importance of post-shock electromechanical dissociation. J Am Coll Cardiol 2002;39:1323–8.

67. Babbs CF, Tacker WA, VanVleet JF, et al. Therapeutic indices for transchest defibrillator shocks: effective,

damaging, and lethal electrical doses. Am Heart J 1980;99:734–8.

68. Wilson CM, Allen JD, Bridges JB, et al. Death and damage caused by multiple direct current shocks: studies in an animal model. Eur Heart J 1988;9: 1257–65.

69. Jones JL, Proskauer CC, Paull WK, et al. Ultrastructural injury to chick myocardial cells in vitro following "electric countershock". Circ Res 1980; 46:387–94.

70. Bun SS, Duytschaever M, Tavernier R. Defibrillation testing can reveal 'concealed' lead fracture. Europace 2013;15:54.

71. Doshi R, Ceballos S, Mendez F. Is high-voltage lead integrity measurement adequate during defibrillator generator replacement? Journal of Innovations in Cardiac Rhythm Management 2012;3:1016–9.

72. Shah P, Singh G, Chandra S, et al. Failure to deliver therapy by a Riata Lead with internal wire externalization and normal electrical parameters during routine interrogation. J Cardiovasc Electrophysiol 2013;24:94–6.

73. Moss AJ, Brown MW, Cannom DS, et al. Multicenter Automatic Defibrillator Implantation Trial-Cardiac Resynchronization Therapy (MADIT-CRT): design and clinical protocol. Ann Noninvasive Electrocardiol 2005;10:34–43.

74. Buxton AE, Fisher JD, Josephson ME, et al. Prevention of sudden death in patients with coronary artery disease: the Multicenter Unsustained Tachycardia Trial (MUSTT). Prog Cardiovasc Dis 1993; 36:215–26.

75. Gold MR, Olsovsky MR, DeGroot PJ, et al. Optimization of transvenous coil position for active can defibrillation thresholds. J Cardiovasc Electrophysiol 2000;11:25–9.

76. Moss AJ, Schuger C, Beck CA, et al, MADIT-RIT Trial Investigators. Reduction in inappropriate therapy and mortality through ICD programming. N Engl J Med 2012;367:2275–83.

77. Wilkoff BL, Williamson BD, Stern RS, et al, PREPARE Study Investigators. Strategic programming of detection and therapy parameters in implantable cardioverter-defibrillators reduces shocks in primary prevention patients: results from the PREPARE (Primary Prevention Parameters Evaluation) study. J Am Coll Cardiol 2008; 52:541–50.

78. Wathen MS, Sweeney MO, DeGroot PJ, et al. Shock reduction using antitachycardia pacing for spontaneous rapid ventricular tachycardia in patients with coronary artery disease. Circulation 2001;104:796–801.

79. Sweeney MO, Wathen MS, Volosin K, et al. Appropriate and inappropriate ventricular therapies, quality of life, and mortality among primary and secondary prevention implantable cardioverter

defibrillator patients: results from the pacing Fast VT Reduces Shocke ThErapies (PainFREE Rx II) Trial [abstract]. Circulation 2005;111:2898–905.

80. Wilkoff BL, Ousdigian KT, Sterns LD, et al. A comparison of empiric to physician-tailored programming of implantable cardioverter-defibrillators: results from the prospective randomized multicenter EMPIRIC trial. J Am Coll Cardiol 2006;48:330–9.

81. deVries JW, Bakker PF, Visser GH, et al. Changes in cerebral oxygen uptake and crebral electrical activity during defibrillation threshold testing. Anesth Analg 1998;87:16–20.

82. Singer I, Edmonds H. Changes in cerebral perfusion during third generation implantable cardioverter defibrillator testing. Am Heart J 1994;127: 1052–7.

83. Vriens EM, Bakker PF, Vries JW, et al. The impact of repeated short episodes of ciruclatory arrest on cerebral function. Electroencephalogr Clin Neurophysiol 1996;98:236–42.

84. de Silva MP, Rivetti LA, Mathias LA, et al. Impact of induced cardiac arrest on cognitive function after implantation of a cardioverter-defibrillator. Rev Bras Anestesiol 2009;59:37–45.

85. Karaoguz R, Altln T, Atbasoglu EC, et al. Defibrillation testing and early neurologic outcome. Int Heart J 2008;49:553–63.

86. Schluter T, Baum H, Plewan A, et al. Effects of implantable cardioverter defibrillator implantation and shock application on biochemical markers of myocardial damage. Clin Chem 2001;47:459–63.

87. Hasdemir C, Shah N, Rao AP, et al. Effect of out-of-hospital implantable cardioverter defibrillator shocks on cardiac troponin I levels [abstract]. Circulation 2000;102(Suppl II):II-622.

88. McPherson CA, Blendea D. Clinical significance of elevated serum Troponin-T after implantable cardioverter defibrillator discharges. Chest 2003;124: 151S–2S.

89. Frame R, Brodman R, Furman S, et al. Clinical evaluation of the safety of repetitive intraoperative defibrillation threshold testing. Pacing Clin Electrophysiol 1992;15:870–7.

90. Toh N, Nishii N, Nakamura K, et al. Cardiac dysfunction and prolonged hemodynamic deterioration after implantable cardioverter-defibrillator shock in patients with systolic heart failure. Circ Arrhythm Electrophysiol 2012;5:898–905.

91. Mollerus M, Naslund L. Myocardial stunning following defibrillation threshold testing. J Interv Card Electrophysiol 2007;19:213–6.

92. Schuger C, Ellengoben KA, Faddis M, et al. Defibrilllation energy requirements in an ICD population receiving cardiac resynchronization therapy. J Cardiovasc Electrophysiol 2006;17:247–50.

93. Frame R, Brodman R, Gross J, et al. Initial experience with transvenous implantable cardioverter

defibrillator lead systems: operative morbidity and mortality. Pacing Clin Electrophysiol 1993;16: 149–52.

94. Russo AM, Verdino RJ, Gerstenfeld E, et al. Contemporary implantable cardioverter defibrillator complications at a University Center. J Am Coll Cardiol 2008;51(10 Suppl A):A25.

95. Alter P, Waldhans S, Plachta E, et al. Complications of implantable cardioverter defibrillator therapy in 440 consecutive patients. Pacing Clin Electrophysiol 2005;28:926–32.

96. Birnie D, Tung S, Simpson C, et al. Complications associated with defibrillation threshold testing: the Canadian experience. Heart Rhythm 2008;5: 387–90.

97. Hammill SC, Stevenson LW, Kadish AH, et al. Review of the registry's first year, data collected, and future plans. Heart Rhythm 2007;4:1260–3.

98. Brignole M, Occhetta E, Bongiorni MG, et al, SAFE-ICD Study Investigators. Clinical evaluation of defibrillation testing in an unselected population of 2,120 consecutive patients undergoing first implantable cardioverter-defibrillator implant. J Am Coll Cardiol 2012;60(11):981–7.

99. Larsen GK, Evans J, Lambert WE, et al. Shocks burden and increased mortality in implantable cardioverter-defibrillator patients. Heart Rhythm 2011;8:1881–6.

100. Poole JE, Johnson GW, Hellkamp AS, et al. Prognostic importance of defibrillator shocks in patients with heart failure. N Engl J Med 2008;359: 1009–17.

101. Daubert JP, Zareba W, Cannom DS, et al, MADIT II Investigators. Inappropriate implantable cardioverter-defibrillator shocks in MADIT II: frequency, mechanisms, predictors, and survival impact. J Am Coll Cardiol 2008;51:1357–65.

102. van Rees JB, Borleffs CJ, de Bie MK, et al. Inappropriate implantable cardioverter-defibrillator shocks: incidence, predictors, and impact on mortality. J Am Coll Cardiol 2011;57:556–62.

103. Aktas MK, Huang DT, Daubert JP, et al. Effect of defibrillation threshold testing on heart failure hospitalization or death in the Multicenter Automatic Defibrillator Implantation Trial-Cardiac Resynchronization Therapy (MADIT-CRT). Heart Rhythm 2013;10:193–9.

104. Bhavnani SP, Kluger J, Coleman CI, et al. The prognostic impact of shocks for clinical and induced arrhythmias on morbidity and mortality among patients with implantable cardioverter-defibrillators. Heart Rhythm 2010;7:755–60.

105. Al-Khatib SM, Hellkamp A, Curtis J, et al. Non-evidence-based ICD implantations in the United States. JAMA 2011;305:43–9.

106. Mehra MR, Yancy CW, Albert NM, et al. Evidence of clinical practice heterogeneity in the use of implantable cardioverter-defibrillators in heart failure and post-myocardial infarction left ventricular dysfunction: findings from IMPROVE HF. Heart Rhythm 2009;6:1727–34.

107. Pires LA, Hull ML, Nino CL, et al. Sudden death in recipients of transvenous implantable cardioverter defibrillator systems: terminal events, predictors, and potential mechanisms. J Cardiovasc Electrophysiol 1999;10:1049–56.

108. Codner P, Nevzorov R, Kusniec J, et al. Implantable cardioverter defibrillator with and without defibrillation threshold testing. Isr Med Assoc J 2012; 14(6):343–6.

109. Michowitz Y, Lellouche N, Contractor T, et al. Defibrillation threshold testing fails to show clinical benefit during long-term follow-up of patients undergoing cardiac resynchronization therapy defibrillator implantation. Europace 2011;13:683–8.

110. Hall B, Jeevanantham V, Levine E, et al. Comparison of outcomes in patients undergoing defibrillation threshold testing at the time of implantable cardioverter-defibrillator implantation versus no defibrillation threshold testing. Cardiol J 2007;14: 463–9.

111. Rubenstein JC, Kim MH, Morady F, et al. The relationship between defibrillation threshold and total mortality. J Interv Card Electrophysiol 2013;38: 203–8.

112. Russo AM, Gerstenfeld EP, Dixit S, et al. Changing patterns of defibrillation testing at the time of implantable cardioverter defibrillator insertion over the past 8 years. J Am Coll Cardiol 2009; 53(Suppl):A134.

113. Bianchi S, Ricci RP, Biscione F, et al. Primary prevention implantation of cardioverter defibrillator without defibrillation threshold testing: 2-year follow-up. Pacing Clin Electrophysiol 2009;32: 573–8.

114. Brignole M, Raciti G, Bongiorni MG, et al. Defibrillation testing at the time of implantation of cardioverter defibrillator in the clinical practice: a nation-wide survey. Europace 2007;9:540–3.

115. Stefano B, Pietro RR, Maurizio G, et al. Defibrillation testing during implantable cardioverter-defibrillator implantation in Italian current practice: the Assessment of Long-term Induction clinical ValuE (ALIVE) project. Am Heart J 2011;162: 390–7.

116. Healey JS, Hohnloser SH, Glikson M, et al. The rationale and design of the Shockless IMPLant Evaluation (SIMPLE) trial: a randomized, controlled trial of defibrillation testing at the time of defibrillator implantation. Am Heart J 2012;164:146–52.

The Totally Subcutaneous Implantable Defibrillator

John Rhyner, MD[a], Bradley P. Knight, MD, FHRS[b],*

KEYWORDS

- Subcutaneous implantable cardioverter-defibrillator • S-ICD • Cardiac arrest • Therapy
- Clinical trial

KEY POINTS

- The subcutaneous implantable cardioverter-defibrillator (S-ICD) system is a new therapeutic option for patients at risk of sudden cardiac arrest.
- The S-ICD is implanted in the lateral thoracic region of the body and uses a tunneled lead to sense and deliver therapy.
- The S-ICD system is entirely outside the vasculature/heart, limiting the risk of systemic infection, vascular/cardiac trauma, and device failure.
- Clinical trials suggest that the S-ICD is effective for the sensing, discrimination, and conversion of spontaneous and induced ventricular tachycardia and ventricular fibrillation.
- The S-ICD may be used for both primary and secondary prevention.

 A video of the S-ICD implantation procedure accompanies this article at http://www.cardiology. theclinics.com/

INTRODUCTION

Cardiovascular disease is the most common cause of death in the Western world, and sudden cardiac death (SCD) represents approximately 60% of all cardiovascular mortality.[1] The implanted cardioverter-defibrillator (ICD) was developed to address this issue, and since 1980 has shown significant mortality benefits for both the primary and secondary prevention of SCD.[2,3] The development of well-substantiated indications for primary prevention in particular has resulted in a large expansion of potentially eligible patients with diverse clinical needs and potential procedural and device-related risks.[4–6]

Initial ICDs involved epicardial patch electrodes and epicardial rate-sense leads requiring a thoracotomy for implantation. The current standard ICD uses transvenous leads, which, compared with epicardial patches, are associated with significantly fewer complications.[7,8]

However, the placement of a transvenous ICD system still involves considerable risk, with a major complication rate of approximately 1.5%.[9] These risks include hemorrhage, infection, pneumothorax, cardiac perforation, and death.[10–14] Additional risks present after the time of implantation as well, including inappropriate device therapy, endocarditis, vessel occlusion (of particular concern with patients in need of catheter-mediated dialysis), lead dislodgment, valvular dysfunction, and intrinsic lead defects.[15,16] Lead failure either generates inappropriate shocks or impedes appropriate therapy.[17–19] Over the long term, lead failure

Disclosures: Dr Bradley P. Knight is a consultant for Boston Scientific, Inc, the manufacturer of the subcutaneous implantable defibrillator.
[a] Division of Cardiology, Department of Medicine, Northwestern University, 303 E Chicago Ave, Chicago, IL 60611, USA; [b] Division of Cardiology, Department of Medicine, Bluhm Cardiovascular Institute of Northwestern, Feinberg School of Medicine, Northwestern University, 251 East Huron Street, Feinberg 8-503E, Chicago, IL 60611, USA
* Corresponding author.
E-mail address: bknight@nmff.org

Cardiol Clin 32 (2014) 225–237
http://dx.doi.org/10.1016/j.ccl.2013.12.001
0733-8651/14/$ – see front matter © 2014 Elsevier Inc. All rights reserved.

remains a significant limitation of transvenous ICDs, despite decades of lead research and development.[9,17,18,20–27] One series showed the rate of lead failure of 8-year-old systems to be up to 20%.[28] Furthermore, management of these complications frequently involves significant complexity, morbidity, mortality, and cost.[28–39] Lead failures and infection frequently require extraction and placement of new systems, and inappropriate therapies often result in significant pain and psychological trauma to the patient.

An ICD system that remains outside the heart and vasculature involves significantly less risk of the aforementioned complications, and complications that may ensue would be more easily managed. This improved safety profile and reduction in the complexity of implantation and management may reduce the barrier to the provision of life-saving devices in a rapidly expanding population of eligible patients.

A subcutaneous format may offer physiologic benefits as well. Although subcutaneous systems require larger defibrillation energies than transvenous systems, the energy is distributed more evenly throughout the myocardium.[40] The uneven energy associated with transvenous systems cause electroporation, which leads to transient myocardial stunning.[41,42] Animal models have shown significant troponin release associated with transvenous delivery of 35 J of energy, whereas the subcutaneous delivery of 80 J of energy did not raise troponin. Additional studies in humans have shown a relationship between transvenous ICD shocks and mortality.[43–46] The relationship between subcutaneous ICD shocks and mortality is yet to be determined.

The original ICD concept was developed by Schuder and colleagues[47] in 1970. Two electrodes were implanted between the pectoralis muscle and the rib cage, 2 sensing electrodes in the chest wall musculature, and a pulse generator and capacitor were implanted into the abdomen (**Fig. 1**). The fully implanted, automatic system was successful in the defibrillation of induced ventricular fibrillation (VF) in all 3 animals into which it was implanted, requiring 1 to 3 shocks of 23 to 37 J to terminate the rhythm.

More recently, studies were published exploring the clinical application of a subcutaneous system. Burke and colleagues[48] investigated a pectoral can with a subcutaneous electrode over the cardiac apex. This and other studies produced promising results, showing reliable defibrillation in acute and chronically defibrillated patients. The primary limitations to clinical use were the lack of a dedicated detection algorithm and commercial production, and US Food and Drug Administration (FDA) approval of a subcutaneous ICD system. The first of these limitation was addressed by Burke and colleagues[48] with the suggestion that surface electrocardiogram signals could differentiate VF from sinus rhythm using detection already developed for transvenous ICDs,[19] and was further supported by Gold and colleagues[49] with the Subcutaneous versus Transvenous Arrhythmia Recognition Testing (START) trial, which showed improved specificity of arrhythmia detection and lower rates of inappropriate defibrillation in S-ICDs relative to single-chamber or dual-chamber transvenous devices. Gold and colleagues[49] also showed that subcutaneous electrodes did not differ significantly in sensitivity from relative to transvenous electrodes. The manufacturing and regulatory challenge was addressed by Cameron Health Incorporated (San Clemente, CA) with the development of a commercial platform.

The S-ICD system, comprising the SQ-RX 1010 pulse generator and Q-TRAK 3010 subcutaneous electrode, was first permanently implanted in 2008 into 6 patients. Fifty-five additional patients underwent implantation during the CE (Conformité Européenne) study,[50] and more than 1300 more thereafter.[51] Devices have been implanted for primary and secondary prevention, with a wide range of ages (10–82 years), and challenging substrates including tetralogy of Fallot, hypertrophic cardiomyopathy, sinus inversus, transposition of the great vessels, Brugada syndrome, and long QT syndrome.

After preclinical and clinical studies, the S-ICD was approved for commercial use by the European Union in June of 2009. The device was approved for commercial use by the FDA on September 28, 2012. The recognized indication for an implant is to provide defibrillation therapy for the treatment of life-threatening ventricular tachyarrhythmias in patients who do not have any of the following:

- Symptomatic bradycardia
- Incessant ventricular tachycardia (VT)
- Spontaneous, frequently recurring VT that is reliably terminated with antitachycardia pacing

The FDA also required, in addition to other adverse event reporting, that a postapproval registry be created to track outcomes of patients and devices for at least 60 months after implantation. The primary safety end point of the registry is the complication-free rate at 60 months. The primary effectiveness end point is the overall shock effectiveness in converting spontaneous discrete episodes of VT/VF through 60 months. Results of

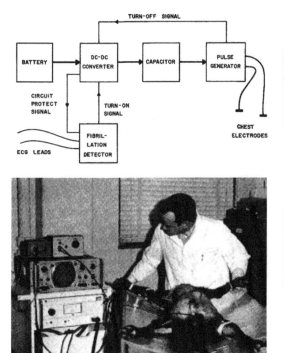

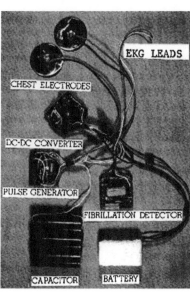

Fig. 1. (*Top left*) Schuder's completely implantable automatic defibrillation system. A battery, on prompting from a fibrillation detector, charges a capacitor, which then delivers energy via a pulse generator to 2 electrodes. (*Right*) Schuder's completely implantable automatic defibrillation system. (*Bottom left*) Schuder with experimental animal with automatic internal ventricular defibrillation system. DC, direct current; ECG/EKG, electrocardiogram. (*From* Schuder JC, Stoeckle H, Gold JH, et al. Experimental ventricular defibrillation with an automatic and completely implanted system. Trans Am Soc Artif Intern Organs 1970;16:207–12; with permission.)

this ongoing study and other clinical trials are reviewed later.

SPECIFICATIONS

Although the modern device has the same rationale as a transvenous device, the specifications are significantly different (**Figs. 2** and **3**). The system consists of a pulse generator placed subcutaneously over the left thorax and a single subcutaneous lead placed along the left side of the sternum. The lead includes a single high-voltage, low-impedance shock coil and 2 low-voltage, high-impedance sensing electrodes. Three distinct sensing vectors are available: proximal ring of electrode to pulse generator, distal tip of electrode to pulse generator, and distal tip of electrode to proximal ring of electrode. The device weighs 145 g and has a volume of 69 mL. Development of a smaller pulse generator is underway. The nominal and maximal deliverable shock is 80 J. The system is capable of delivering 30 seconds of postshock transcutaneous pacing. The

projected longevity of the pulse generator is 5 years, which is significantly shorter than most currently available transvenous devices, which are anticipated to last up to 10 years.

PATIENT SELECTION

The S-ICD is indicated for primary or secondary prevention of sudden cardiac arrest in all individuals without the need for pacing, cardiac resynchronization therapy, or antitachycardia pacing for termination of clinically documented VT. Devices have been used successfully in patients with various indications and challenging substrates as described earlier.

Certain populations are likely to benefit particularly from an S-ICD as opposed to a transvenous system. Children with dilated cardiomyopathy, hypertrophic cardiomyopathy, arrhythmogenic right ventricular cardiomyopathy, long or short QT syndrome, Brugada syndrome, catecholaminergic polymorphic VT, and congenital heart disease are at increased risk of sudden cardiac arrest.[52–55]

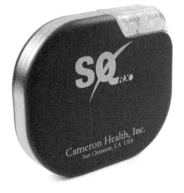

SQ-RX® Pulse Generator Specifications

Physical	
Dimensions (HxWxD)	78.2 × 65.5 × 15.7 mm
Mass	145 g
Volume	69.9 cc
Longevity	Normal use: 5.1 years*
Electrode compatibility	Requires Cameron Health Q-TRAK® electrode
Automatic functions	
Sensing configuration	Optimal sensing configuration automatically selected during Auto Setup
Gain selection	Optimal gain selection automatically selected during Auto Setup
Rhythm discrimination	Rate and morphology automatically operate when the Conditional Shock Zone is activated
Polarity	Automatically selected based on history of successful shocks
Internal warning system	Audible tone alerts patient to elective replacement indicator, electrode impedance out of range, prolonged charge times, failed device integrity check
Smart Charge™	Adjusts arrhythmia detection to prevent shocks for non-sustained VT
Programmable parameters	
Shock Zone	170 bpm – 250 bpm (steps of 10 bpm)
Conditional Shock Zone	Off, 170 bpm – 240 bpm (minimum 10 bpm less than Shock Zone)
S-ICD System Therapy	Off, Manual, Auto
Post-shock pacing	On, Off
Delivered Energy (Induction Only)	10 – 80 j (steps of 5 j)
Non-programmable parameters	
Induction testing	50 Hz, 200 mA waveform
Delivered Energy	80 j
Diagnostics	
Episode storage	Treated episodes 128 s of annotated S-ECG (up to 24 episodes)
	Untreated episode 68 s of annotated S-ECG (up to 20 episodes)
Other data	Electrode impedance System status (remaining battery life, patient alerts, etc.)

* Defined as 3 full-energy capacitor charges per year.

Fig. 2. The Cameron Health S-ICD pulse generator, appearance and specifications. The device has a volume of 70 mL, weighs 145 g, and is only compatible with the Cameron Health Q-TRAK electrode. The maximal delivered energy is 80 J. The device is capable of providing brief postdefibrillation on-demand pacing, but cannot provide chronic pacing. (*Courtesy of* Cameron Health, San Clemente, CA; with permission.)

Furthermore, in these patients prophylactic ICD is the primary recommended therapeutic option.[56,57] Transvenous systems are particularly problematic in such patients because of structural heart disease, variable access to the right ventricle, small somatic and/or venous size, and potential for future growth.[58] The S-ICD may also be particularly appealing for patients with a temporally limited indication for an ICD, such as those awaiting cardiac transplantation, experiencing myocarditis, or immediately after myocardial infarction. The S-ICD may have cosmetic advantages, with an axillary implant preferred anecdotally, particularly by women.

Patients in whom the S-ICD is less favorable include those with recurrent monomorphic VT (antitachycardia pacing may be effective to terminate this rhythm and obviate a shock[59]) and those patients who prefer home monitoring, because this service is not currently available for the S-ICD. The S-ICD is a poor choice for those with bradycardia requiring pacing or cardiac resynchronization therapy (CRT).

De Bie and colleagues[60] retrospectively assessed the proportion of patients receiving a traditional ICD who might be appropriate for the S-ICD. At their tertiary care center in the Netherlands, 1345 patients who received a single-chamber or dual-chamber ICD from 2002 to 2011 who did not require cardiac pacing or cardiac resynchronization therapy were included. Suitability of an ICD was assessed at 1 and 5 years after implantation.

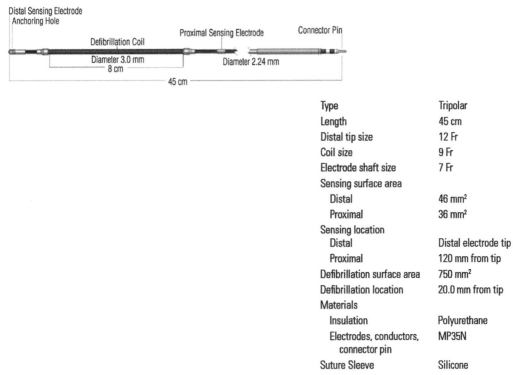

Type	Tripolar
Length	45 cm
Distal tip size	12 Fr
Coil size	9 Fr
Electrode shaft size	7 Fr
Sensing surface area	
Distal	46 mm²
Proximal	36 mm²
Sensing location	
Distal	Distal electrode tip
Proximal	120 mm from tip
Defibrillation surface area	750 mm²
Defibrillation location	20.0 mm from tip
Materials	
Insulation	Polyurethane
Electrodes, conductors, connector pin	MP35N
Suture Sleeve	Silicone

Fig. 3. Cameron Health electrode. The electrode is 45 cm in length, and includes a proximal sensing electrode, defibrillation coil, and distal sensing electrode. (*Courtesy of* Cameron Health, San Clemente, CA; with permission.)

Suitability was defined as not reaching one of the following end points: atrial and/or right ventricular pacing indication, successful antitachycardia pacing without a subsequent shock, or upgrade to a CRT with a defibrillator (CRT-D) device. Initial device programming parameters followed a standard protocol. During a mean follow-up of 3.4 years, 34% of the patients met an end point, and the cumulative incidence of ICD recipients suitable for an initial S-ICD implantation was 56% at 5 years (**Fig. 4**). Significant independent predictors for the unsuitability of an S-ICD were secondary prevention, severe heart failure, and prolonged QRS duration.

Before all implantations, a screening 3-lead surface electrocardiogram must be recorded in the supine and upright positions, and electrocardiographic R waves, T waves, and the ratio of R-wave to T-wave amplitudes are assessed. The cutaneous electrodes are placed in the same position as the planned subcutaneous electrodes would be to confirm that the signals are sufficient for the S-ICD to adequately sense cardiac potentials and not double count the T wave. If these signals are insufficient, the patient is deemed not to be a candidate for an S-ICD implant for concern of inappropriate sensing.

SURGICAL TECHNIQUE AND PERIOPERATIVE MANAGEMENT

Appropriate patient preparation is critical to a successful implant. For optimal results, all anticoagulation is discontinued before the procedure, although there is no absolute contraindication to performance of the procedure on anticoagulation. If anticoagulation must be continued, warfarin with International Normalized Ratio as low as possible within the therapeutic range or bridging with unfractionated heparin are preferred rather than low-molecular-weight heparin or novel oral anticoagulants. Analgesia may be provided with moderate sedation or general anesthesia depending on patient and implanter preference. Implantation at our institution is generally performed under general anesthesia. The procedure may be performed without the use of fluoroscopy.

The patient is prepped for the procedure with normal sterile technique. Because the implant location is not conventional and because the implantation involves a large part of the chest, physician involvement in the preparation is critical during the early experience with the procedure. After administration of antibiotic prophylaxis, local anesthetic is applied to a previously marked incision line from

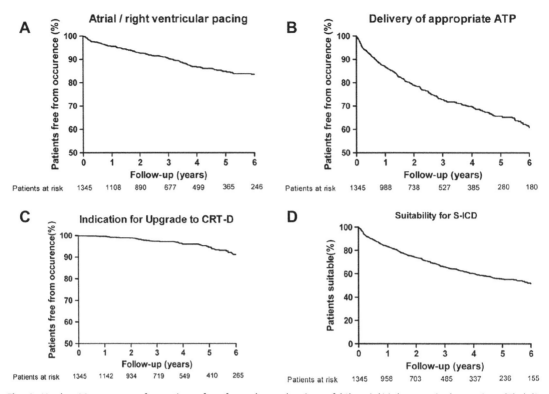

Fig. 4. Kaplan-Meyer curves for patients free from the end points of (A) atrial/right ventricular pacing, (B) delivery of appropriate ATP, and (C) indication for upgrade to CRT-D. These end points are deemed contraindications to S-ICD implants. (D) Kaplan-Meyer curve for suitability for S-ICD graphed against time from implant. At the conclusion of the study, 56% of the patients met an end point indicating unsuitability for an S-ICD system. (*From* de Bie MK, Thijssen J, van Rees JB, et al. Suitability for subcutaneous defibrillator implantation: results based on data from routine clinical practice. Heart 2013;99(14):1018–23; with permission.)

the anterior axillary line to the midaxillary line over the sixth rib (Video 1) usually along the inframammary crease. With a combination of sharp and blunt dissection as well as electrocautery, the plane of incision is extended through the subcutaneous tissue until the fascia is visualized. A pocket is created lateral to the incision to accommodate the pulse generator. A second, smaller incision is then made 1 to 2 cm to the left of the sternum at the level of the xiphoid with dissection to the periosteal fascia. Using a tunneling tool, the lead is tunneled from the first to the second incision. Then, another vertical incision is made 1 to 2 cm left of the sternum at the level of manubriosternal junction. Dissection is performed down to the fascia. The lead is tunneled from the second to the third incision. The lead tip is sutured to the muscle/fascia at the base of the third incision. Using a suture sleeve, the lead is also sutured down at the base of incision 2. The lead is then secured into the pulse generator and the generator is placed into the pocket. All pockets and incisions are copiously irrigated with antibiotic solution and hemostasis is obtained. The pulse generator is sutured to the base of the pocket. Incisions are

closed in layers with absorbable suture. Defibrillation threshold testing was required as part the initial clinical trial and remains recommended since commercial availability. The mean duration of the procedure among operators who have performed at least 3 implantations is 55 ± 23 minutes.[50]

Device parameters including sensing, impedance, and pacing capture thresholds are assessed via wireless communication with a programmer console.[50] The appropriate vector for rhythm detection and avoiding double QRS counting and T-wave oversensing is automatically selected (**Fig. 5**). All device settings are automated with the exception of on/off options for the following:

- Shock therapy
- Pacing after a shock (asystole for >3.5 shocks prompts pacing at 50 beats per minute for 30 seconds)
- Conditional discrimination of supraventricular tachycardia (a conditional discrimination zone can be programmed from 170 to 240 beats per minute to distinguish supraventricular tachycardia from VT)

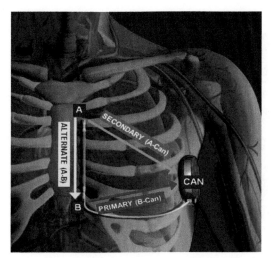

Fig. 5. Three sensing vectors are possible with the S-ICD system: distal electrode (A) to can, distal electrode to proximal electrode (B), and proximal electrode to can. The orientation most suitable for detecting malignant arrhythmia and simultaneously minimizing the risk of double QRS counting and T-wave oversensing is automatically selected at the time of implantation. (*Courtesy of* Cameron Health, San Clemente, CA; with permission.)

The upper-rate cutoff for the conditional shock zone (between 170 and 240 beats per minute) is also programmable.

Patients generally stay in house overnight under observation status. One additional dose of prophylactic antibiotic is provided. The following morning, bandages are removed and wounds assessed. If wounds are healing appropriately, patients may be discharged home.

Postprocedure care is similar to that of patients receiving a transvenous ICD. Patients are instructed to keep incisions dry for 7 days. A bruise or mild swelling is expected and may take several weeks to heal. Patients are to notify their provider if they observe an increase in swelling, drainage, bleeding, or fever. Restrictions are often placed on movement and load bearing performed with the left arm, although these restrictions are not likely to be as important as for those patients undergoing implantation of a transvenous ICD. Patients return to the clinic in 7 days for the incisions to be inspected (**Fig. 6**).

Ongoing S-ICD telemetry control is provided by the programmer console. The device allows review and/or programming of all S-ICD diagnostics including therapy and postshock pacing activation, conditional shock VT and shock VF activation zones, stored arrhythmic events, shock therapies, battery status, and shock coil integrity.[61]

CLINICAL OUTCOMES

The initial clinical experience of the current paradigm of S-ICD was described by Bardy and colleagues[50] in 2010. A total of 49 patients underwent simultaneous implantation of a temporary subcutaneous and permanent commercially available transvenous ICD. Four different vector orientations of electrode and pulse generator were assessed acutely at the time of temporary device implantation, arriving on the aforementioned orientation. This format permitted the lowest defibrillation threshold of those tested, with a mean value of 32.5 ± 17.0 J (95% confidence interval [CI], 27.8–37.3 J). Comparison of the temporary S-ICD with the transvenous ICD was then performed. The mean defibrillation threshold was 11.1 ± 8.5 J (95% CI, 8.6–13.5) with the transvenous ICD and 36.6 ± 19.8 J (95% CI, 31.1–42.5) with the subcutaneous ICD ($P<.001$). The transvenous device in 1 patient and the subcutaneous device in another patient failed to terminate induced VF at maximum device output. In the patient whose subcutaneous ICD failed, the parasternal electrode had been incorrectly positioned 6 cm to the left of the sternum, beyond the left lateral margin of the heart.

Following these proof-of-concept studies, the S-ICD was permanently implanted in 6 individuals. The mean age of the patients was 60 ± 11 years with a mean weight of 99.0 ± 12.0 kg. One patient had a secondary prevention indication, whereas the others had primary prevention indications. All 6 patients underwent successful implantation, and in all patients defibrillation with 65-J shocks was successful in terminating 2 consecutive episodes of induced VF (**Fig. 7**). After 488 ± 2 days of follow-up (95 patient-months of therapy), all patients were well, with no device-related complications or inappropriate shocks. The S-ICD was then implanted into 55 additional patients. Of 137 episodes of induced VF, 100% were appropriately detected. In 52 of the 53 patients in whom VF was able to be induced, defibrillation was successful with 65 J delivered by the S-ICD. In the 53rd patient, defibrillation at 65 J was effective during the first induction, but not during the second induction. A total of 12 episodes of spontaneous VT were detected and successfully treated in 3 patients after device implantation. All patients were treated before the onset of syncope.

Clinically significant adverse events included 2 pocket infections and 4 lead revisions. The leads that migrated were not initially anchored to the chest wall, a practice that is now standard. There were no cases of pocket erosion, lead fractures, or generator migration. In 1 patient, oversensing occurred secondary to inadequate placement of

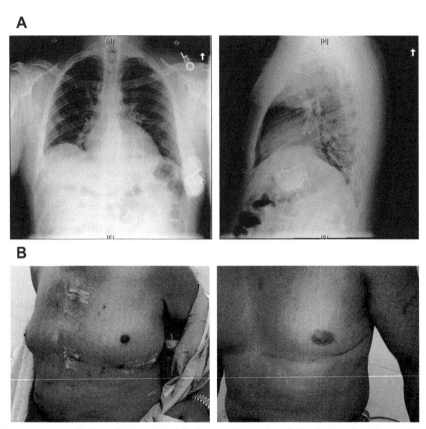

Fig. 6. (A) Posteroanterior (*left*) and lateral (*right*) chest radiographs of the first patient to receive the S-ICD at Northwestern Memorial Hospital, postprocedure day 1. (B) The third patient to receive an S-ICD at Northwestern Memorial Hospital, 1 week after the procedure (*left*). The first patient to receive an S-ICD at Northwestern Memorial Hospital, 3 months after the procedure (*right*).

the electrode pin in the pulse generator header. The device was revised with complete resolution of the sensing failure. Inappropriate sensing caused by muscle noise occurred in 3 patients, which was successfully managed with reprogramming. One patient placed on new drug therapy experienced a change in QRS morphology from a narrow to a right bundle branch block pattern, resulting in double detection. The detection algorithm was revised, and the problem alleviated. No shocks were delivered inappropriately.

Jarman and colleagues[62] reported their experience implanting 16 devices in 2012. The median age of implanted patients was 20 years (range, 10–48 years). Twelve patients, including pediatric patients, had primary electrical disease, whereas 4 had congenital structural heart disease. There were no operative complications and defibrillation testing was successful in all cases. During a median follow-up of 9 months (range, 3–15 months), 3 children required reoperation. A total of 18 shocks were delivered in 6 patients. Ten of these shocks in 4 patients were inappropriate,

secondary to T-wave oversensing. Of the 8 shocks for a ventricular arrhythmia, 3 were delivered for VF, among which 2 had a delay in detection with times to therapy of 24 and 27 seconds. Compared with an age-matched and disorder-matched control group, there were no statistically significant differences in the frequency of reoperation or appropriate or inappropriate shocks.

Olde Nordkamp and colleagues[63] described the first 118 Dutch patients who underwent implantation of S-ICD. Patients were selected if they had a guideline class I or IIa indication for primary or secondary prevention of SCD. All consecutive patients from 4 high-volume centers implanted between December 2008 and April 2011 were included. The mean age of patients was 50 ± 14 years. Seventy-one percent of patients bore a primary indication and 39% a secondary indication for an ICD. After a mean 18 ± 7 months of follow-up, 8 patients received 45 successful shocks (98% first-shock efficacy). Fifteen patients (13%) received inappropriate shocks, mostly associated with T-wave oversensing that was

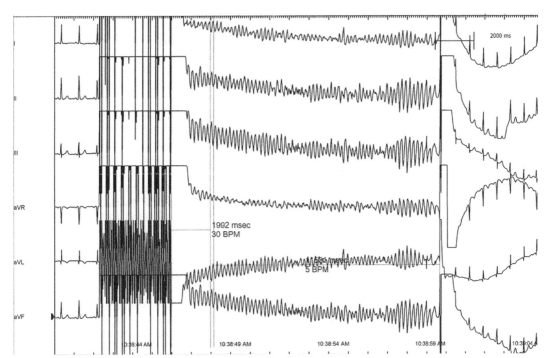

Fig. 7. Electrocardiogram in a patient who underwent defibrillation testing immediately after placement of an S-ICD. VF was induced by 50-Hz pacing, which was promptly recognized and definitively treated by the device with a single shock, resulting in sinus rhythm.

overcome with programming changes. No sudden deaths occurred. Clinically significant ICD complications, defined as events requiring surgical correction or hospitalization, occurred in 16 patients (14%). Dislocation of the subcutaneous lead occurred in 3 patients. In all cases, the parasternal segment of the lead migrated caudally, which prompted the introduction of an additional suture sleeve at the xiphoid level, after which dislocation was no longer observed. Two patients had skin erosion at the location of the generator requiring surgical revision. Seven patients developed an infection necessitating extraction. The rates of inappropriate shocks and complications decreased significantly as centers gained more experience.

Köbe and colleagues[64] reported their experience with 69 patients compared with sex-matched and age-matched patients with conventional ICDs. Implants were performed in 3 German centers. Fifty-nine percent of patients bore a primary prevention indication. The predominant underlying heart disease was ischemic cardiomyopathy in 16%, dilated cardiomyopathy in 36%, and hypertrophic cardiomyopathy in 15%. The S-ICD procedure was performed under general anesthesia for 88% and conscious sedation for 12% of patients, whereas transvenous implantation was performed under general anesthesia for 79% of patients.

Mean implantation time was 70.8 ± 27.9 minutes for the S-ICD and 65.2 ± 30.9 minutes for the transvenous ICD. Conversion rates of induced VF were 89.5% at 65 J, and 95.5% including reversed shock wave polarity in the study group. Termination of induced VF was successful in 90.8% (10-J safety margin) in the traditional ICD group. Complications between the two arms were similar. During a mean follow-up of 217 ± 138 days, 3 patients with S-ICDs were appropriately treated for ventricular arrhythmias. Three inappropriate shocks occurred (5.2%) in 3 patients with S-ICDs because of T-wave oversensing. One patient with an S-ICD developed a hematoma requiring surgical revision.

Weiss and colleagues[65] performed a prospective, nonrandomized multicenter trial comprising adult patients with a standard indication for an ICD. The results of this trial led to FDA approval of the S-ICD. Patients requiring pacing or those with documented pace-terminable VT were excluded. The primary effectiveness end point was the induced defibrillation conversion rate compared with a prespecified goal of 88%. The primary safety end point was the 180-day S-ICD complication-free rate compared with a prespecified goal of 79%. Detection and conversion of spontaneous episodes, as well as time to therapy for induced episodes, incidence of appropriate postshock pacing, postconversion creatinine and creatine phosphokinase levels, spontaneous arrhythmia episodes, and chronic conversion of induced VF were reported as well. The study population was 74% male with a mean age of 52 ± 16 years and a mean ejection fraction of 36 ± 16%. Implantation was attempted in 321 patients and failed in 7. Of the 314 remaining patients, 21 left the study (11 underwent explantation, 8 expired, and 2 withdrew with the device remaining implanted). Both primary end points were met: the 180-day system complication-free rate was 99%, and the sensitivity analysis of the acute VF conversion rate was greater than 90%. Forty-one patients (13%) received an inappropriate shock. Supraventricular tachycardia in the high-rate zone (no discriminators), in which the rate alone determines whether a shock is delivered, was the cause in 16 patients (5.1%). The use of a conditional zone (rate plus discriminators) was associated with significantly fewer inappropriate shocks for oversensing (56% relative reduction) or supraventricular tachycardia (70% relative reduction). Thirty-eight discrete spontaneous episodes of VT/VF occurred in 21 patients (7%), all of which were successfully converted. Eighteen total suspected or confirmed infections occurred. Four infections required explantation. There were no infections requiring explantation in the final two-thirds of the patients enrolled in the study.

COMPLICATIONS AND CONCERNS

Despite the inherent benefits of a system that stays outside the heart, significant concerns regarding the safety and suitability of the S-ICD remain. The aforementioned clinical trials identify the risks of hematoma, infection, need for lead revision, inappropriate sensing of skeletal muscle myopotentials or T-wave oversensing leading to inappropriate shocks, undersensing leading to delays in or withholding of therapy, higher defibrillation thresholds, and erosion at the generator site. Many of these complications became less frequent as the device was improved with hardware modifications, evolution of the surgical technique, and programming improvements.

A legitimate concern is how many patients who undergo implantation of an S-ICD subsequently develop an indication for a therapy that cannot be provided by an S-ICD and require implantation of a transvenous system. These indications include the need for antibradycardia pacing, antitachycardia pacing, or cardiac resynchronization therapy. No patient in the US investigational device exemption trial published by Weiss and colleagues[65] required conversion to a transvenous device during the trial.

SUMMARY

The S-ICD represents a novel tool for the prevention of sudden cardiac arrest. The benefits compared with a traditional ICD include simplified implantation requiring fewer operative resources, and avoidance or mitigation of significant complications inherent in the placement of hardware within the vasculature and heart. These complications include bleeding, infection, loss of future vascular access, pneumothorax, cardiac perforation, and tamponade. Although the S-ICD has been found to be effective in the discrimination and defibrillation of malignant arrhythmias, limited data are available related to the efficacy of the S-ICD for spontaneous events and in specific patient populations, and no prospective randomized controlled trials comparing the safety or efficacy of transvenous ICDs with the S-ICD exist.

Although the S-ICD is capable of providing brief on-demand pacing following defibrillation, the device does not have long-term pacing capability. This limitation is significant, because a considerable proportion of patients with traditional ICDs develop an indication for atrial and/or ventricular pacing, antitachycardia pacing, or CRT within 5 years of implantation of a traditional ICD. Significant independent predictors for the unsuitability of an S-ICD are secondary prevention, severe heart failure, and prolonged QRS duration. Patients most likely to benefit from the S-ICD are young individuals with a normal ejection fraction and without electrical dyssynchrony. Patients with congenital heart disease or limited vascular access may also be especially appropriate for the S-ICD. Future studies are needed to evaluate the long-term clinical safety, efficacy, and suitability of the S-ICD relative to traditional ICDs.

SUPPLEMENTARY DATA

Supplementary data related to this article can be found online at http://dx.doi.org/10.1016/j.ccl.2013.12.001.

REFERENCES

1. Smith TW, Cain ME. Sudden cardiac death: epidemiologic and financial worldwide perspective. J Interv Card Electrophysiol 2006;17(3):199–203.
2. Bardy GH, Lee KL, Mark DB, et al. Amiodarone or an implantable cardioverter-defibrillator for congestive heart failure. N Engl J Med 2005;352(3):225–37.
3. Moss AJ, Zareba W, Hall WJ, et al. Prophylactic implantation of a defibrillator in patients with myocardial infarction and reduced ejection fraction. N Engl J Med 2002;346(12):877–83.

4. Moss AJ, Hall WJ, Cannom DS, et al. Improved survival with an implanted defibrillator in patients with coronary disease at high risk for ventricular arrhythmia. Multicenter Automatic Defibrillator Implantation Trial Investigators. N Engl J Med 1996; 335(26):1933–40.

5. Buxton AE, Lee KL, Fisher JD, et al. A randomized study of the prevention of sudden death in patients with coronary artery disease. Multicenter Unsustained Tachycardia Trial Investigators. N Engl J Med 1999;341(25):1882–90.

6. Anvari A, Stix G, Grabenwoger M, et al. Comparison of three cardioverter defibrillator implantation techniques: initial results with transvenous pectoral implantation. Pacing Clin Electrophysiol 1996; 19(7):1061–9.

7. Saksena S. Defibrillation thresholds and perioperative mortality associated with endocardial and epicardial defibrillation lead systems. The PCD investigators and participating institutions. Pacing Clin Electrophysiol 1993;16(1 Pt 2):202–7.

8. Curtis JP, Luebbert JJ, Wang Y, et al. Association of physician certification and outcomes among patients receiving an implantable cardioverter-defibrillator. JAMA 2009;301(16):1661–70.

9. Kleemann T, Becker T, Doenges K, et al. Annual rate of transvenous defibrillation lead defects in implantable cardioverter-defibrillators over a period of >10 years. Circulation 2007;115(19): 2474–80.

10. Alter P, Waldhans S, Plachta E, et al. Complications of implantable cardioverter defibrillator therapy in 440 consecutive patients. Pacing Clin Electrophysiol 2005;28(9):926–32.

11. Grimm W, Menz V, Hoffmann J, et al. Complications of third-generation implantable cardioverter defibrillator therapy. Pacing Clin Electrophysiol 1999;22(1 Pt 2):206–11.

12. van Rooden CJ, Molhoek SG, Rosendaal FR, et al. Incidence and risk factors of early venous thrombosis associated with permanent pacemaker leads. J Cardiovasc Electrophysiol 2004;15(11): 1258–62.

13. Epstein AE, Baker JH 2nd, Beau SL, et al. Performance of the St. Jude Medical Riata leads. Heart Rhythm 2009;6(2):204–9.

14. Khairy P, Landzberg MJ, Gatzoulis MA, et al. Transvenous pacing leads and systemic thromboemboli in patients with intracardiac shunts: a multicenter study. Circulation 2006;113(20):2391–7.

15. Gold MR, Peters RW, Johnson JW, et al. Complications associated with pectoral implantation of cardioverter defibrillators. World-Wide Jewel Investigators. Pacing Clin Electrophysiol 1997;20(1 Pt 2):208–11.

16. Kron J, Herre J, Renfroe EG, et al. Lead- and device-related complications in the antiarrhythmics versus implantable defibrillators trial. Am Heart J 2001;141(1):92–8.

17. Dorwarth U, Frey B, Dugas M, et al. Transvenous defibrillation leads: high incidence of failure during long-term follow-up. J Cardiovasc Electrophysiol 2003;14(1):38–43.

18. Ellenbogen KA, Wood MA, Shepard RK, et al. Detection and management of an implantable cardioverter defibrillator lead failure: incidence and clinical implications. J Am Coll Cardiol 2003; 41(1):73–80.

19. Tung R, Zimetbaum P, Josephson ME. A critical appraisal of implantable cardioverter-defibrillator therapy for the prevention of sudden cardiac death. J Am Coll Cardiol 2008; 52(14):1111–21.

20. Hauser RG, Kallinen LM, Almquist AK, et al. Early failure of a small-diameter high-voltage implantable cardioverter-defibrillator lead. Heart Rhythm 2007; 4(7):892–6.

21. Danik SB, Mansour M, Singh J, et al. Increased incidence of subacute lead perforation noted with one implantable cardioverter-defibrillator. Heart Rhythm 2007;4(4):439–42.

22. Hauser RG, Almquist AK. Learning from our mistakes? Testing new ICD technology. N Engl J Med 2008;359(24):2517–9.

23. Hauser RG, Maron BJ. Lessons from the failure and recall of an implantable cardioverter-defibrillator. Circulation 2005;112(13):2040–2.

24. Sohail MR, Uslan DZ, Khan AH, et al. Management and outcome of permanent pacemaker and implantable cardioverter-defibrillator infections. J Am Coll Cardiol 2007;49(18):1851–9.

25. Maisel WH, Moynahan M, Zuckerman BD, et al. Pacemaker and ICD generator malfunctions: analysis of Food and Drug Administration annual reports. JAMA 2006;295(16):1901–6.

26. Lelakowski J, Majewski J, Malecka B, et al. Retrospective analysis of reasons for failure of DDD pacemaker implantation in patients operated on between 1993 and 2005. Cardiol J 2007;14(2):155–9.

27. Sherrid MV, Daubert JP. Risks and challenges of implantable cardioverter-defibrillators in young adults. Prog Cardiovasc Dis 2008;51(3):237–63.

28. Eckstein J, Koller MT, Zabel M, et al. Necessity for surgical revision of defibrillator leads implanted long-term: causes and management. Circulation 2008;117(21):2727–33.

29. Schoenfeld MH. The "natural" history of implantable defibrillators under advisory. Heart Rhythm 2008;5(12):1682–4.

30. Maisel WH. Implantable cardioverter-defibrillator lead complication: when is an outbreak out of bounds? Heart Rhythm 2008;5(12):1673–4.

31. Gould PA, Gula LJ, Champagne J, et al. Outcome of advisory implantable cardioverter-defibrillator

replacement: one-year follow-up. Heart Rhythm 2008;5(12):1675–81.

32. Ellenbogen KA, Wood MA, Swerdlow CD. The Sprint Fidelis lead fracture story: what do we really know and where do we go from here? Heart Rhythm 2008;5(10):1380–1.

33. Farwell D, Green MS, Lemery R, et al. Accelerating risk of Fidelis lead fracture. Heart Rhythm 2008; 5(10):1375–9.

34. Cannom DS, Fisher J. The Fidelis recall: how much pressure can the ICD world bear? Pacing Clin Electrophysiol 2008;31(10):1233–5.

35. Maisel WH. Semper fidelis–consumer protection for patients with implanted medical devices. N Engl J Med 2008;358(10):985–7.

36. Wilkoff BL. Lead failures: dealing with even less perfect. Heart Rhythm 2007;4(7):897–9.

37. Corrado A, Gasparini G, Raviele A. Lead malfunctions in implantable cardioverter defibrillators: where are we and where should we go? Europace 2009;11(3):276–7.

38. Duray GZ, Schmitt J, Cicek-Hartvig S, et al. Complications leading to surgical revision in implantable cardioverter defibrillator patients: comparison of patients with single-chamber, dual-chamber, and biventricular devices. Europace 2009;11(3):297–302.

39. Byrd CL, Wilkoff BL, Love CJ, et al. Intravascular extraction of problematic or infected permanent pacemaker leads: 1994-1996. U.S. Extraction Database, MED Institute. Pacing Clin Electrophysiol 1999;22(9):1348–57.

40. Lerman BB, Deale OC. Relation between transcardiac and transthoracic current during defibrillation in humans. Circ Res 1990;67(6):1420–6.

41. Walcott GP, Killingsworth CR, Ideker RE. Do clinically relevant transthoracic defibrillation energies cause myocardial damage and dysfunction? Resuscitation 2003;59(1):59–70.

42. Crozier I. The subcutaneous defibrillator will replace the transvenous defibrillator. J Interv Card Electrophysiol 2011;32(1):73–7.

43. Daubert JP, Zareba W, Cannom DS, et al. Inappropriate implantable cardioverter-defibrillator shocks in MADIT II: frequency, mechanisms, predictors, and survival impact. J Am Coll Cardiol 2008;51(14):1357–65.

44. van Rees JB, Borleffs CJ, de Bie MK, et al. Inappropriate implantable cardioverter-defibrillator shocks: incidence, predictors, and impact on mortality. J Am Coll Cardiol 2011;57(5):556–62.

45. Dorian P, Hohnloser SH, Thorpe KE, et al. Mechanisms underlying the lack of effect of implantable cardioverter-defibrillator therapy on mortality in high-risk patients with recent myocardial infarction: insights from the Defibrillation in Acute Myocardial

Infarction Trial (DINAMIT). Circulation 2010;122(25): 2645–52.

46. Poole JE, Johnson GW, Hellkamp AS, et al. Prognostic importance of defibrillator shocks in patients with heart failure. N Engl J Med 2008; 359(10):1009–17.

47. Schuder JC, Stoeckle H, Gold JH, et al. Experimental ventricular defibrillation with an automatic and completely implanted system. Trans Am Soc Artif Intern Organs 1970;16:207–12.

48. Burke MC, Coman JA, Cates AW, et al. Defibrillation energy requirements using a left anterior chest cutaneous to subcutaneous shocking vector: implications for a total subcutaneous implantable defibrillator. Heart Rhythm 2005;2(12):1332–8.

49. Gold MR, Theuns DA, Knight BP, et al. Head-to-head comparison of arrhythmia discrimination performance of subcutaneous and transvenous ICD arrhythmia detection algorithms: the START study. J Cardiovasc Electrophysiol 2012;23(4):359–66.

50. Bardy GH, Smith WM, Hood MA, et al. An entirely subcutaneous implantable cardioverter-defibrillator. N Engl J Med 2010;363(1):36–44.

51. S-ICD system commercial implants analysis, Q2 2012. Data on file. San Clemente (CA): Cameron Health, Inc.

52. Daliento L, Turrini P, Nava A, et al. Arrhythmogenic right ventricular cardiomyopathy in young versus adult patients: similarities and differences. J Am Coll Cardiol 1995;25(3):655–64.

53. Probst V, Denjoy I, Meregalli PG, et al. Clinical aspects and prognosis of Brugada syndrome in children. Circulation 2007;115(15):2042–8.

54. Priori SG, Schwartz PJ, Napolitano C, et al. Risk stratification in the long-QT syndrome. N Engl J Med 2003;348(19):1866–74.

55. Colan SD, Lipshultz SE, Lowe AM, et al. Epidemiology and cause-specific outcome of hypertrophic cardiomyopathy in children: findings from the Pediatric Cardiomyopathy Registry. Circulation 2007; 115(6):773–81.

56. Alexander ME, Cecchin F, Walsh EP, et al. Implications of implantable cardioverter defibrillator therapy in congenital heart disease and pediatrics. J Cardiovasc Electrophysiol 2004;15(1):72–6.

57. Berul CI, Van Hare GF, Kertesz NJ, et al. Results of a multicenter retrospective implantable cardioverter-defibrillator registry of pediatric and congenital heart disease patients. J Am Coll Cardiol 2008;51(17):1685–91.

58. Berul CI. Defibrillator indications and implantation in young children. Heart Rhythm 2008;5(12):1755–7.

59. Sweeney MO, Sherfesee L, DeGroot PJ, et al. Differences in effects of electrical therapy type for ventricular arrhythmias on mortality in implantable

cardioverter-defibrillator patients. Heart Rhythm 2010;7(3):353–60.

60. de Bie MK, Thijssen J, van Rees JB, et al. Suitability for subcutaneous defibrillator implantation: results based on data from routine clinical practice. Heart 2013;99(14):1018–23.

61. Lupo PP, Pelissero G, Ali H, et al. Development of an entirely subcutaneous implantable cardioverter-defibrillator. Prog Cardiovasc Dis 2012; 54(6):493–7.

62. Jarman JW, Lascelles K, Wong T, et al. Clinical experience of entirely subcutaneous implantable cardioverter-defibrillators in children and adults: cause for caution. Eur Heart J 2012;33(11):1351–9.

63. Olde Nordkamp LR, Dabiri Abkenari L, Boersma LV, et al. The entirely subcutaneous implantable cardioverter-defibrillator: initial clinical experience in a large Dutch cohort. J Am Coll Cardiol 2012;60(19):1933–9.

64. Köbe J, Reinke F, Meyer C, et al. Implantation and follow-up of totally subcutaneous versus conventional implantable cardioverter-defibrillators: a multicenter case-control study. Heart Rhythm 2013;10(1):29–36.

65. Weiss R, Knight BP, Gold MR, et al. Safety and efficacy of a totally subcutaneous implantable-cardioverter defibrillator. Circulation 2013;128(9): 944–53.

The Modern EP Practice
EHR and Remote Monitoring

Suneet Mittal, MD[a], Colin Movsowitz, MBChB[b],
Niraj Varma, MA, DM, FRCP[c],*

KEYWORDS

- Defibrillators • Patient monitoring • Follow-up • Remote monitoring guidelines

KEY POINTS

- The follow-up of cardiac implantable electronic devices (CIEDs) is transitioning from scheduled routine in-office visits to remote monitoring and alert-driven, unscheduled in-office visits.
- Remote monitoring of wireless CIEDs permits early access to clinically valuable information about system integrity, arrhythmias, and heart failure parameters.
- Clinical trials have substantiated the safety and efficacy of remote monitoring in clinical practice.
- It is imperative that barriers that have limited enrollment of patients into remote monitoring systems and for patients to remotely transmit information on a reliable basis be overcome.
- New work flows have to be developed that facilitate the effective capture and communication of information acquired from remote monitoring systems to ensure maximal clinical benefit for patients.

INTRODUCTION

The implantation of cardiac implantable electronic devices (CIEDs) has increased exponentially during the last decade in response to widening indications. Subsequent monitoring is an integral part of both device and patient care. However, follow-up schedules vary according to facility, physician preference, and available resources.[1] A review of recent US Medicare beneficiaries revealed that almost a quarter of patients were not seen in the year after the implant.[2] This finding represents a quality-of-care deficit, highlighted by the comparative survival advantage gained by those patients who did adhere to the prescribed follow-up.[3] To address this problem, professional organizations have advocated the institution of regular periodic assessments for patients receiving CIEDs.[4] However, frequent in-office evaluation generates a large service commitment and challenges patient compliance, and its efficacy has remained unappraised until recently. Such a system is further stressed in response to product advisories or recalls or with unscheduled encounters (eg, shock therapy or elective replacement indicator [ERI] status). A major limitation of this conventional follow-up method, which is based on patient presentation, is that no monitoring takes place between office visits (ie, most of the time). This lack of monitoring will miss important events, especially if asymptomatic (eg, regarding system integrity or onset of arrhythmias, such as atrial

Disclosures: Consultant to Biotronik, Boston Scientific, Medtronic, Scottcare, and St Jude Medical (S. Mittal); Consultant to Biotronik, Boston Scientific, Scottcare, and St Jude Medical (C. Movsowitz); Research/speaker to Biotronik, Boston Scientific, Medtronic, and St Jude Medical (N. Varma).

[a] Electrophysiology Laboratory, The Valley Hospital Health System, Ridgewood, NJ 07450, USA; [b] Cardiology Consultants of Philadelphia, Einstein Medical Center Montgomery, 609 West Germantown Pike, East Norriton, PA 19403, USA; [c] Heart and Vascular Institute, J2-2 Cardiac Pacing and Electrophysiology, Cleveland Clinic, 9500 Euclid Avenue, Cleveland, OH 44195, USA
* Corresponding author.
E-mail address: varman@ccf.org

fibrillation [AF]). Their early detection is critical to optimal patient care.

Remote Follow-up and Remote Monitoring

Remote monitoring is a potential mechanism for performing intensive device and patient surveillance. Different functions are identified. Remote follow-up involves scheduled automatic device interrogation, which replaces in-office visits aimed at assessing device function (eg, battery status, thresholds, and so forth). The interrogations can be performed automatically in patients implanted with modern wireless devices and manually using wanded home transmitters if the implanted device is not enabled with wireless technology. Remote monitoring involves automatic unscheduled transmission of alert events (eg, AF, abnormal lead impedance, and so forth). This feature is possible in all modern wireless devices. Patient-initiated interrogations are nonscheduled follow-ups initiated manually by patients as a result of a real or perceived clinical event.

Remote Technologies

The platforms available for remote monitoring of CIEDs differ. Wand-based (inductive) systems require patient-driven downloads relayed via telephone connections to tracking facilities.[5,6] These systems are becoming obsolete because they demand coordination with a device clinic on a calendar-based schedule, are cumbersome to use, challenge compliance, and increase service

burden without offering gain.[7,8] Important diagnostic data may be overwritten because device diagnostics have finite memory. Early detection is limited. Thus, when used to follow up a pacemaker population, clinically actionable events took several months to be discovered, and only 66% of data were transmitted.[9] In contrast, automatic (wireless or landline) transmission mechanisms are fully independent of patient and physician interaction (**Fig. 1**), which makes them particularly suitable for children[10] and the elderly. Data may be reviewed securely via the Internet. This system was pioneered by Home Monitoring (HM) (Biotronik, Berlin, Germany), with excellent reliability and early notification ability.[11] Ninety percent of transmitted data were received within 5 minutes, with greater than 99% data fidelity. Implantable cardioverter-defibrillator (ICD) generators were shown to self-declare problems promptly regardless of interrogation schedules or associated symptoms.[12,13] System operation is not energy costly.[14] This technology has the ability to maintain surveillance and rapidly bring to attention significant data, enabling clinically appropriate intervention. These potentials have been tested prospectively in recent trials.

Clinical Trials

The first large remote monitoring trial was the Lumos-T Safely Reduces Routine Office Device Follow-up (TRUST).[12,15] In this trial, 1500 patients were randomized to remote management with HM or conventional face-to-face evaluations

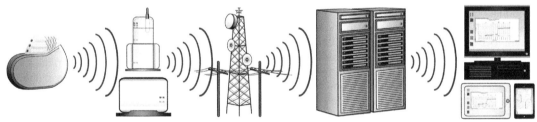

Fig. 1. Automatic remote monitoring technology: transmission steps associated with the Biotronik Home Monitoring system. A very-low-power radiofrequency transmitter circuitry integrated within the pulse generator wirelessly transmits stored data daily to a mobile transceiver (typically placed bedside at night). The data are relayed via landline or wirelessly to a service center that generates customized summaries available online via secure Internet access. Thus, patients are monitored daily, and trend analysis information is compiled from typical follow-up data (eg, battery status, lead impedance, and sensing function). Processing is fully automatic, bypassing potential delays (and errors) associated with manual processing. Critical event data may be transmitted immediately and flagged for attention on the Web page. Automatic alerts occur for silent but potentially dangerous events. These alerts include transmission of intracardiac electrograms (IEGM-online snapshots) similar to those available during office-based device interrogations. This technology provides the ability for early detection and enables prompt clinical intervention, if necessary. Daily transmission load had no effect on battery longevity in the Lumos-T Safely Reduces Routine Office Device Follow-up trial. (*From* Varma N, Ricci RP. Telemedicine and cardiac implants: what is the benefit? Eur Heart J 2012;34:1885–95, with permission; and *Data from* Varma N, Michalski J, Epstein A, TRUST Investigators. Long term preservation of battery longevity (despite daily transmission load) with home monitoring: the TRUST trial. Europace 2013;Suppl:Abstract.)

(Fig. 2, *top left*). HM promoted greater adherence to long-term follow-up without compromising safety. (This safety end point was endorsed in the ECOST [Effectiveness and Cost Of ICD follow-up Schedule with Telecardiology] trial during longer follow-up.[16]) When inclusive of all patient encounters (ie, scheduled and unscheduled), health care utilization was reduced by approximately 50% (see **Fig. 2**, *top right*). The second important result of TRUST was demonstration of early detection ability of clinical events during continuous remote monitoring. Despite the extension of intervals between face-to-face encounters to yearly, event the onset to physician evaluation of combined first AF, ventricular tachycardia (VT), and fibrillation (VF) events in HM was median 1 day, dramatically less than in conventional care (>1 month) despite frequent face-to-face encounters (see **Fig. 2**, *bottom left*). Importantly, early detection was maintained for silent problems (see **Fig. 2**, *bottom right*). (This ability was inconceivable even a few years previously with wanded remote systems when detection at 5.7 months

was considered early.[9]) Similar benefits were seen in pacemaker recipients in the COMPAS (COMPArative follow-up Schedule with home monitoring) trial.[17] The HomeGuide Registry confirmed that the high quality of remotely acquired data since the majority (>80%) of clinically meaningful events were remotely detected (sensitivity 84%; positive predictive value 97%).[18]

The CONNECT (Clinical Evaluation of Remote Notification to Reduce Time to Clinical Decision) trial followed up to TRUST with a similar study design but with a different wireless remote technology (Medtronic CareLink Network, Medtronic, Inc, Minneapolis, MN) in a separate ICD population.[19] The results confirmed that remote interrogation effectively substituted for in-office visits and provided early detection capability. However, safety was not assessed. Furthermore, the susceptibility of this technology platform to transmission failure with negative effects of multiple transmission attempts on battery longevity is significant.[20] When alert transmissions for some conditions were successful, manual reset was

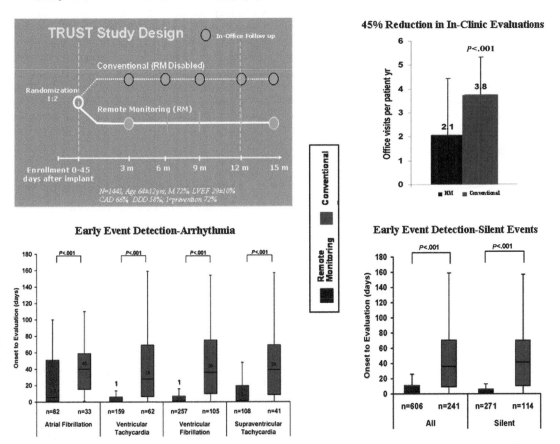

Fig. 2. TRUST study. (*Top left*) Study design: remote monitoring versus conventional care; (*Top right*) effect on clinic volumes per year; (*Bottom left*) early detection of arrhythmias; (*Bottom right*) early detection of silent problems. (*From* Varma N, Epstein A, Irimpen A, et al, TRUST Investigators. Efficacy and safety of automatic remote monitoring for ICD follow-up: the TRUST trial. Circulation 2010;122:325–32; with permission.)

required to reactivate this notification ability (ie, the ability for further notification in the interim was lost until an otherwise unnecessary in-person encounter could be arranged). This design, depending on patient interaction and single transmissions vulnerable to failure, limits its role as an early warning mechanism. Technology reliability remains unreported with the Boston Scientific Latitude (Boston Scientific Corporation, Natick, MA) and the St Jude Merlin.net (St Jude Medical, Inc, St Paul, MN) systems.

DEVICE MANAGEMENT

Remote monitoring with the capability for same-day discovery of problems (even when asymptomatic), when appropriate technology and clinic infrastructure are in place,[21] may profoundly affect patient management. Although HM does not supplant the first postimplant in-person evaluation[4] important for the assessment of wound healing, determination of chronic thresholds, and setting of final pacing parameters, subsequent device follow-up may be better achieved with remote monitoring,[13,22] especially for components subject to advisories. This postulate underlied the original announcements from professional societies for "device manufacturers use wireless and remote monitoring technologies to identify device malfunctions in a timely manner and to increase the accuracy of detecting and reporting device

malfunctions",[23] carrying the expectation of early detection and correction of device malfunction.[23,24] TRUST confirmed that conventional monitoring methods underreport device-related problems (**Fig. 3**).[13] Automatic remote monitoring, in contrast, enhanced the discovery of system problems (even when asymptomatic) and enabled prompt clinical decisions regarding conservative versus surgical management. Most ICD system malfunctions could be identified within 24 hours of occurrence even though performance problems were often asymptomatic.[21] (In contrast, these would remain quiescent with conventional follow-up or even wanded remote systems.) The ECOST trial[16] showed that clinical reactions enabled by early detection resulted in a large reduction in the number of actually delivered shocks (−72%), the number of charged shocks (−76%), the rate of inappropriate shocks (−52%) and, at the same time, exerted a favorable impact on battery longevity.

Recalls and Advisories

Managing components under advisory notices poses several daunting challenges. **Fig. 4** illustrates the benefit of HM for the management of recalled components.[23,25] Advisories encompass disintegration of high-voltage circuitry, battery depletion, and lead failure—almost all of which are captured by currently evaluated event triggers.[26,27] In comparison, conventional detection

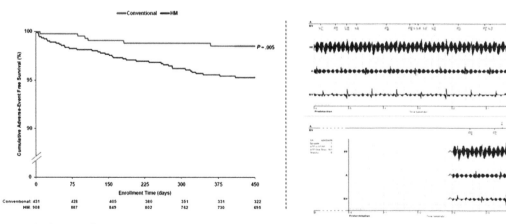

Fig. 3. (*Left*) Event-free survival rates in HM patients compared with conventional-care group. The observed time to the first event was shorter in the HM group. Although the incidence of patients developing system problems was similar in both groups, these incidents were considerably underreported with conventional care. (*Right*) Event notification received for an aborted shock detected at 7:16 PM. The accompanying automatic, wirelessly transmitted electrogram shows gross artifact on both atrial and ventricular leads. The patient was asymptomatic but, in response to the notification, was seen in the office within 24 hours. The observation of nonphysiologic signals simultaneously on both leads suggests the presence of electromagnetic interference. (*From* Varma N, Michalski J, Epstein AE, et al. Automatic remote monitoring of implantable cardioverter-defibrillator lead and generator performance: the Lumos-T Safely Reduces Routine Office Device Follow-up (TRUST) trial. Circ Arrhythm Electrophysiol 2010;3:428–36; with permission.)

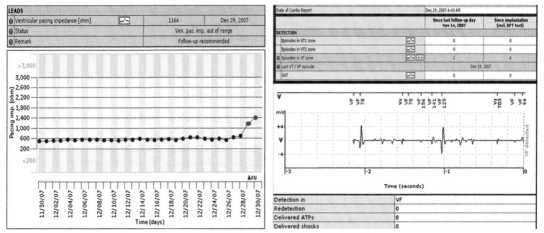

Fig. 4. A Biotronik HM–enabled generator coupled to a Sprint Fidelis (Medtronic 6949) ICD lead transmitted 2 event notifications immediately on occurrence of a lead fracture, occurring silently during sleep at 4:43 AM, 6 weeks after last clinic follow-up on November 14. (*Left*) Lead impedance alert triggered on sudden increase from prior stable trend (600 Ω). (*Right*) A separate notification response to the same event, indicating 2 occurrences of detection in VF zone (*top*) and flagged (*red exclamation mark on yellow background*). The accompanying wirelessly transmitted electrogram demonstrated irregular sensed events (coupling intervals as short as 78 ms) with VF detection (*marked*). No therapy was delivered, indicating spontaneous event termination. ATP, antitachycardia pacing; FU, follow-up. (*From* Varma N. Remote monitoring for advisories: automatic early detection of silent lead failure. Pacing Clin Electrophysiol 2009;32:525–27; with permission.)

methods, such as increasing the frequency of office visits,[28] are impractical, burdensome, and likely to miss dangerous interim problems. Patient alert mechanisms, such as beeps, are insensitive and prone to false-positive evaluations.[29] In contrast, HM generators trigger immediate alerts when data deviate from established trends. This capability reduces the burden both for patients who frequently monitor their own devices and for clinics who are responsible for large cardiac patient populations that have a low incidence of typically silent problems. The ability to collect detailed, device-specific data and to assess component function daily and automatically archive the information sets a precedent for the long-term evaluation of lead and generator performance. Technology differences may affect early detection capability. Early discovery can be improved with repeated messaging in the instance that the initial clinic notification was missed.[21]

Remote monitoring for device function has great benefits for patients. It may facilitate the management of unscheduled encounters provoked by device-related symptoms.[30] For example, an appropriate or phantom ICD shock could be managed simply with a reassuring telephone conversation. However, an in-person evaluation may be recommended if the physician and/or patients expressed any reservation regarding reconciliation of stated symptoms with remotely acquired data. There is increasing patient concern regarding the

function of their implanted devices, despite the great overall reliability of implantable technology in general. Patients who have received inappropriate shocks or informed of recalled components may be particularly apprehensive. In this regard, remote monitoring (rather than remote follow-up at preset intervals) is especially assuring.

DISEASE MANAGEMENT
AF

AF event notifications are commonly received during automatic remote surveillance. These data may influence important clinical decisions to treat or prevent stroke, ventricular arrhythmias, and heart failure (HF). However, diagnosing AF events is challenging. The ability to detect this evanescent and largely asymptomatic arrhythmia early, by automatic remote monitoring, may permit early treatment,[11] such as starting anticoagulants, controlling heart rate for rapid ventricular rates that may elicit inappropriate shock therapy or lead to HF, or reversion to normal sinus rhythm. There may be a potential benefit for stroke risk reduction.[31] The interaction of AF and HF is particularly deleterious. One large multicenter study (1193 patients with cardiac resynchronization therapy-defibrillator [CRT-D] from 44 Italian centers) reported significantly higher freedom from the composite end point of death or heart transplantation or HF hospitalization in patients in sinus rhythm than in those with AF.[32] AF associated with periods of rapid ventricular conduction reduces the benefits of CRT.[33] Withdrawal of ventricular pacing in CRT-D is immediately notified during remote monitoring.

HF

In patients with HF, nonimplantable technologies, depending on patient compliance and following nonspecific parameters, have been unhelpful.[34] Preliminary signals indicate a benefit from remote monitoring (eg, the significant shortening of hospital length of stay and reduced overall hospital costs).[19] Device-based physiologic information and diagnostics indicate that several interdependent cardiovascular factors (arrhythmias and paced burden shifts, intrathoracic impedance, vagal withdrawal, intracardiac hemodynamics) may change several days to weeks before ultimate hospitalization.[35] A combined risk score incorporating all of these individual factors may improve their predictive value,[36] creating an opportunity for early preemptive intervention. Success will depend on accurate longitudinal parameter trends (preferably updated daily) and early notification for out-of-bounds parameter groups. This function can be efficiently delivered by remote monitoring. Preliminary results from a large multicenter trial (IN-TIME [Influence of Home Monitoring on the clinical status of heart failure patients]) indicated that remotely managed patients with HF suffered fewer HF hospitalizations and their mortality was reduced.[37]

Mega-Cohort Studies

Remote monitoring collects a wealth of data from large numbers of patients that is not subject to saturation or overwritten memory counters within any implantable device. These databases provide an opportunity to better understand system function, patient condition, and disease progression in real-world patients, as opposed to more narrowly defined enrollees in relatively short-term trials. Long-term parameter trends derived from these databases will provide important measures of system performance (eg, generator and lead survival). Automatically archived data will also permit an accurate follow-up of patient morbidities. For example, AF is difficult to characterize in practice; but remote monitoring permits clinicians to interpret arrhythmia patterns, absolute AF burden, degree of temporal dispersion, and progression to persistent arrhythmia. These factors may help clinicians to understand the risks this condition poses and to optimize its management. These questions are being addressed, in

particular by the ALTITUDE committee, which observed that networked patients derived a survival benefit.[38]

BARRIERS TO ENROLLING IN REMOTE MONITORING

The rationales for instituting remote monitoring of patients with CIEDs as a routine part of the modern electrophysiology practice seem, on the surface, to be self-evident. There is a wealth of scientific data supporting the clinical value to remote monitoring in patients with CIEDs. In addition to the early management of important arrhythmias (eg, AF, VT, and VF), reductions in hospitalizations and strokes related to atrial arrhythmias, reductions in inappropriate and appropriate ICD shocks, an increase in battery longevity, and decreased mortality have all been demonstrated.[12,16,17,38] As an early notification system, remote monitoring is well aligned with the ongoing health care reform in the United States. For example, the Affordable Care Act of 2010 required the Department of Health and Human Services to establish a readmission-reduction program. Toward that end, remote patient monitoring may significantly reduce the likelihood of readmission by heading off small problems before they become critical. These problems may be related to the device, leads, arrhythmias, or a patient's HF status (**Box 1**). Virtually all CIED devices are capable of

---

Box 1
The promises of remote monitoring

Device related

- ERI or end of life

Lead related

- Significant Δ in pacing Ω
- Significant increase in pacing thresholds
- Significant increase in the percentage of right ventricular pacing
- Significant decrease in the percentage of left ventricular pacing

Arrhythmia related

- New onset of atrial tachycardia/fibrillation (AT/AF)
- Rapid ventricular rates during ongoing AT/AF
- Nonsustained or sustained VT/VF, including information about antitachycardia pacing and delivery of ICD shocks

HF related

remote follow-up; increasingly, devices are wireless, which allows them to provide remote monitoring on a continuous basis. Finally, at least in the United States, there is a defined reimbursement policy that permits monthly reimbursement for the monitoring of implantable cardiac monitors and HF parameters and quarterly reimbursement for monitoring of pacemakers, defibrillators, and CRT devices (**Box 2**).

However, despite these rationales, the reality is that a significant number of patients are never enrolled in remote monitoring despite undergoing implantation of a CIED fully capable of such monitoring. Data from the Medtronic CareLink system show that, in 2010, only 66% of eligible patients were enrolled into remote monitoring; by 2013, the enrollment rate had actually decreased to 55%. Thus, there seems to be a disparity between the scientific data supporting the clinical value of remote monitoring and the ability/willingness of health care providers to actually implement this for their patients. Furthermore, even when patients are enrolled into a remote monitoring system, only a trivial number of patients are actually undergoing quarterly remote monitoring.

The authors have identified 5 major barriers that preclude universal enrollment of patients into a remote monitoring program.[39] The greatest barrier is technology. Many patients are unable to correctly connect the remote monitoring system once it arrives to their home. The need to connect to an analog phone line has been particularly problematic. Some patients do not take the initiative of splitting their analog phone line to connect their remote monitoring system; for others, the use of a cable or voice-over-Internet-protocols telephone system in their home precludes seamless operation of the remote systems. Importantly, the Biotronik HM system overcomes this limitation; HM requires that patients connect the unit into a power outlet but is otherwise completely automatic. Data transmission then occurs seamlessly over a Global System for Mobile (GSM) cellular network. Although other vendors also offer a GSM-based option, this may not be fully automatic, and patients needs to bear the monthly charge for cellular service. This charge is something many patients are unwilling to accept, especially older patients on fixed incomes. To date, individual practices are unable and hospital systems unwilling to absorb this additional cost on behalf of their patients, despite the efficiencies that ensue from large-scale adoption of remote monitoring.

A second important barrier is the inability of patients to grasp the difference between remote monitoring and remote follow-up. The latter can obviate some in-office visits but cannot completely eliminate these visits. Most patients welcome the increased convenience of remote follow-up; however, a minority dislikes the concept because they prefer face-to-face contact with their physician. Thus, patients need further education on the value of continuous surveillance to optimize their device and disease management.

Another issue is to understand the role and belief of the referring cardiologist. Some cardiologists accept the responsibility for remote follow-up and/or monitoring but lack the infrastructure in their practice to execute reliably; others specifically discourage their patients from remote monitoring or follow-up, typically citing the absence of clinical guidelines. Finally, in a small number of patients, a language barrier precludes them from understanding the available literature from vendors on remote systems because there is very little information available in a language other than English.

Box 2
Reimbursement for remote monitoring

Technical reimbursement

- 93296 ($36)

    Interrogation device evaluations remote, up to 90 days; single, dual, or multiple lead permanent pacemaker (PPM) or ICD system, remote data acquisitions, receipt of transmissions and technician review, technical support and distribution of results

Professional reimbursement

- 93294 ($37; once per 90 days)

    Interrogation device evaluations (remote), up to 90 days; single, dual, or multiple lead PPM system with interim physician analysis, reviews, and reports

- 93295 ($66; once per 90 days)

    Interrogation device evaluations (remote), up to 90 days; single, dual, or multiple lead ICD system with interim physician analysis, reviews, and reports

- 93297 ($26; once per 30 days)

    Interrogation device evaluations (remote), up to 30 days; implantable cardiovascular monitor system, including analysis of 1 or more recorded physiologic cardiovascular data elements from all internal or external sensors, physician analysis, reviews, and reports

THE FOLLOW-UP CLINIC IN THE ERA OF REMOTE MONITORING

Best-Case Scenario

The safe and effective replacement of the bulk of routine in-clinic evaluations demonstrated in TRUST (see **Fig. 2**) has potential implications for resource utilization. Although demanding a restructuring of work-flow patterns, especially for alert notifications, this was balanced by the reduction of routine nonactionable in-person evaluations, as demonstrated by Ricci and colleagues using HM.[18,40] Before the implementation of HM, all involved personnel, including patients, were primed to the process and expectations. The results were astonishing: the median committed monthly manpower was 55.5 minutes of health personnel per 100 patients with a range of CIEDs. This efficiency was based on a cooperative interaction between a reference nurse and a responsible physician with an agreed list of respective tasks and responsibilities. Although demanding extra resources, nurse-based remote patient management improves follow-up quality, generates manpower efficiencies, and directs only problematic remote assessments (which occur infrequently) to physicians otherwise released to their other assignments.

Current Reality

The promise suggested earlier has been difficult to translate to most modern electrophysiology practices. The best-case scenario has emerged as a result of 3 fundamental assumptions. The first is that all patients have been enrolled into a remote monitoring system and have successfully established a connection to the monitoring center. Although the Biotronik HM system is a plug-and-play model, systems from other vendors have required an additional connection to an analog phone line, which has been difficult for some patients (as described earlier). Second, all patients were monitored using the Biotronik HM system. In reality, most electrophysiologists work within a universe that includes remote monitoring systems from several device manufacturers; it remains unproven whether all remote monitoring systems can deliver the same benefits as the Biotronik HM system. Third, in the studies to date, there was no requirement for written communication of all remote interrogations to patients' health care providers. This is necessary if all of the patients' health care providers are either not part of the same practice or do not share the same electronic medical record (EMR) and, thus, have no access to the remotely acquired information.

To understand the impact of remote monitoring on the manpower requirements and revenues, the authors performed a comprehensive 1-year review of all patients with CIEDs followed in one of their (SM) practices. A total of 1148 patients with CIEDs generated 3194 device checks (either remote or in the office). The principal responsibility of the device follow-up was assigned to a single advanced nurse practitioner (ANP); she spent 20% of her time exclusively on remote monitoring of patients and another 20% of her time on purely administrative (nonclinical) responsibilities related to scheduling and billing of patients with CIEDs. Most pacemaker checks were performed as in-office checks; although a greater portion of ICD checks were performed remotely, most were still also performed in the office. Unfortunately, with a single ANP responsible for all of the authors' device checks (in the office and remote), they were unable to achieve their goal of monthly remote checks of implantable cardiac monitors and quarterly remote checks of pacemakers and ICDs. (Of note, during this period, there was no systematic attempt made to monitor HF status on appropriate patients on a monthly basis.) Not surprisingly, this incomplete adherence to a desired remote monitoring had a marked adverse financial impact on the authors' practice (**Fig. 5**). In the authors' opinion, practices need to appreciate that remote monitoring requires a staff dedicated to this service (adopted in the practice of NV); to expect that it can simply be tagged onto an in-office service line is inherently unrealistic without devoting significant resources to hire and train additional staff.

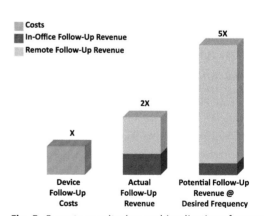

Fig. 5. Remote monitoring and implications for revenues. The costs and revenues in one of the authors' practices (SM) were evaluated over the course of a single calendar year. The salary of the ANP, the rent for the office space, and purchase of required supplies accounted for the cost (X) of running the device clinic. Although the device clinic yielded revenues of 2X, it was possible to earn 5X with adherence to the desired remote monitoring schedule.

FUTURE DIRECTIONS

In constructing an electrophysiology practice in 2013 and beyond, the following facts need to be accepted. There is an ever-growing number of patients with CIEDs, and this number will continue to grow for the foreseeable future. CIEDs store valuable data related to system integrity, arrhythmias, and HF parameters. Wireless technology allows for the near-continuous transmission of these data without patient intervention, and the Internet allows for worldwide access to these data. There is evidence that remote monitoring allows early access to the clinically valuable data stored in wireless CIEDs and that access to these data impacts patient care, improves outcomes, and decreases mortality. In the future, it is likely that these devices will provide better information about diseases, such as HF (eg, data from pulmonary artery and direct left atrial pressure sensors) as well as additional disease states (eg, sleep apnea). Future devices may also alert patients directly of changes in their condition, thus, encouraging them to participate in their own therapy. Eventually, it seems inevitable that devices with closed-loop systems will render obsolete much of the current monitoring requirements of device parameters. Automatic threshold testing and output adjustments have already eliminated what used to be the main reason for in-office device follow-up.

The goal of the modern electrophysiology practice is to access the data stored in CIEDs in a timely fashion, mine this data for clinically valuable information, and present this information in a contextual and relevant format to the device-following physician and EMR system (**Fig. 6**). The immediate challenge is one of data management. How does one create a new work flow that will take the issues presented earlier into consideration and yet continue to be flexible enough to accommodate the rapidly changing landscape of patient care?

Shared Labor Force Model

Scottcare/Ambucor is an example of a software and personal service company that attempts to address the unmet need within a modern electrophysiology practice to maximize the clinical utility of remote patient monitoring (**Box 3**, see **Fig. 6**). Currently, this enterprise operates only within the United States. Ambucor provides a virtual shared labor force for employment by individual electrophysiology practices. This labor force is composed of certified technicians, ANPs, and physician assistants who provide continuous coverage from its operational center in Wilmington, Delaware. The service operates under the direct supervision of the electrophysiology physician and is bound by individual and customized agreements between the electrophysiology provider/practice and the Ambucor workforce. The electrophysiology practice can directly incorporate Ambucor services, avoiding the issues of fee splitting inherent to a relationship with an independent diagnostic testing facility. Furthermore, this relationship provides the practice with complete

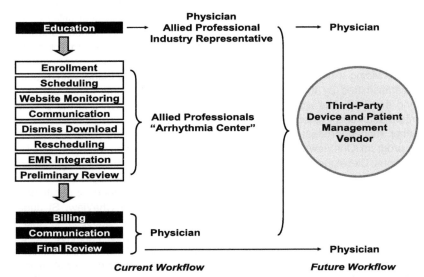

Fig. 6. Current and proposed future work flow for remote patient monitoring and follow-up. (*From* Movsowitz C, Mittal S. Remote patient management using implanted devices. J Interv Card Electrophysiol 2011;31:81–90; with permission.)

transparency and oversight over the tests administered. Ambucor essentially provides a shared workforce for practices, thereby eliminating the need to employ additional staff to provide continuous monitoring. The Ambucor workforce plays a pivotal role in providing a human interface between the data transmitted by the CIEDs to the Web portals and the EMR. The workforce mines the data for information and presents processed information rather than unprocessed data to a data repository program (OneView; Scottcare Cardiovascular Solutions, Cleveland, OH) or the EMR.

OneView is a device-neutral, Web-based platform for the capture, display, and reporting of both remote and in-clinic CIED interrogations. OneView retrieves data from the various proprietary Web portals and provides a central workstation for reporting and data analysis. Reports in the form of PDF files can be exported to EHRs that have been configured to be interfaced with OneView. Alternatively, discrete data elements can be exported to interfaced EMRs with device

follow-up templates. The only other data repository system currently available is the Medtronic Paceart system (Medtronic Inc, Minneapolis, MN). However, as compared with Paceart, OneView offers 2 distinct advantages. First, it can also be a data repository for ambulatory external electrocardiogram monitoring (eg, Holter monitoring, patient-activated event monitoring, automatically triggered loop monitoring, and ambulatory cardiovascular telemetry monitoring). Second, the platform is Web based. This benefit is particularly advantageous for practices that deliver care to device patients in various locations because the data can be accessed over any personal computer that is connected to the Internet.

The modern electrophysiology practice must accommodate the Health Information Technology for Economic and Clinical Health Act, which was signed into law in 2009 by President Obama as part of the American Recovery and Reinvestment Act in 2009. This act essentially mandates that practices institute EMR systems; the rationale for the EMR is that it will reduce medical errors and the cost of caring for patients (eliminating duplicative tests and services). Most electrophysiology practices, which incorporate electrophysiologists, allied health professionals, and in-office support staff, are already overwhelmed with EMR implementation; the need to incorporate remote monitoring data presents an additional challenge. To make matters worse, at the current time, there are multiple device companies and many EMR systems. Historically, device companies have been incentivized to create products with proprietary features to maintain a competitive advantage over rivals. To optimize the clinical utility of the EMR, interoperability across device vendors is necessary; this goal does not seem achievable in the near future. In the interim, companies like Scottcare/Ambucor are working with practices to create the necessary interfaces between the various vendors, OneView, and the practices' particular EMR system.

Device companies are also trying to provide a direct connection between the CIED data (acquired either from their programmer or Web portal) and the practices' EMR in an attempt to minimize or eliminate the need for additional staff or use of middleware like OneView. St Jude Medical has achieved some success in this endeavor by adhering to industry-defined standards (Implantable Device Cardiac Observation profile) on its Web portal (Merlin.net) for all incoming data from its programmers and wireless CIEDs. Additionally, St Jude Medical has created interfaces between its proprietary Web portal (Merlin.net) and several

EHRs, thus, forgoing the need for middleware. Although on the surface it would seem that this direct interface is ideal, in actuality, this model has its own issues. CIEDs generate a great deal of data, much of which is not of clinical significance. Exporting all these data into the EMR slows it down, making it more time consuming to even open a patient's chart.

Creating an Integrated Remote Monitoring Center

Although the available scientific data supports the clinical utility of routine remote monitoring of patients with CIEDs, the reality is that only one-half of all eligible patients are being enrolled into remote monitoring and only a rare patient is actually transmitting data on a quarterly basis. This reality suggests the need to reexamine our current work flow, which largely leaves the responsibility of managing remote monitoring to individual practices. It remains unclear whether the expertise exists within these practices to expeditiously manage device advisories, optimize pacing and tachyarrhythmia detection and therapy programing, determine which atrial high-rate episodes are clinically meaningful, manage inappropriate and inappropriate ICD shocks, and recognize impending HF.

The Scottcare/Ambucor model provides an opportunity to explore a different patient care model. Its technicians monitor for arrhythmias and HF and alert the electrophysiology physician based on prespecified criteria. In this model, data gleaned from remote monitoring of CIEDs are mined for information that is interfaced into the patients' EMR where the patients' physician acts on the acquired data. In the future, as physicians become hospital employees, it stands to reason that large centralized remote monitoring centers may emerge in lieu of the smaller centers taking place in individual practices.

Role of Remote Interrogation in Other Health Care Settings

Patients with CIEDs frequently present to the emergency department, need to go the operating room for a surgical procedure, need magnetic resonance imaging, or are admitted to hospital. At that time, patients frequently need to have their CIEDs interrogated to examine the stored data, which may shed light on the clinical presentation. The days of device representatives being available to interrogate devices anywhere at anytime are likely coming to an end as all device companies continue to contract their sales force in response to the financial constraints being observed in today's health care

system. This work is likely to be replaced by remote device interrogation systems.

All device vendors have developed or are actively developing proprietary universal and agnostic interrogators (with respect to devices manufactured by a given vendor) capable of performing inductive downloads of device data to the company's Web proprietary portal. These interrogators will ultimately be placed in the radiology suite, operating rooms, emergency departments, and on hospital floors where they will allow for timely interrogations that will be transmitted to a central Web site and interpreted by trained technical staff. This work flow promises to be more time efficient and will alleviate the unremunerated service burden currently placed on the device companies.

The first 2 vendors that have entered this market are Medtronic and St Jude Medical. Medtronic made the first foray into testing the commercial viability of this approach. The CareLink Express system is available for implementation in hospitals using several different financial models. The inductive monitors can be placed in emergency departments, postanesthesia care units, and on the hospital inpatient floors. Downloads made by the hospital staff to the CareLink site are available to the hospital staff for interpretation at no cost. Alternatively, the hospital can enter into a business arrangement with Medtronic whereby the hospital pays Medtronic for providing around-the-clock skilled technicians to interpret downloads and communicate the results to the hospital staff. CareLink Express is advertised to save the hospital money by improving triage in the emergency department by reducing the average wait time for representative interrogation from 84 minutes to less than 15 minutes with CareLink Express.[41] While this article was in development, St Jude Medical was completing their New Technology Assessment testing of their Merlin OnDemand product.

Remote Reprogramming

Remote reprogramming seems to be a natural extension of the function of a remote monitoring center. Remote programing is not currently a feature in any CIED. Remote reprogramming is intriguing in that it could provide efficiencies in the management of patients with CIEDs. Remote interrogation/monitoring is a passive intervention where data are collected. It does not change how the device delivers therapy and, therefore, has been accepted by patients and physicians.

Remote reprogramming implies an active change in the device function. This change could include deactivation of device therapy. Patients and physicians understandably have misgivings with regard to remote reprogramming with perceived loss of control. Patients envisage potential inappropriate reprogramming with life-threatening consequences. This potential has led many patients to dispense with this idea without any further consideration.

Remote programing cannot be viewed as an all-or-none feature. Firstly, it is important to examine which device parameters are reprogrammed and when and where this reprogramming takes place. Device automaticity has largely eliminated the need for reprogramming outputs and sensitivity. Devices most frequently need to be reprogrammed after therapy delivery to make adjustments to improve therapy efficacy or to help prevent inappropriate therapy. Device therapy commonly needs to be temporarily disabled to prevent inappropriate therapy for electromagnetic interference in the hospital setting. Mass device reprogramming is required when the device vendor, to either improve device function or serve as a fix for device malfunction, releases a software upgrade.

Remote reprogramming limited to specific parameters and delivered with checks and balances may address the concerns and still allow for workflow efficiencies. Reprogramming should only go into effect once the remote programmer can verify that the device has received the programing instruction. Remote reprogramming will need to be coordinated by a device company center manned by an around-the-clock staff to verify the patients and the requests for reprogramming. In the case of therapy deactivation, reprogramming could be time limited.

SUMMARY

A paradigm shift in the follow-up of CIEDs is underway. Remote monitoring of wireless devices and alert-driven office visits are replacing scheduled in-office well-baby visits. This shift in care has been driven by trials demonstrating the clinical superiority of remote monitoring and by financial constraints in the health care system.

Device companies are coming to terms with the financial impact of a sharp decrease in the price of their devices and their substantially longer battery life. These changes have rendered the sales representative service model unsustainable. To maintain a profitable business, device companies need to reduce costs by changing the service model. Remote monitoring is an attractive solution to this problem. Physicians need to be cognizant of this change.

The new health care system is rapidly taking shape and, although no one can predict how it is going to evolve, it does seem for now that the fee-for-service reimbursement model is likely to be replaced with capitated and pay-for-performance models that will emphasize reduced hospital stays and office visits. Physicians are being encouraged to adjust their practice patterns to deliver value-based care in order to cut costs and improve care under the Affordable Care Act. Remote monitoring is tailor made to achieve these goals, having been demonstrated to reduce scheduled office visits and reduce hospital admissions for HF. Remote monitoring may prove to be a key solution for many of the challenges faced by the modern electrophysiology practice.

REFERENCES

1. Marinskis G, van Erven L, Bongiorni MG, et al. Practices of cardiac implantable electronic device follow-up: results of the European Heart Rhythm Association survey. Europace 2012;14:423–5.
2. Al-Khatib SM, Mi X, Wilkoff BL, et al. Follow-up of patients with new cardiovascular implantable electronic devices: are experts' recommendations implemented in routine clinical practice? Circ Arrhythm Electrophysiol 2012;6:108–16.
3. Hess PL, Mi X, Curtis LH, et al. Follow-up of patients with new cardiovascular implantable electronic devices: is adherence to the experts' recommendations associated with improved outcomes? Heart Rhythm 2013;10:1127–33.
4. Wilkoff BL, Auricchio A, Brugada J, et al. HRS/EHRA expert consensus on the monitoring of cardiovascular implantable electronic devices (CIEDs): description of techniques, indications, personnel, frequency and ethical considerations. Heart Rhythm 2008;5:907–25.
5. Schoenfeld MH, Compton SJ, Mead RH, et al. Remote monitoring of implantable cardioverter defibrillators: a prospective analysis. Pacing Clin Electrophysiol 2004;27:757–63.
6. Joseph GK, Wilkoff BL, Dresing T, et al. Remote interrogation and monitoring of implantable cardioverter defibrillators. J Interv Card Electrophysiol 2004;11:161–6.
7. Cronin E, Ching EA, Varma N, et al. Remote monitoring of cardiovascular devices: a time and activity analysis. Heart Rhythm 2012;9:1947–51.
8. Al-Khatib SM, Piccini JP, Knight D, et al. Remote monitoring of implantable cardioverter defibrillators versus quarterly device interrogations in clinic: results from a randomized pilot clinical trial. J Cardiovasc Electrophysiol 2010;21:545–50.
9. Crossley GH, Chen J, Choucair W, et al. Clinical benefits of remote versus transtelephonic monitoring

of implanted pacemakers. J Am Coll Cardiol 2009; 54:2012–9.

10. de Asmundis C, Ricciardi D, Namdar M, et al. Role of home monitoring in children with implantable cardioverter defibrillators for Brugada syndrome. Europace 2013;15:i17–25.

11. Varma N, Stambler B, Chun S. Detection of atrial fibrillation by implanted devices with wireless data transmission capability. Pacing Clin Electrophysiol 2005;28(Suppl 1):S133–6.

12. Varma N, Epstein A, Irimpen A, et al, TRUST Investigators. Efficacy and safety of automatic remote monitoring for ICD follow-up: the TRUST trial. Circulation 2010;122:325–32.

13. Varma N, Michalski J, Epstein AE, et al. Automatic remote monitoring of implantable cardioverter-defibrillator lead and generator performance: the Lumos-T Safely Reduces Routine Office Device Follow-up (TRUST) trial. Circ Arrhythm Electrophysiol 2010;3:428–36.

14. Varma N, Michalski J, Epstein A, TRUST Investigators. Long term preservation of battery longevity (despite daily transmission load) with home monitoring-The TRUST trial. Europace 2013;(Suppl). Abstract.

15. Varma N. Rationale and design of a prospective study of the efficacy of a remote monitoring system used in implantable cardioverter defibrillator follow-up: the Lumos-T reduces routine office device follow-up study (TRUST) study. Am Heart J 2007; 154:1029–34.

16. Guedon-Moreau L, Lacroix D, Sadoul N, et al. A randomized study of remote follow-up of implantable cardioverter defibrillators: safety and efficacy report of the ECOST trial. Eur Heart J 2012;34: 605–14.

17. Mabo P, Victor F, Bazin P, et al. A randomized trial of long-term remote monitoring of pacemaker recipients (the COMPAS trial). Eur Heart J 2012;33: 1105–11.

18. Ricci RP, Morichelli L, D'Onofrio A, et al. Effectiveness of remote monitoring of CIEDs in detection and treatment of clinical and device-related cardiovascular events in daily practice: the HomeGuide registry. Europace 2013;15(7):970–7. http://dx.doi.org/10.1093/europace/eus440.

19. Crossley G, Boyle A, Vitense H, et al. The Clinical Evaluation of Remote Notification to Reduce Time to Clinical Decision (CONNECT) trial: the value of wireless remote monitoring with automatic clinician alerts. J Am Coll Cardiol 2011;57:1181–9.

20. Medtronic I. Clinician manual supplement Protecta XT/Protecta projected service life information related to remote monitoring. 2010; Manual no: M945739A001A.

21. Varma N, Pavri BB, Stambler B, et al. Same-day discovery of implantable cardioverter defibrillator dysfunction in the TRUST remote monitoring trial: influence of contrasting messaging systems. Europace 2013;15:697–703.

22. Varma N. Automatic remote home monitoring of ICD lead and generator function-a system that tests itself everyday. Europace 2013;15:i26–31.

23. Carlson MD, Wilkoff BL, Maisel WH, et al. Recommendations from the Heart Rhythm Society task force on device performance policies and guidelines endorsed by the American College of Cardiology Foundation (ACCF) and the American Heart Association (AHA) and the International Coalition of Pacing and Electrophysiology organizations (COPE). Heart Rhythm 2006;3:1250–73.

24. Maisel WH, Hauser RG, Hammill SC, et al. Recommendations from the Heart Rhythm Society task force on lead performance policies and guidelines: developed in collaboration with the American College of Cardiology (ACC) and the American Heart Association (AHA). Heart Rhythm 2009;6:869–85.

25. Varma N. Remote monitoring for advisories: automatic early detection of silent lead failure. Pacing Clin Electrophysiol 2009;32:525–7.

26. Maisel WH, Sweeney MO, Stevenson WG, et al. Recalls and safety alerts involving pacemakers and implantable cardioverter-defibrillator generators. JAMA 2001;286:793–9.

27. Maisel WH, Stevenson WG, Epstein LM. Changing trends in pacemaker and implantable cardioverter defibrillator generator advisories. Pacing Clin Electrophysiol 2002;25:1670–8.

28. Medtronic physician advisory letter: urgent medical device information Sprint Fidelis lead patient management recommendations. Available at: http://www.medtronic.com/product-advisories/physician/sprint-fidelis/PROD-ADV-PHYS-OCT.htm. 2007. Accessed February 3, 2014.

29. Kallinen LM, Hauser RG, Lee KW, et al. Failure of impedance monitoring to prevent adverse clinical events caused by fracture of a recalled high-voltage implantable cardioverter-defibrillator lead. Heart Rhythm 2008;5:775–9.

30. Burri H. Remote follow-up and continuous remote monitoring, distinguished. Europace 2013;15: i14–6.

31. Ricci RP, Morichelli L, Gargaro A, et al. Home monitoring in patients with implantable cardiac devices: is there a potential reduction of stroke risk? Results from a computer model tested through Monte Carlo simulations. J Cardiovasc Electrophysiol 2009;20: 1244–51.

32. Santini M, Gasparini M, Landolina M, et al. Device-detected atrial tachyarrhythmias predict adverse outcome in real-world patients with implantable biventricular defibrillators. J Am Coll Cardiol 2011; 57:167–72.

33. Koplan BA, Kaplan AJ, Weiner S, et al. Heart failure decompensation and all-cause mortality in relation to percent biventricular pacing in patients with heart failure: is a goal of 100% biventricular pacing necessary? J Am Coll Cardiol 2009;53:355–60.

34. Chaudhry SI, Mattera JA, Curtis JP, et al. Telemonitoring in patients with heart failure. N Engl J Med 2010;363:2301–9.

35. Varma N, Wilkoff B. Device features for managing patients with heart failure. Heart Fail Clin 2011;7: 215–25.

36. Whellan DJ, Ousdigian KT, Al-Khatib SM, et al. Combined heart failure device diagnostics identify patients at higher risk of subsequent heart failure hospitalizations: results from PARTNERS HF (Program to Access and Review Trending Information and Evaluate Correlation to Symptoms in Patients With Heart Failure) study. J Am Coll Cardiol 2010; 55:1803–10.

37. Hindricks G. The INTIME trial. Available at: http://www.escardio.org/about/press/esc-congress-2013/press-conferences/Documents/slides/hindricks.pdf. 2013. ESC Hotline Session. Accessed February 3, 2014.

38. Saxon LA, Hayes DL, Gilliam FR, et al. Long-term outcome after ICD and CRT implantation and influence of remote device follow-up: the ALTITUDE survival study. Circulation 2010;122:2359–67.

39. Bonnell S, Mittal S. Clinical guidelines for remote monitoring. In: Asirvatham SJ, Venkatachalam KL, Kapa S, editors. Remote monitoring and physiologic sensing technologies (Cardiac Electrophysiology Clinics). Philadelphia: Elsevier; 2013. p. 283–92.

40. Varma N, Ricci RP. Telemedicine and cardiac implants: what is the benefit? Eur Heart J 2012;34: 1885–95.

41. Mitchell M. Emerging applications for remote monitoring. EP Lab Digest 2012;12:30–2.

The Role of the Wearable Cardioverter Defibrillator in Clinical Practice

Mina K. Chung, MD[a,b,c,*]

KEYWORDS

- Wearable cardioverter defibrillator • Clinical practice • Implantable cardioverter defibrillator
- Sudden cardiac arrest

KEY POINTS

- The wearable cardioverter defibrillator (WCD) is an effective option for external monitoring and defibrillation in patients at risk for sudden cardiac arrest caused by ventricular tachycardia or ventricular fibrillation and who are not candidates for or who refuse an implantable cardioverter defibrillator (ICD).
- The device has been used when a patient's condition delays or prohibits ICD implantation, or as a bridge during periods when an indicated ICD must be explanted, such as for treatment of infection.
- The WCD has been increasingly used for primary prevention of sudden cardiac death during the high risk gap periods early after myocardial infarction, coronary revascularization with coronary artery bypass graft or percutaneous coronary intervention, or new diagnosis of heart failure, when its use is as a protective bridge to ICD or left ventricular improvement.
- The WCD can also provide monitoring with backup defibrillation protection during diagnosis and risk stratification periods.
- Although compliance and absence of pacing capability are limitations, shock efficacy and overall survival seem similar with a WCD compared with ICDs, and studies have reported satisfactory overall compliance.

Although implantable cardioverter defibrillators (ICDs) have been well established to reduce the risk of sudden cardiac death (SCD) in high-risk patients, there remain situations of significant risk in which an implantable device may not be indicated or accepted. In these situations, an external wearable cardioverter defibrillator (WCD) may be used to bridge this gap.

DESCRIPTION

The WCD (LifeVest, ZOLL Lifecor, Pittsburgh, PA) is composed of 4 dry nonadhesive capacitive rhythm monitoring electrodes, which provide 2 channels of monitoring, and 3 self-gelling defibrillation electrodes. Electrodes are imbedded in a vest garment and connected to a monitoring and defibrillation unit, which can be carried on a belt or shoulder strap (**Fig. 1**). The WCD can be sized to fit chest circumferences of 66.0 to 142.2 cm (26–56 in). The unit must be fitted properly to achieve satisfactory skin contact for best reduction of noise and resulting alarms.

The WCD is capable of automatic detection of ventricular tachycardia (VT) or ventricular fibrillation (VF) and can then deliver up to 5 shocks, with a maximum of 150 J of biphasic shock energy. On detection of a ventricular arrhythmia,

[a] Department of Molecular Cardiology, Lerner Research Institute, Cleveland Clinic, 9500 Euclid Avenue, J2-2, Cleveland, OH 44195, USA; [b] Cleveland Clinic Lerner College of Medicine of Case Western Reserve University, 9500 Euclid Avenue, Cleveland, OH 44195, USA; [c] Department of Cardiovascular Medicine, Heart & Vascular Institute, Cleveland Clinic, 9500 Euclid Avenue, Cleveland, OH 44195, USA
* Department of Molecular Cardiology, Lerner Research Institute, Cleveland Clinic, 9500 Euclid Avenue, J2-2, Cleveland, OH 44195.
E-mail address: chungm@ccf.org

Cardiol Clin 32 (2014) 253–270
http://dx.doi.org/10.1016/j.ccl.2013.11.002
0733-8651/14/$ – see front matter © 2014 Elsevier Inc. All rights reserved.

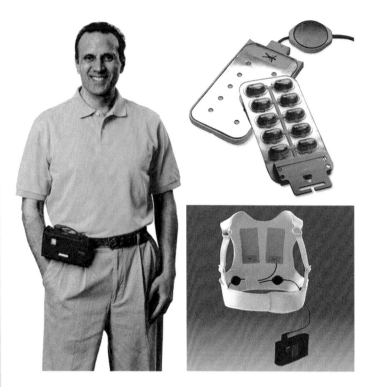

Fig. 1. WCD components. The Life-Vest WCD is composed of: 4 dry nonadhesive electrodes, providing 2 channels of monitoring; self-gelling defibrillation electrodes; a monitor unit capable of providing 150-J biphasic shocks and electrocardiographic storage; and response buttons that can inhibit shocks if patient is awake. (*Courtesy of* ZOLL, Pittsburgh, PA; with permission.)

vibration, visual illuminating response buttons, and increasingly louder siren alerts are activated. A patient-audible prompt states "Electrical shock possible," gel is extruded from the defibrillation electrode surfaces, and a bystander-audible prompt states "Do not touch patient," after which the treatment shock is delivered. Unlike an implanted ICD, the patient may abort this sequence at any time by pressing a response button, which serves as a test of consciousness. Current WCDs have no pacing capabilities for treatment of asystole. The devices are also incapable of delivering antitachycardic pacing.

PROGRAMMING AND DETECTION

Ventricular tachyarrhythmia detection requires a ventricular rate exceeding a programmed detection rate and morphology that does not match a baseline template. Heart rate is assessed using a 4-electrode, 2-lead configuration. Electrocardiographic (ECG) signal frequencies are analyzed using a fast Fourier transform algorithm to determine the strongest frequency, indicating heart rate. The detection algorithm applies logical weights to inputs for heart rate determination, based on comparing leads, signal quality, and historical rates. If the rate exceeds the programmed detection rate, the algorithm proceeds to a morphology analysis, which compares a baseline template obtained during device setup with a current

vectorcardiogram. The vectorcardiogram is formed from 2 orthogonal leads (anterior-posterior, right-left lateral) positioned by the vest at approximately the level of the xiphoid. Failing to match the real time vectorcardiogram to the baseline morphology templates contributes to determining a treatable arrhythmia. If the signal quality of one of the leads is unreliable, then morphology analysis is not used, and heart rate, stability, and onset criteria are used. Stability criteria measures differences in R-R intervals, and onset criteria are triggered by rapid changes in heart rate. To decide on treatment of an arrhythmia, the algorithm also applies a confidence level, calculated as the sum of the individual weighted input factors of heart rate, morphology, signal quality, spectral analysis, and response button use. Unreliable factors are decreased in weight. If the confidence interval decreases lower than a specified level, then the treatment sequence is terminated and monitoring for a new arrhythmia is resumed.

VF detection is programmable between 120 and 250 bpm, with detection delays programmable from 25 to 55 seconds. VT detection is programmable between 120 and the VF detection rate. Detection of an arrhythmia typically requires 5 to 6 seconds, and an additional 10 seconds meeting criteria are required before the treatment sequence alarms begin. The arrhythmia confirmation time reduces the incidence of false arrhythmia alarms. The WCD detection algorithm is designed to treat a ventricular tachyarrhythmia within 1 minute of detection. Delays of 60 to 180 seconds can also be programmed. Additional delays to 30 seconds can be programmed during sleep.

Up to 5 biphasic shocks may be programmed, with shock energies from 75 to 150 J. VT shocks can be synchronized, if R wave synchronization is identified, but unsynchronized if an R wave is not identified.

MONITORING CAPABILITIES

The monitor can store ECGs and automatically captures ECGs from 30 seconds before VT or VF events until 15 seconds after alarms stop. The device also records bradycardic events, including asystole, when heart rates decrease lower than 20 bpm, storing 5 minutes of ECG data before asystole events. The device can store up to 75 minutes of ECG recordings.

Surface ECG signal quality can be affected by skin factors, movement, and electromagnetic interference (EMI). Monitoring of interference or poor electrode-skin contact uses the 2-lead configuration to discard poor input from either lead. When interference common to all electrodes is detected, as from EMI, a driven ground returns a filtered result onto the skin. Both analog and digital filters are used to reduce frequencies outside usual ECG ranges. Signal voltage interference, or clipping, can also be detected and cause the algorithm to place no weight on that lead.

In addition, compliance during daily use is recorded by determination of electrode-skin contact using microampere alternating current signals through the ground electrode, which can be detected at each electrode. If the signal is lower than expected or not detected, then the algorithm places no weight on that signal for detection of arrhythmias. Compliance can be derived by determining the time that at least 1 monitoring electrode is in contact with skin with the electrode monitor connected and device activated. Rhythm strips, compliance, therapies, alarm history, noise occurrence, monitor-electrode connection times, and device on/off switching times are transmitted by a modem to the manufacturer's network and can be accessed by clinicians on a secure password-protected Web site (https://wcdnet.lifecor.com/wcd/default.asp). An example of an appropriate detection and shock is shown in **Fig. 2**.

CURRENT APPROVED INDICATIONS FOR WCD USE

The LifeVest WCD is currently approved for use in the United States, Europe, Israel, and Japan. It has been approved by the US Food and Drug Administration (FDA) for use in the United States since 2001 and is indicated for adult patients who are at risk for sudden cardiac arrest (SCA) and who are not candidates for or who refuse an implantable defibrillator. These indications include patients with a transient high risk for cardiac arrest, such as patients awaiting cardiac transplantation without an ICD or those needing a temporary removal of an infected ICD and requiring a course of antibiotics before reimplantation because of concern for ongoing infection (**Table 1**). The WCD has been used for primary prevention of SCD in high-risk patients with reduced left ventricular (LV) function (LV ejection fraction [LVEF] $\leq$35%) early after cardiac events, such as after recent acute myocardial infarction (MI) during the 40-day period under which ICD implantation is not indicated or deferred, before and after coronary artery bypass graft (CABG) or percutaneous coronary intervention (PCI) during the 90-day ICD waiting period, or recently diagnosed nonischemic cardiomyopathy during the 3-month to 9-month period awaiting LV improvement or ICD implantation. In these situations, the WCD may be used as a bridge to LV improvement or, if LV function remains reduced, ICD implantation. It has also been used in some patients with New York Heart Association (NYHA) class IV heart failure, in which an ICD is contraindicated unless used as part of a cardiac resynchronization therapy strategy, or patients at high risk of cardiac arrest with a terminal disease with life expectancy less than 1 year.

WCD INDICATIONS IN GUIDELINES AND EXPERT CONSENSUS STATEMENTS

WCD use has been covered under several clinical practice documents.

- The *American College of Cardiology (ACC)/American Heart Association (AHA)/European Society of Cardiology (ESC) 2006 Guidelines for Management of Patients with Ventricular Arrhythmias and Prevention of Sudden Cardiac Death*[1] note that the WCD has been approved in the United States by the FDA for cardiac patients with a transient high risk for VF, such as those awaiting cardiac transplantation, patients at very high risk after a recent MI or invasive cardiac procedure, or those needing temporary removal of an infected ICD and requiring a course of antibiotics before reimplantation.
- The *2006 International Society for Heart and Lung Transplantation Guidelines for the Care*

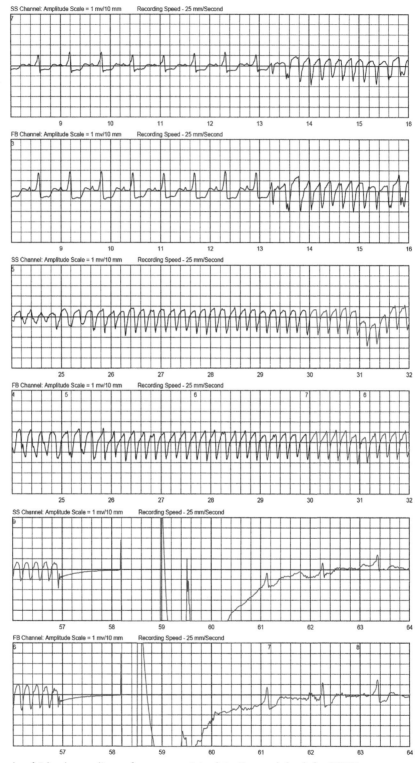

Fig. 2. Example of 2-lead recordings of an appropriate detection and shock for VT/VF.

Table 1
Indications for WCD use

FDA Indication: Adult Patients Who Are at Risk for SCA and Are Not Candidates for or Who Refuse an Implantable Defibrillator

Condition	Typical Usage Period	End Points Indicating End of WCD Usage
LVEF ≤35% with recent MI	40 d–3 mo	LV improvement or ICD implantation
LVEF ≤35% after recent CABG or PCI	3 mo	LV improvement or ICD implantation
LVEF ≤35% with recent diagnosis of cardiomyopathy	3–9 mo	LV improvement or ICD implantation
Bridge to heart transplant	Variable	Heart transplantation
NYHA class IV heart failure	Variable	Indefinite, CRT, transplantation, ICD implantation
Terminal disease with life expectancy <1 y	Variable	Indefinite
Genetic risk for life-threatening arrhythmia	Variable	Indefinite, ICD implantation
Deferred ICD after SCA, VT/VF	Variable	Improvement in comorbidity, ICD implantation
Explantation of ICD (eg, for infection)	1–3 mo	Completion of antibiotics, reimplantation of ICD
Refusal of indicated ICD	Variable	Indefinite
High-risk syncope	1–3 mo	Completion of risk stratification, lowered SCA risk, ICD implantation

Abbreviations: CABG, coronary artery bypass graft; CRT, cardiac resynchronization therapy; LV, left ventricular; LVEF, left ventricular ejection fraction; MI, myocardial infarction; NYHA, New York Heart Association; PI, percutaneous intervention.

of Cardiac Transplant Candidates[2] state a class I recommendation for ICD implantation or WCD use for status 1B patients discharged home.

- The *Transvenous Lead Extraction: Heart Rhythm Society Expert Consensus on Facilities, Training, Indications, and Patient Management*[3] document suggests that a wearable defibrillator can be an alternative to early reimplantation of ICDs when there is concern for ongoing infection.
- The *2013 American College of Cardiology Foundation/AHA Guideline for the Management of ST-Elevation Myocardial Infarction*[4] notes that the usefulness of a WCD in high-risk patients during the first 4 to 6 weeks after ST-elevation myocardial infarction (STEMI) is under investigation.

THE WCD USAGE IN CLINICAL PRACTICE

Although the WCD can be worn long-term, the WCD is most useful in patients at risk for SCD requiring temporary coverage. The device has been useful as a bridge to heart transplant, bridge during temporary interruption ICD therapy, such as after ICD lead extraction for infection, or other inability or refusal of ICD implantation.

The manufacturer maintains a database of WCD users, and in a postmarket report of WCD use from the database published in 2010,[5] indications in 2731 patients included the following: ICD explantation with delayed reimplantation, such as for extended antibiotic therapy for infections (23% of WCD users); delays in ICD implantation, such as for comorbidities, after a VF or sustained VT event (16.1%); delays in ICD implantation for genetic arrhythmogenic syndromes or congenital heart disease (0.4%); before ICD evaluation after MI with LVEF 35% or less (12.5%); before ICD evaluation after revascularization with LVEF 35% or less and past MI (8.9%); before ICD evaluation after diagnosis with nonischemic cardiomyopathy and LVEF 35% or less (20.0%); unspecified cardiomyopathy with LVEF 35% or less (8.1%); MI with an LVEF greater than 35% or unspecified (3.8%); and other temporary or fluctuating SCD risk conditions, including as a bridge to cardiac transplant (6.8%).

In recent years, WCD usage has increased significantly, and most of the use has been during waiting periods of high risk in patients with LV dysfunction after MI, after coronary revascularization, or after a new diagnosis of cardiomyopathy, as a bridge to LV function improvement or ICD implantation. From the manufacturer's database, as of September, 2013, more than 100,000 patients have worn the LifeVest, with an average duration of use between 2 and 3 months, and median daily use of 22.5 h/d. Recorded WCD indications (**Fig. 3**) show that nearly three-quarters of WCDs are used as a bridge early after cardiac events, with 26% being used in patients with recent MI, 8% after recent CABG, and 37% early after diagnosis of nonischemic cardiomyopathy. Other uses include class IV congestive heart failure (CHF) (2%), SCA/VT/VF before ICD implant (9%), genetic predisposition to SCD (1%), ICD explants (8%), other SCA risk (7%), and unspecified (1%).

ICD VERSUS WCD USE FOR PRIMARY PREVENTION OF SCD

ICDs have been shown to improve survival in certain patient populations with ischemic or nonischemic cardiomyopathy and reduced LV function. The indications for ICD implantation are based on evidence from randomized controlled trials. However, entry criteria of these clinical trials tended to exclude patients early after MI, coronary revascularization (CABG or PCI) (**Table 2**), or new diagnosis of heart failure. MADIT (Multicenter Automatic Defibrillator Implantation Trial)[6] excluded patients within 3 weeks after MI, 2 months after CABG, and 3 months after percutaneous transluminal coronary angioplasty. MADIT-2[7] excluded patients within 1 month of MI and 3 months after revascularization. SCD-HeFT (Sudden Cardiac Death-Heart Failure Trial),[8] which included patients with ischemic or nonischemic cardiomyopathy, required a history of heart failure of at least 3 months duration. In contrast, MUSTT (Multicenter Unsustained Tachycardia Trial)[9] included patients after only 4 days after MI or revascularization, and CABGPatch (Coronary Artery Bypass Graft [CABG] Patch)[10] implanted ICDs at the time of CABG. DEFINITE (Defibrillators in Non-Ischemic Cardiomyopathy Treatment Evaluation),[11]

a study in nonischemic cardiomyopathy, did not specify timing of ICD implantation.

Based on these primary prevention studies, current guidelines[12] support the implantation of ICDs after MI in coronary artery disease with LVEF 30% or less (MADIT II[7]) or LVEF 40% or less with nonsustained VT and inducible sustained VT/VF (MADIT,[6] MUSTT[9]), and for ischemic or nonischemic cardiomyopathy with NYHA functional class 2 or 3 and LVEF 35% or less (SCD-HeFT[8]). However, ICDs are generally not reimbursed by health insurance or US Center for Medicare Services (CMS) within 40 days after MI, 3 months after revascularization, or 3 to 9 months after new diagnosis of heart failure. Nevertheless, these gap periods can be high-risk periods and are discussed further next.

EARLY AFTER MI WITH LV DYSFUNCTION

In the acute to subacute period after acute MI, arrhythmia substrate is dynamic. LV function may improve in up to 70%. However, the risk of SCD after MI is highest in the first 30 days after MI. However, this period is further complicated, in that SCD may occur from not only arrhythmic, but nonarrhythmic, mechanical causes, limiting benefits from an implanted device. The WCD may provide protection from SCD during the early period after MI until arrhythmic risk may be reduced after improvement in LVEF or until ICD implantation can be performed for those with persistently reduced LVEF.

Risk of SCD Early After MI

The HEART (Healing and Early Afterload Reducing Therapy) study showed the changing substrate after MI.[13] In 352 patients with Q wave anterior MI treated with reperfusion therapy and ramipril, only 3.4% had normal LV function on day 1. By day 90, 66% had improvement in LVEF, with a mean improvement of 4.5% and complete recovery in 22%. However, despite advances in

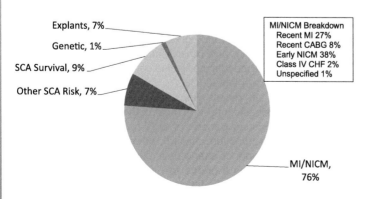

Fig. 3. WCD orders by indication, cumulative as of October, 2013. (*Courtesy of ZOLL, Pittsburgh, PA; with permission.*)

Table 2
Timing in entry criteria for major ICD trials for primary prevention of SCD: ischemic cardiomyopathy

Study/Year	N	Design	Population	Timing	Mortality HR (ICD)
MADIT, 1996	196	ICD vs conventional medical treatment	Previous MI; LVEF ≤35%; NSVT; inducible nonsuppressible sustained VT/VF at EPS	>3 wk after MI >2 mo after CABG >3 mo after PTCA	0.46 (P = .009)
MUSTT, 1999	704	EP-guided treatment with AADs or ICD or no AA treatment	CAD; LVEF ≤40%; Asx NSVT; inducible sustained ventricular tachyarrhythmia	≥4 d after MI or revascularization	0.40 (P<.001)
MADIT2, 2002	1232	3:2 ICD vs conventional medical treatment	Previous MI; LVEF ≤30%	>1 mo after MI >3 mo after revascularization	0.69 (P = .016)
SCD-HeFT, 2005	2521	ICD vs amiodarone vs placebo	NYHA FC II-III; LVEF ≤35%	>3 mo HF	0.77 (P = .007)
CABGPatch, 1997	900	EPI ICD vs no ICD	CABG; LVEF ≤35%; abnormal SAECG	At time of CABG	1.07 (NS)
DINAMIT, 2004	674	ICD vs no ICD	Recent MI; LVEF ≤35%; ↓ HRV or average HR ≥80 bpm	6–40 d after MI	1.08 (P = .66)
IRIS, 2009	898	ICD vs no ICD	Recent MI; LVEF ≤40% and HR >90 bpm or NSVT >150 bpm	3–31 d after MI	1.04 (P = .78)

Abbreviations: AAD, antiarrhythmic drug; ASX, asymptomatic; CAD, coronary artery disease; EP, electrophysiology; EPI, epicardial; EPS, electrophysiology study; HR, heart rate; HRV, heart rate variability; NS, not significant; NSVT, nonsustained VT; NYHA FC, NYHA functional class; PTCA, percutaneous transluminal coronary angioplasty; SAECG, signal averaged electrocardiogram.
　Data from Refs.[6–10,21,22,34]

revascularization and medical therapies that have reduced mortality after acute MI, the risk of SCD remains high early after an MI, especially in patients with reduced LVEF (2.3%/mo in patients with LVEF ≤30%).[14,15] Bunch and colleagues,[16] from the Intermountain Heart Rhythm Specialists and the Intermountain Medical Center, reported that LVEF 35% or less and right bundle branch block or left bundle branch block conduction system disease were associated with higher mortality; survival curves had the sharpest declines in the first 30 days after MI. Another study of SCD and all-cause mortality after MI among residents of Olmsted County, MN, showed that among 2997 patients with MI and a median follow-up of 4.7 years, there were 1160 deaths, including 282 SCDs.[17] The 30-day SCD rate was 1.2%, whereas the rate was 1.2%/y thereafter. In VALIANT,[14] a trial of 14,609 patients with acute MI and LV dysfunction or CHF, the rate of sudden death or resuscitated cardiac arrest was highest in the first month, at 1.4%, and 2.5% in months 1 to 6. The risk decreased over 2 years to 0.14%/mo. Survival curves showed a sharp decline initially, which plateaued between 6 and 12 months, with higher mortality seen with lower LVEF.[14,18] In the first month, the cause of sudden death was more because of recurrent MI or rupture, but by 3 months, the proportion caused by presumed arrhythmic death was higher.[19]

Role of an ICD Early After MI

A subanalysis of SCD-HeFT in 712 patients with previous MI reported no differential mortality benefit from ICDs as a function of time after implant, concluding that the benefit of an ICD was not restricted only to remote MIs.[20] However, SCD-HeFT required heart failure duration of more than 3 months for study entry.

The recognized early risk of sudden death after MI led to 2 randomized trials of ICD therapy early after MI. In DINAMIT,[21] 674 patients within 6 to 40 days after MI with LVEF 35% or less and impaired cardiac autonomic function (decreased heart rate variability or increased heart rate on Holter monitoring) were randomized to ICD versus no ICD. The mean time to randomization was 18 days, and ICDs were implanted 18 to 25 days after MI. There was no significant difference in the primary outcome of all-cause mortality ($P = .66$). However, there was a significantly lower risk of death from arrhythmia ($P = .009$) in the ICD group, but this was counterbalanced by a higher risk of nonarrhythmic causes of death ($P = .02$). Similarly in IRIS, 898 patients were enrolled 5 to 31 days after MI with LVEF 40% or less, heart rate 90 bpm or greater on first ECG or nonsustained VT 150 bpm or greater on Holter monitoring.[22] Patients were randomized to ICD or medical therapy. Again, there was no significant difference in all-cause death ($P = .76$), with a significantly lower risk of SCD in the ICD group ($P = .049$), counterbalanced by a significantly higher risk of non-SCD ($P = .001$).

Thus, early ICD implantation 6 to 40 days after acute MI in patients with LVEF 35% or less does not improve overall mortality despite a reduction in arrhythmic death, because of a higher risk of nonarrhythmic deaths, resulting in similar overall mortality. Therefore, current guidelines do not recommend ICD implantation for primary prevention of SCD within 40 days of acute MI.[12]

The reasons for the higher risks of nonarrhythmic death in the ICD groups in DINAMIT and IRIS and whether the invasive surgical nature of ICD implantation contributed remain unclear. Similar lack of efficacy findings were also found in CABG-Patch,[10] which randomized patients to epicardial ICD systems or no ICD at the time of CABG. Such studies help to rationalize use of a noninvasive strategy, such as the WCD, to protect patients early after MI in hopes of avoiding the higher risk of nonarrhythmic death.

Role of the WCD Early After MI

WEARIT/BIROAD (Wearable Defibrillator Investigative Trial/Bridge to ICD in Patients at Risk of Arrhythmic Death) studied 289 patients with either symptomatic NYHA functional class III or IV heart failure with LVEF less than 30% (WEARIT) or at high risk for SCD after MI or CABG not receiving an ICD for up to 4 months (BIROAD).[23] Over a mean WCD use duration of 3 months, 6 successful defibrillations occurred in 4 patients (1.4%). Experience with the WCD early after MI has also been studied from data using the national WCD database.[5] In this analysis, 341 patients with recent MI and LVEF 35% or less wore the WCD. There were 12 events in 10 patients for an event rate of 2.9%. Eight of 10 patients survived. In a more recent analysis of WCD use in patients perceived to be at high risk early after MI, 8435 patients with recent MI and LVEF 35% or less or *International Classification of Diseases, Ninth Revision* code for acute MI and matched to device-recorded data were studied from September, 2005 to July, 2011.[24] Shocks were received in 1.6% of patients; 75% of shocks occurred in the first 1 month and 96% within the first 3 months. The median time from MI to first shock was 16 days and mean time 30 days. There was 91% survival. The 1.6% event rate is comparable with the 1.4% first 30-day sudden death rate in VALIANT; however, all of these events in the WCD group were arrhythmic and could reflect a change in SCD substrate toward higher arrhythmic and less mechanical risk with current therapies for acute MI.

Whether the WCD can improve sudden death mortality after MI is the subject of the VEST study (ClinicalTrials.gov NCT01446965), which is enrolling patients with recent acute MI and LVEF 35% or less identified in the hospital or within 7 days of discharge. Patients are being randomized 2:1 to a WCD versus no WCD for the primary outcome of sudden death mortality. Target enrollment is 1900, with estimated study completion in 2015.

Recommendations

The current strategy for management of sudden death risk in patients with low LVEF early after MI includes reevaluation of LVEF 1 to 3 months after MI. Approximately 30% may still have a low LVEF. If LVEF remains 35% or less, ICD implantation is indicated. Because mortality from SCD early after MI may exceed 2%/mo, in patients with reduced LVEF, the WCD may offer protection early after MI as a bridge to LV improvement or ICD implantation.

EARLY AFTER CORONARY REVASCULARIZATION WITH LV DYSFUNCTION

After coronary revascularization, LV function may improve. Persistent LV dysfunction after CABG in patients with LVEF 35% or less has been reported in 25% to 74%.[25,26] Imaging studies, such as nuclear imaging, positron emission tomography or cardiac magnetic resonance imaging with late gadolinium enhancement, may help predict improvement in patients with significant preoperative ischemia or hibernating myocardium. However, identification of such patients remains challenging and imprecise at best. For example, in the STICH trial,[27] identification of preoperative viability failed to identify a survival benefit of CABG versus medical therapy alone.

Risk of Mortality Early After Coronary Revascularization

The risk of mortality is highest early after coronary revascularization in patients with LV dysfunction. Patients with significant LV dysfunction have higher 30-day mortality after CABG or PCI than patients with normal LV function. Although the risk of arrhythmic death may be higher, they are also at risk for nonarrhythmic causes of death. Survival data from the Society of Thoracic Surgeons Adult Cardiac Surgery Database linked to CMS databases (ASCERT study) in 348,341 patients older than 65 years who underwent isolated CABG showed that early hazard for death is particularly higher for patients with reduced LV function (LVEF <30%).[28] After PCI, the CADILLAC trial[29] identified factors predictive of high risk of mortality during recovery from revascularization. Low LVEF, age older than 65 years, Killip class 2/3, anemia, renal insufficiency, triple-vessel disease, and postprocedure TIMI (Thrombolysis in Myocardial Infarction) flow grade 2 were identified as strong risk factors for 1-year mortality. The National Cardiovascular Database Registry CathPCI registry linked survival from CMS databases in 343,466 patients and showed high early mortality in patients with low LVEF with or without STEMI.[30] Overall mortality in patients undergoing PCI with STEMI was 12% at 3 months and 16% at 1 year, and in patients with LVEF less than 30% was 32% at 3 months and 38% at 1 year. Predictors of mortality included low LVEF, renal insufficiency, and multivessel disease.

Role of the ICD Early After Coronary Revascularization

The CABGPatch trial[10] randomized patients with LVEF 35% or less undergoing CABG to epicardial ICD implantation at the time of CABG versus no ICD and did not report a survival benefit from ICD implantation. Most other randomized trials of ICD implantation for primary prevention of SCD excluded patients within 1 to 3 months after coronary revascularization (see **Table 1**). Thus, the benefit of ICD placement for primary prevention of SCD early after revascularization has not been well established, and ICDs may not be reimbursed by health insurers during this early period.

Role of the WCD

Early mortality risk in a large single-center cohort of 4149 patients who underwent CABG or PCI with LVEF 35% or less at the Cleveland Clinic was compared with a cohort from the national database of 809 WCD users who had the WCD prescribed for low LVEF after CABG or PCI.[31] Early mortality hazard was prominent within the first 3 months in the no-WCD cohorts, but less early mortality was observed in WCD users (2% vs 7%, P<.0001). Cox proportional hazards modeling identified WCD use as an independent predictor of better survival after both CABG and PCI. This early mortality difference remained significant in propensity score–matched cohorts (**Fig. 4**); 90-day mortality was 2% among WCD patients and 10% in no-WCD users (P<.0001). Survival curves continued to show better survival after 90 days in the WCD users, mainly driven by worse mortality in the post-PCI group who did not use a WCD (**Fig. 5**). In the total cohort of WCD users, there were 18 successful appropriate defibrillations in 11 patients; 1.3% of the WCD group received appropriate therapies. There were 3 asystolic events, of which 2 were fatal. After wearing the WCD, 32% of CABG and 30% of the PCI WCD users subsequently received an ICD. Thus, survivors of coronary revascularization with LVEF 35% or less have higher early compared with late mortality. The higher early-phase mortality observed after revascularization was less marked in the WCD group. These differences appeared most marked after PCI. Factors in addition to defibrillation from the WCD likely also contributed to mortality differences. The WCD may facilitate better follow-up and risk stratification, particularly in the post-PCI population. Nondefibrillation alarms triggering early evaluation were not collected in this study, but may have also contributed to differences in early survival.

In another study of 354 patients in Germany wearing the WCD, approximately 90 wore the WCD early after CABG.[15] During 3 months of use, 7% were shocked for ventricular arrhythmias. In the postmarketing study of 3569 patients in the United States using the WCD, 9% used the WCD early after coronary revascularization. Over a mean follow-up of 47 days, 0.8% of patients received appropriate shocks for ventricular arrhythmias.[5,32]

Recommendations

The current strategy for prevention of SCD in patients with low LVEF within 90 days of revascularization includes early ICD implantation for survivors of sustained VT/VF (secondary prevention of SCD). For primary prevention of SCD, ICD implantation is reasonable in patients who have LVEF 35% or less and who have documented need for device implantation for antibradycardic pacing.

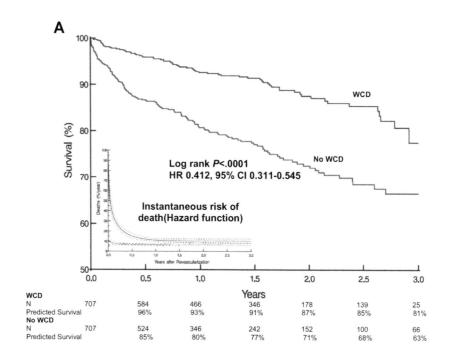

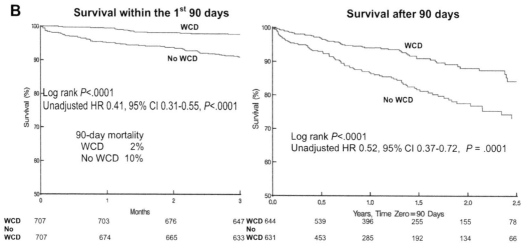

Fig. 4. Survival after CABG or PCI in patients with LVEF ≤35%. Propensity score–matched groups from a no-WCD cohort are compared with a WCD cohort. N = 707, each group. (*A*) Long-term Kaplan-Meier survival. (*Inset*) Hazard function curves: instantaneous risk of death (hazard function) stratified by WCD use. Solid lines are parametric hazard estimates enclosed within dashed 68% confidence bands equivalent to 1 standard deviation. (*B*) Survival in the first 90 days (*left*) and after 90 days (*right*). Blue: WCD patients; red: no-WCD patients. CI, confidence interval; HR, hazard ratio. (*From* Zishiri ET, Williams S, Cronin EM, et al. Early risk of mortality after coronary artery revascularization in patients with left ventricular dysfunction and potential role of the wearable cardioverter defibrillator. Circ Arrhythm Electrophysiol 2013;6(1):124; with permission.)

However, in others with low LVEF, early WCD use can have a reasonable role in bridging to LV improvement or ICD implantation. LVEF should be reassessed 3 months after revascularization, and if LVEF remains 35% or less, ICD implantation is indicated.

EARLY AFTER RECENT DIAGNOSIS OF CARDIOMYOPATHY

Improvement in LV function after new diagnosis of cardiomyopathy may be expected in many patients with institution of medical therapies or recovery from reversible causes of

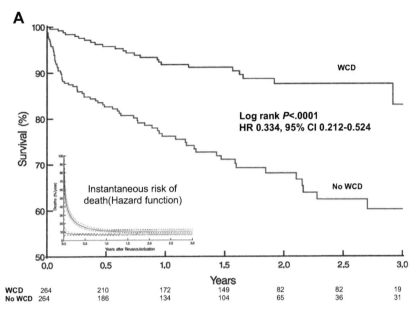

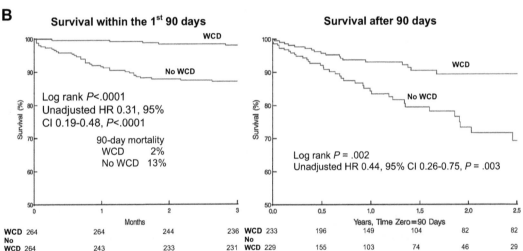

Fig. 5. Survival after PCI in patients with LVEF ≤35%. Propensity score–matched groups from a no-WCD cohort are compared with a WCD cohort. N = 264, each group. (*A*) Long-term Kaplan-Meier survival. (*Inset*) Hazard function curves: instantaneous risk of death (hazard function) stratified by WCD use. Solid lines are parametric hazard estimates enclosed within dashed 68% confidence bands equivalent to 1 standard deviation. (*B*) Survival in the first 90 days (*left*) and after 90 days (*right*). Blue: WCD patients; red: no-WCD patients. CI, confidence interval; HR, hazard ratio. (*From* Zishiri ET, Williams S, Cronin EM, et al. Early risk of mortality after coronary artery revascularization in patients with left ventricular dysfunction and potential role of the wearable cardioverter defibrillator. Circ Arrhythm Electrophysiol 2013;6(1):126; with permission.)

cardiomyopathy. However, identification of these patients remains challenging, and arrhythmic risk may persist even if LVEF improves to greater than 35%. In DEFINITE, 37% of patients had follow-up LVEF greater than 35%. There were fewer arrhythmic events with improved LV function, but 5.7% had significant ventricular arrhythmias, even after LVEF improved to greater than 35%.[33]

Role of an ICD Early After Diagnosis of Heart Failure

Current device implantation guidelines recommend ICD implantation for nonischemic cardiomyopathy with LVEF 35% or less after exclusion of reversible causes of LV dysfunction and assessing response to optimal medical therapy.[12] These guidelines do not specify a waiting period.

However, the CMS and other US health care insurers require a 3-month period of optimal medical therapy before reimbursement for ICD placement, primarily based on SCD-HeFT,[8] which showed a benefit of ICD implantation for ischemic and nonischemic cardiomyopathy, but included only patients with a history of heart failure greater than 3 months.[34] In contrast, DEFINITE[11] enrolled 458 patients with nonischemic cardiomyopathy to ICD versus medical therapy and did not specify a duration of heart failure for inclusion, but did exclude potentially reversible causes of CHF. Mean time from cardiomyopathy diagnosis to randomization in DEFINITE was 2.9 ± 4 years, but a subsequent analysis divided patients into recent versus remote diagnosis using cut points of 3 and 9 months.[35] There were no significant differences between ICD benefit in recent versus remote diagnosis groups, but patients with recently diagnosed cardiomyopathy who received an ICD had better survival than standard therapy at both cut points ($P = .049$ <3 months; $P = .058$ <9 months), whereas no significant differences were seen between ICD and standard therapy in patients with remote diagnosis greater than 3 months or greater than 9 months.

Similar conclusions regarding the difficulty of the 9-month CMS time qualifier were reached in another study of 131 patients with nonischemic cardiomyopathy and LVEF 35% or less who had an ICD implanted.[36] Similar high occurrences of treated and potentially lethal arrhythmias were observed, irrespective of diagnosis duration.

Experience with the WCD

In the postmarketing study of the WCD,[5] 546 wore the WCD with recently diagnosed nonischemic cardiomyopathy with LVEF 35% or less. Over a mean follow-up of 57 days, there were 4 shock events, with 0.7% of patients receiving shocks for a ventricular arrhythmia.[5,32]

Recommendations

Management of newly diagnosed heart failure can be problematic, given the gap period in current reimbursement guidelines. ICDs remain recommended and reimbursed for secondary prevention of SCD in patients who have survived sustained VT/VF. For primary prevention of SCD, device-based therapy guidelines do not specify wait times, but insurers often exclude reimbursement for ICDs implanted in the first 3 months. Likelihood of LVEF improvement may guide some approaches. The WCD can be useful in high-risk patients after new diagnosis of

cardiomyopathy while undergoing trials of optimal medical therapy, particularly in patients with potentially reversible causes, such as tachycardia-induced cardiomyopathy or myocarditis. For these patients, the WCD can provide bridge protection while awaiting improvement in LV function, ICD implantation, or advanced therapies for heart failure.

SEVERE HEART FAILURE
Bridge to Heart Transplantation

Patients with severe cardiac dysfunction awaiting heart transplantation are at particularly high risk for SCD, especially if patients are discharged home to await transplantation. Although they often have indications for ICD implantation, NYHA functional class IV in the absence of cardiac resynchronization therapy or life expectancy less than 1 year are typical exclusions for ICD implantation. The WCD can serve as a useful bridge to transplantation, particularly if waiting times are expected to be short with certain blood types.

Experience with the WCD

In a study of 91 United Network for Organ Sharing status 1B heart transplant candidates receiving home inotrope infusion, 25 had an ICD and 13 used a WCD. There were 2 sudden deaths at home: 1 who declined a WCD and 1 who was not wearing the WCD. In 13 wearing the WCD, 3 asymptomatic events were recorded, with 1 shock delivered for atrial fibrillation with rapid ventricular response.[37] In 354 WCD patients in Germany, 6% used the WCD as a bridge to transplantation, with 11% experiencing ventricular arrhythmias.[15] In the WEARIT study,[23] of 177 patients with NYHA class III or IV heart failure, 1 patient received 2 successful defibrillations.

Use with Ventricular Assist Devices

Although circulatory support from ventricular assist devices (VADs) can be adequate even in the presence of VF, hemodynamics may be more optimal with prompt defibrillation.[2] Also, the presence of an ICD was associated with improved survival in 1 study of patients with VADs.[38] Whether the WCD could provide similar benefits and appropriate sensing has not been studied.

Recommendations

Heart and lung transplantation guidelines list a class I recommendation for ICD implantation or WCD use for status 1B patients discharged home.[2] The WCD may also be useful in patients with anticipated short waiting times to transplantation (ie, blood types A and B).[2]

BRIDGE TO INDICATED ICD THERAPY

Instances in which an ICD is indicated, but deferred, include infection, recovery from acute illness or surgery, or lack of vascular access. ICD therapy may also be interrupted by system extraction caused by device infection or endocarditis and need for clearance of infection after a course of antibiotics. A WCD has been used as a bridge to indicated first or reimplanted ICD. Although WCD use after ICD extraction previously accounted for 23% of WCD use, more recent surveys with growth in WCD use for other indications show that overall, approximately 8% of WCD use has been for ICD explants. However, in the original national database survey, this group accounted for most of the VT/VF shocked events (49 events in 33/638 patients, or 5.2% of patients).[5] The use of a WCD in hospital inpatients at high risk for cardiac arrest, such as cardiac arrest survivors who are recovering in a hospital but at risk for recurrence, is being considered for investigation. Such therapy may yield shorter VF to shock times than routine hospital floor telemetry monitoring.

Recommendations

In patients who have traditional ICD indications, but who must defer ICD implantation or interrupt ICD therapy, event rates may be significant. A WCD can provide bridge protection until the ICD can be implanted. The use of a WCD for high-risk hospitalized patients warrants further study.

HIGH-RISK SYNCOPE MONITORING

Patients presenting with syncope without documented VT/VF, but who have high-risk factors for VT/VF/SCA as a cause of the syncope, may be at high risk for recurrence while being evaluated. The WCD may provide active monitoring and treatment of VT/VF during this evaluation period. In a study of 354 patients in Germany using the WCD,[15] 18% wore the WCD (average use 106 days) during diagnostic evaluation periods, including for syncope or after cardiac arrest, and 13% of these patients had ventricular arrhythmias requiring a shock.

Recommendations

The WCD may be useful for monitoring and protection in patients at high risk for cardiac arrest until arrhythmia risk can be determined, improved, or treated.

EFFECTIVENESS OF THE WCD

The effectiveness of the WCD is dependent on patient compliance, appropriate device use, patient selection, appropriate management of VT/VF, and avoidance of inappropriate shocks.

Compliance

Patient compliance and usage are recorded by the device by determination of the time of electrode-skin contact. In the WEARIT/BIROAD study,[23] 23% withdrew early, mainly because of size and weight of the monitor. Improved compliance and acceptance of the WCD seem to be reported with newer devices, which are 40% smaller in size and weight. In a German study, 72% had excellent compliance, with usage at 22 to 24 h/d and 13% had good compliance with 20 to 22 h/d; mean daily use was 21.3 hours.[15] In the US survey of the postmarketing national WCD database,[5] mean duration of use was 52.6 days (median 36 days), with median and mean daily use time of 21.7 and 19.9 hours, respectively. Use was more than 90% in 52% of patients and more than 80% in 71% of patients. WCD use was stopped early in 14%, mainly because of comfort issues and size or weight of the WCD. More recent data report median usage compliance of 22.5 h/d (http://lifevest.zoll.com).

Efficacy

In clinical trials and postmarket studies, the WCD has shown efficacy in successful detection and termination of VT/VF (summarized in **Table 3**). An early study performed in the electrophysiology laboratory reported successful detection and termination of VT/VF, with 100% first shock success by the WCD.[39] Subsequent studies, including the WEARIT/BIROAD studies,[23] a German study by Klein and colleagues,[15] and the US experience gleaned from the national database of postmarket WCD users kept by the manufacturer,[5,24] report 75% to 100% success rates for conversion of VT/VF. In the WEARIT/BIROAD study,[23] 6 of 8 shocks were successful (75%), with the 2 failures caused by electrode misplacement (eg, pads reversed and not directed to the skin). These occurrences seem to have been minimized with awareness since this early study was published in 2004. In the US postmarket study of 3569 patients,[5] in 80 VT/VF events, first shock success was 100% in unconscious patients and 99% for all patients. The single failure was in a conscious patient who prevented shock for 10 minutes by use of the response button. Survival after successful conversion of unconscious VT/VF was 86%,

Table 3
Published series on use of the WCD

Study/Year	N	Indications	Mean Duration of Use (mo)	Successful Treatment of VT/VF Events	Deaths	Inappropriate Shocks	Premature Discontinuation
Auricchio et al, 1998	10	Clinical testing of device for treating induced VT/VF	N/A	9/10 (90%) (1 pt erroneously discontinued sensing electrode so VT could not be detected)	None	N/A	N/A
Reek et al, 2003	12	Clinical testing of newer generation of WCD for treating induced VT/VF	N/A	22/22 (100%)	None	N/A	N/A
Lang et al, 2003	13	Status 1B on heart transplant list	0.8	No VT/VF events while wearing the WCD	1 died on inotropes while not wearing WCD	1 shock for atrial fibrillation	Not reported
Feldman et al, 2004 WEARIT/ BIROAD	289	WEARIT NYHA FC III, IV HF BIROAD after MI/CABG	3.4 WEARIT 2.6 BIROAD	6/8 (75%) (2 failures caused by electrode malplacement)	6 nonsudden 5 sudden (not wearing WCD) 1 sudden (reversed leads)	6 (0.67%/mo)	30% WEARIT 11% BIROAD
Klein et al, 2010	354	Various: Early after MI (39%) After CABG (25%) Risk stratification (18%) ICD explants (10%) Pretransplant (6%) Delay/refusal of ICD (2%)	3.5	246 events in 27 pts (5 NSVT, 3 ST/SVT), 2 asystole (both died); 139 in 1 pt with LQTS, all but 6 terminated spontaneously while patient withheld shock; first shock success 95% in rest	16: 2 with asystole, 1 caused by misplaced electrodes	3 (0.8%)	11 (3.1%)

Chung et al, 2010	3569	Various	1.75	79/80 (99%)	28 (4 recurrent VT/VF, 1 bystander prevention of therapy, 2 ECG disruption, 1 unipolar PM inhibition; 3 no WCD events recorded; 17 asystole)	67 (1.9%, 1.4%/mo)	N/A
Dillon et al, 2010	2105	Various Evaluation of effectiveness of arrhythmia detection algorithm in patients who wore device in 2006	1.2	53/54 (98%)	1 (caused by unipolar pacemaker interference with arrhythmia detection)	34 (0.99 per 100 patient months of use)	Not reported
Rao et al, 2011	162	CSHD (43) IA (119)	Median 0.9 CSHD 0.97 IA	0 CSHD 3 in 2 pts (100%) IA	4 (2.5%, 2 in each group) (2 noncompliant, 1 N/A, 1 intra-abdominal viscous rupture)	0 CSHD 7 in 4 pts (3%, 63/100 pt-y) IA	9% both groups
Saltzberg et al, 2012	266	107 PPCM 159 matched NIDCM women	4.1 PPCM 3.2 NIDCM	0 events in PPCM 2/2 in 1 pt (100%) with NIDCM	0 PPCM 11 NIDCM	0 PPCM 0 NIDCM	15 (14%) PPCM 14 (9%) NIDCM
Zishiri et al, 2013	809	After CABG, PCI (compared with 4149 without WCD)	2.6 CABG; 2.7 PCI	18 in 11 pts (1.3%); successful in 12/18 shocks (1 pt required 8 shocks for 2 VT episodes)	90-d mortality 2% (compared with 7% no WCD)	13	Not reported
Epstein et al, 2013	8453	Recent MI with LVEF ≤35%	2.3	146 events in 133 pts (1.6%), 91% survival	4% 3 mo, 6% 6 mo, 7% 12 mo mortality; 0.4% died of bradycardia or asystole	114 in 91 pts (0.006 shocks/pt-mo)	Not reported

Abbreviations: CSHD, congenital structural heart disease; IA, inherited arrhythmia; LQTS, long QT syndrome; N/A, not available; NIDCM, nonischemic dilated cardiomyopathy; NSVT, nonsustained VT; NYHA FC, NYHA functional class; PM, pacemaker; PPCM, peripartum cardiomyopathy; ST, sinus tachycardia; SVT, supraventricular tachycardia.

Data from Refs.[5,15,23,24,31,37,39,48–51]; and *Adapted from* Zishiri ET, Chung MK. The role of the wearable cardioverter-defibrillator in contemporary clinical practice. J Innovations in Cardiac Rhythm Management 2011;2:307–16.

with 4 deaths occurring because of recurrent VT/ VF after initial recovery and arrival of emergency personnel, 1 because of bystander interference preventing therapy, 2 because of ECG disruption from a fall, and 1 from unipolar permanent pacemaker pacing inhibiting detection. These occurrences highlight the importance of patient instruction in use of the WCD. Nevertheless, this study also reported that long-term survival was similar in WCD users compared with a cohort of first ICD implant patients.[5]

Inappropriate Shocks

The response buttons present on the WCD act as a test of consciousness and can prevent inappropriate shocks caused by noise, malfunction, or supraventricular arrhythmias higher than the rate criteria. Reported rates of inappropriate shocks from the WCD typically range from 0.4% to 1.9%/mo (see **Table 3**). In comparison, inappropriate shocks from ICDs are reported to occur in 0.2% to 2.3% of patients/mo.[11,40–46]

LIMITATIONS OF THE WCD

The major limitations of the WCD include the absence of pacemaker function and the requirement for patient compliance.

Absence of Pacemaker Function

In the German study,[15] asystole occurred in 2 patients wearing the WCD, and both died. In the US postmarketing study,[5] 23 patients experienced asystole (0.6%), with mortality of 74%. In the US study of WCD use after recent MI,[24] 0.4% died of bradycardia or asystole. The lack of pacing also means that the WCD cannot deliver antitachycardic pacing.

Compliance

The WCD provides no protection when it is not worn, including while bathing. Patients should be advised that caregivers or other persons should be nearby during periods when the WCD is not worn. Patients may also reduce use in warm weather or request premature removal because of discomfort or weight of the system. Although the monitoring leads are dry, some patients have reported pruritus or rash limiting use. These have been the main issues leading to premature termination of use. The rate of premature discontinuation was 11% to 30% in the WEARIT/BIROAD study, but in more recent reports including the smaller monitoring device, it has been reported to range from 3% to 14% (see **Table 3**).

USE IN CHILDREN

Reported experience in children is limited, because in the United States, the FDA indication is for adult use, and the minimum chest circumference required is typically 66 cm (26 in). One study of WCD use in 4 children aged 9 to 17 years reported difficulty with compliance and requirement for refitting of the vest to achieve better contact and noise reduction, although no inappropriate shocks were delivered.[47] A 14-year-old patient had a VF arrest that was not detected because of an unfastened vest but was resuscitated by emergency personnel. Extra attention to compliance and fitting and further study are obviously needed in children.

SUMMARY

The WCD is an effective option for external monitoring and defibrillation in patients at risk for SCA caused by VT/VF and who are not candidates for or who refuse an ICD. Compliance and absence of pacing capability are limitations. However, shock efficacy and overall survival seem similar with a WCD compared with ICDs, and studies have reported satisfactory overall compliance. The WCD also provides monitoring with backup defibrillation protection during diagnosis and risk stratification periods. The device has been used when a patient's condition delays or prohibits ICD implantation, or as a bridge during periods when an indicated ICD must be explanted, such as for treatment of infection. The WCD has been increasingly used for primary prevention of SCD during the high-risk gap periods early after MI, coronary revascularization with CABG or PCI, or new diagnosis of heart failure, when its use is as a protective bridge to ICD or LV improvement.

REFERENCES

1. Zipes DP, Camm AJ, Borggrefe M, et al. ACC/AHA/ ESC 2006 guidelines for management of patients with ventricular arrhythmias and the prevention of sudden cardiac death: a report of the American College of Cardiology/American Heart Association Task Force and the European Society of Cardiology Committee for Practice Guidelines (Writing Committee to Develop Guidelines for Management of Patients With Ventricular Arrhythmias and the Prevention of Sudden Cardiac Death). J Am Coll Cardiol 2006;48(5):e247–346.
2. Gronda E, Bourge RC, Costanzo MR, et al. Heart rhythm considerations in heart transplant candidates and considerations for ventricular assist devices: International Society for Heart and Lung Transplantation guidelines for the care of cardiac

transplant candidates–2006. J Heart Lung Transplant 2006;25(9):1043–56.

3. Wilkoff BL, Love CJ, Byrd CL, et al. Transvenous lead extraction: Heart Rhythm Society expert consensus on facilities, training, indications, and patient management: this document was endorsed by the American Heart Association (AHA). Heart Rhythm 2009;6(7):1085–104.

4. O'Gara PT, Kushner FG, Ascheim DD, et al. 2013 ACCF/AHA guideline for the management of ST-elevation myocardial infarction: a report of the American College of Cardiology Foundation/American Heart Association Task Force on Practice Guidelines. J Am Coll Cardiol 2013;61(4):e78–140.

5. Chung MK, Szymkiewicz SJ, Shao M, et al. Aggregate national experience with the wearable cardioverter-defibrillator: event rates, compliance, and survival. J Am Coll Cardiol 2010;56(3):194–203.

6. Moss AJ, Hall WJ, Cannom DS, et al. Improved survival with an implanted defibrillator in patients with coronary disease at high risk for ventricular arrhythmia. Multicenter Automatic Defibrillator Implantation Trial Investigators. N Engl J Med 1996;335(26):1933–40.

7. Moss AJ, Zareba W, Hall WJ, et al. Prophylactic implantation of a defibrillator in patients with myocardial infarction and reduced ejection fraction. N Engl J Med 2002;346(12):877–83.

8. Bardy GH, Lee KL, Mark DB, et al. Amiodarone or an implantable cardioverter-defibrillator for congestive heart failure. N Engl J Med 2005;352(3):225–37.

9. Buxton AE, Lee KL, Fisher JD, et al. A randomized study of the prevention of sudden death in patients with coronary artery disease. Multicenter Unsustained Tachycardia Trial Investigators. N Engl J Med 1999;341(25):1882–90.

10. Bigger JT Jr. Prophylactic use of implanted cardiac defibrillators in patients at high risk for ventricular arrhythmias after coronary-artery bypass graft surgery. Coronary Artery Bypass Graft (CABG) Patch Trial Investigators. N Engl J Med 1997;337(22):1569–75.

11. Kadish A, Dyer A, Daubert JP, et al. Prophylactic defibrillator implantation in patients with nonischemic dilated cardiomyopathy. N Engl J Med 2004; 350(21):2151–8.

12. Epstein AE, DiMarco JP, Ellenbogen KA, et al. ACC/AHA/HRS 2008 Guidelines for Device-Based Therapy of Cardiac Rhythm Abnormalities: a report of the American College of Cardiology/American Heart Association Task Force on Practice Guidelines (Writing Committee to Revise the ACC/AHA/NASPE 2002 Guideline Update for Implantation of Cardiac Pacemakers and Antiarrhythmia Devices): developed in collaboration with the American Association for Thoracic Surgery and Society of Thoracic Surgeons. Circulation 2008;117(21):e350–408.

13. Solomon SD, Glynn RJ, Greaves S, et al. Recovery of ventricular function after myocardial infarction in the reperfusion era: the healing and early afterload reducing therapy study. Ann Intern Med 2001; 134(6):451–8.

14. Solomon SD, Zelenkofske S, McMurray JJ, et al. Sudden death in patients with myocardial infarction and left ventricular dysfunction, heart failure, or both. N Engl J Med 2005;352(25):2581–8.

15. Klein HU, Meltendorf U, Reek S, et al. Bridging a temporary high risk of sudden arrhythmic death. Experience with the wearable cardioverter defibrillator (WCD). Pacing Clin Electrophysiol 2010;33(3): 353–67.

16. Bunch TJ, May HT, Bair TL, et al. Trends in early and late mortality in patients undergoing coronary catheterization for myocardial infarction: implications on observation periods and risk factors to determine ICD candidacy. Heart Rhythm 2011;8(9):1460–6.

17. Adabag AS, Therneau TM, Gersh BJ, et al. Sudden death after myocardial infarction. JAMA 2008; 300(17):2022–9.

18. Goldberger JJ, Passman R. Implantable cardioverter-defibrillator therapy after acute myocardial infarction: the results are not shocking. J Am Coll Cardiol 2009;54(22):2001–5.

19. Pouleur AC, Barkoudah E, Uno H, et al. Pathogenesis of sudden unexpected death in a clinical trial of patients with myocardial infarction and left ventricular dysfunction, heart failure, or both. Circulation 2010;122(6):597–602.

20. Piccini JP, Al-Khatib SM, Hellkamp AS, et al. Mortality benefits from implantable cardioverter-defibrillator therapy are not restricted to patients with remote myocardial infarction: an analysis from the Sudden Cardiac Death in Heart Failure Trial (SCD-HeFT). Heart Rhythm 2011;8(3):393–400.

21. Hohnloser SH, Kuck KH, Dorian P, et al. Prophylactic use of an implantable cardioverter-defibrillator after acute myocardial infarction. N Engl J Med 2004;351(24):2481–8.

22. Steinbeck G, Andresen D, Seidl K, et al. Defibrillator implantation early after myocardial infarction. N Engl J Med 2009;361(15):1427–36.

23. Feldman AM, Klein H, Tchou P, et al. Use of a wearable defibrillator in terminating tachyarrhythmias in patients at high risk for sudden death: results of the WEARIT/BIROAD. Pacing Clin Electrophysiol 2004; 27(1):4–9.

24. Epstein AE, Abraham WT, Bianco NR, et al. Wearable cardioverter-defibrillator use in patients perceived to be at high risk early post myocardial infarction. J Am Coll Cardiol 2013;62(21):2000–7.

25. Nageh MF, Kim JJ, Chung J, et al. The role of implantable cardioverter defibrillators in high-risk CABG patients identified early post-cardiac surgery. Europace 2011;13(1):70–6.

26. John JM, Hussein A, Imran N, et al. Underutilization of implantable cardioverter defibrillators post

coronary artery bypass grafting in patients with systolic dysfunction. Pacing Clin Electrophysiol 2010;33(6):727–33.

27. Bonow RO, Maurer G, Lee KL, et al. Myocardial viability and survival in ischemic left ventricular dysfunction. N Engl J Med 2011;364(17):1617–25.

28. Shahian DM, O'Brien SM, Sheng S, et al. Predictors of long-term survival after coronary artery bypass grafting surgery: results from the Society of Thoracic Surgeons Adult Cardiac Surgery Database (the AS-CERT study). Circulation 2012;125(12):1491–500.

29. Halkin A, Singh M, Nikolsky E, et al. Prediction of mortality after primary percutaneous coronary intervention for acute myocardial infarction: the CADILLAC risk score. J Am Coll Cardiol 2005;45(9):1397–405.

30. Weintraub WS, Grau-sepulveda MV, Weiss JM, et al. Prediction of long-term mortality after percutaneous coronary intervention in older adults: results from the National Cardiovascular Data Registry. Circulation 2012;125(12):1501–10.

31. Zishiri ET, Williams S, Cronin EM, et al. Early risk of mortality after coronary artery revascularization in patients with left ventricular dysfunction and potential role of the wearable cardioverter defibrillator. Circ Arrhythm Electrophysiol 2013;6(1):117–28.

32. Verdino RJ. The wearable cardioverter-defibrillator: lifesaving attire or "fashion faux pas?". J Am Coll Cardiol 2010;56(3):204–5.

33. Schliamser JE, Kadish AH, Subacious H, et al. Significance of follow-up left ventricular ejection fraction measurements in the Defibrillators in Non-Ischemic Cardiomyopathy Treatment Evaluation trial (DEFINITE). Heart Rhythm 2013;10(6):838–46.

34. Bardy GH. The sudden cardiac death-heart failure trial (SCD-HeFT). In: Woosley RL, Singh SN, editors. Arrhythmia treatment and therapy: evaluation of clinical trial evidence. New York: Marcel Dekker; 2000. p. 323–42.

35. Kadish A, Schaechter A, Subacius H, et al. Patients with recently diagnosed nonischemic cardiomyopathy benefit from implantable cardioverter-defibrillators. J Am Coll Cardiol 2006;47(12):2477–82.

36. Makati KJ, Fish AE, England HH, et al. Equivalent arrhythmic risk in patients recently diagnosed with dilated cardiomyopathy compared with patients diagnosed for 9 months or more. Heart Rhythm 2006;3(4):397–403.

37. Lang CC, Hankins S, Hauff H, et al. Morbidity and mortality of UNOS status 1B cardiac transplant candidates at home. J Heart Lung Transplant 2003;22(4):419–26.

38. Cantillon DJ, Tarakji KG, Kumbhani DJ, et al. Improved survival among ventricular assist device recipients with a concomitant implantable cardioverter-defibrillator. Heart Rhythm 2010;7(4):466–71.

39. Auricchio A, Klein H, Geller CJ, et al. Clinical efficacy of the wearable cardioverter-defibrillator in acutely terminating episodes of ventricular fibrillation. Am J Cardiol 1998;81(10):1253–6.

40. Sweeney MO, Wathen MS, Volosin K, et al. Appropriate and inappropriate ventricular therapies, quality of life, and mortality among primary and secondary prevention implantable cardioverter defibrillator patients: results from the Pacing Fast VT Reduces Shock Therapies (PainFREE Rx II) trial. Circulation 2005;111(22):2898–905.

41. Poole JE, Johnson GW, Hellkamp AS, et al. Prognostic importance of defibrillator shocks in patients with heart failure. N Engl J Med 2008;359(10):1009–17.

42. Daubert JP, Zareba W, Cannom DS, et al. Inappropriate implantable cardioverter-defibrillator shocks in MADIT II: frequency, mechanisms, predictors, and survival impact. J Am Coll Cardiol 2008; 51(14):1357–65.

43. Klein RC, Raitt MH, Wilkoff BL, et al. Analysis of implantable cardioverter defibrillator therapy in the Antiarrhythmics Versus Implantable Defibrillators (AVID) Trial. J Cardiovasc Electrophysiol 2003;14(9):940–8.

44. Wilkoff BL, Ousdigian KT, Sterns LD, et al. A comparison of empiric to physician-tailored programming of implantable cardioverter-defibrillators: results from the prospective randomized multicenter EMPIRIC trial. J Am Coll Cardiol 2006;48(2):330–9.

45. Wilkoff BL, Williamson BD, Stern RS, et al. Strategic programming of detection and therapy parameters in implantable cardioverter-defibrillators reduces shocks in primary prevention patients: results from the PREPARE (Primary Prevention Parameters Evaluation) study. J Am Coll Cardiol 2008;52(7):541–50.

46. Wilkoff BL, Hess M, Young J, et al. Differences in tachyarrhythmia detection and implantable cardioverter defibrillator therapy by primary or secondary prevention indication in cardiac resynchronization therapy patients. J Cardiovasc Electrophysiol 2004; 15(9):1002–9.

47. Everitt MD, Saarel EV. Use of the wearable external cardiac defibrillator in children. Pacing Clin Electrophysiol 2010;33(6):742–6.

48. Reek S, Geller JC, Meltendorf U, et al. Clinical efficacy of a wearable defibrillator in acutely terminating episodes of ventricular fibrillation using biphasic shocks. Pacing Clin Electrophysiol 2003; 26(10):2016–22.

49. Dillon KA, Szymkiewicz SJ, Kaib TE. Evaluation of the effectiveness of a wearable cardioverter defibrillator detection algorithm. J Electrocardiol 2010;43(1):63–7.

50. Rao M, Goldenberg I, Moss AJ, et al. Wearable defibrillator in congenital structural heart disease and inherited arrhythmias. Am J Cardiol 2011; 108(11):1632–8.

51. Saltzberg MT, Szymkiewicz S, Bianco NR. Characteristics and outcomes of peripartum versus nonperipartum cardiomyopathy in women using a wearable cardiac defibrillator. J Card Fail 2012;18(1):21–7.

Does Atrial Fibrillation Detected by Cardiac Implantable Electronic Devices Have Clinical Relevance?

Taya V. Glotzer, MD[a],*, Paul D. Ziegler, MS[b]

KEYWORDS

• Atrial fibrillation • Stroke • Implantable device • Continuous monitoring

KEY POINTS

- The precise role atrial fibrillation (AF) plays in increasing the risk of stroke is not well understood, and this is especially true for the implanted device population.
- Current cardiac implanted electronic devices have a very high sensitivity and specificity for true AF detection.
- It does not seem to matter if the AF episode is proximal to the stroke event, and risk seems to be increased by relatively brief AF episodes.
- The appearance of new atrial high-rate episodes increases thromboembolic event rates.
- Until larger trials or registries are conducted, it is important to follow established guidelines regarding anticoagulation.

The current evidence suggests the prevalence of atrial fibrillation (AF) detected by cardiac implanted electronic devices (CIEDs) is considerable, and the presence of this device-detected AF increases the risk of thromboembolism. The AF burden threshold which confers this increased thromboembolism risk is not precisely defined, but may be as brief as several minutes or as long as several hours. The advent of novel oral anticoagulation (NOAC) medications, which offer the promise of improved efficacy along with superior safety profiles, may warrant more aggressive identification of patients who may benefit from these therapies.

Over the last 10 years it has been learned that symptoms are an unreliable indicator of the presence of atrial arrhythmias. Page and colleagues[1] were among the first to demonstrate this lack of correlation by reporting that for each episode of symptomatic paroxysmal AF, patients were likely to experience 12 episodes of asymptomatic AF. Subsequent studies with implanted devices confirmed more than 90% of stored atrial arrhythmia episodes were asymptomatic.[2,3] Furthermore, it was demonstrated that symptoms thought to be caused by AF, actually correlated with AF in only about 20% of cases.[2–4] This lack of correlation of AF with symptoms led to the repurposing of the term "silent AF," which is now commonly used to describe device-detected AF.

PART 1: SENSITIVITY AND SPECIFICITY OF AF DETECTION BY IMPLANTED DEVICES

To assess the stroke risk of device-detected AF accurately, one must first evaluate the sensitivity and specificity of the detected AF, to be certain the implanted devices are accurately classifying and quantifying AF. AF detection algorithms are

a Hackensack University Medical Center, Hackensack, NJ 07601, USA; b Medtronic Cardiac Rhythm Disease Management Division, Medtronic Inc, 8200 Coral Sea St. NE, Mounds View, MN 55112, USA
* Corresponding author. Electrophysiology Associates of Northern New Jersey, 20 Prospect Avenue, Suite 701, Hackensack, NJ 07601.
E-mail address: TayaVG@aol.com

Cardiol Clin 32 (2014) 271–281
http://dx.doi.org/10.1016/j.ccl.2013.11.001
0733-8651/14/$ – see front matter © 2014 Elsevier Inc. All rights reserved.

designed based on their intended application. To avoid rapid pacing in the ventricle, antibradycardia devices must detect atrial arrhythmias quickly to permit mode-switching to a nontracking pacing mode. Devices that deliver atrial tachyarrhythmia therapies, such as implantable cardioverter defibrillators (ICDs), must be highly specific to ensure only true atrial arrhythmias are being treated. If these therapies are delivered erroneously, there can be negative consequences such as proarrhythmia. These devices rely on both rate and pattern information to make accurate detection decisions. Pacemakers and ICDs have sensing leads in the atrium that deliver real-time bipolar intracardiac electrogram information to the implanted device, which make their sensitivity and specificity quite high.

Insertable cardiac monitors (ICMs) have recently been developed to provide continuous arrhythmia monitoring capabilities to patients who do not have an indication for a cardiac rhythm management device. These devices do not have an atrial lead and must detect AF from subcutaneously sensed patterns of ventricular irregularity and incoherence.

AF Detection Based on Mode-Switching

Dual-chamber pacemakers and ICDs that do not deliver atrial therapies have historically used mode-switch detection algorithms to detect AF and prevent ventricular tracking of the rapidly activating atrium. AF detection via mode-switching occurs very quickly and is very sensitive. Details regarding the operation of various mode-switching algorithms have been previously described,[5] but, in general, involve switching from an atrial tracking mode during sinus rhythm to a nontracking mode during atrial arrhythmias. A representative sample of the atrial intracardiac electrogram is typically stored in the device memory for clinicians to examine and adjudicate.

Passman and colleagues[6] reported a sensitivity and specificity for atrial tachyarrhythmia episode detection of 98.1% and 100%, respectively. In this evaluation, they also showed 98.9% of the overall duration of AF was detected accurately. Similarly, De Voogt and colleagues[7] found 99.9% of atrial tachycardia (AT)/AF duration was detected accurately. In contrast, other studies have reported instances of repetitive non-reentrant VA synchrony, which are frequently caused by long programmed AV delays[8] or interactions with AF suppression algorithms,[9] resulting in higher rates of false atrial tachyarrhythmia detection. This repetitive non-reentrant VA synchrony phenomenon contributed to positive predictive values

(PPV) of 59.7% across all episodes, 82.7% for episodes greater than 6 minutes in duration, and 96.7% for episodes greater than 6 hours in duration in the ASSERT (ASymptomatic atrial fibrillation and Stroke Evaluation in pacemaker patients and the atrial fibrillation Reduction atrial pacing Trial) trial.[9] These results are consistent with the finding of Pollak and colleagues,[10] who found episodes greater than 5 minutes in duration had a high correlation with true AF and atrial flutter.

AF Detection Based on Rate and Pattern

High specificity for AF detection in devices that deliver atrial therapies (including most ICDs and some pacemakers) has been achieved by the use of more sophisticated detection algorithms. These algorithms often combine atrial rate information with pattern-based algorithms to recognize an atrial tachyarrhythmia when there is greater than 1:1 Atrial:Ventricular conduction, while rejecting far-field R-wave oversensing on the atrial sensing channel.

Purerfellner and colleagues[11] reported greater than 95% of AF episodes detected by both ICDs and pacemakers with atrial therapy capabilities were true episodes and 100% of sustained atrial arrhythmias observed on Holter recordings were detected appropriately by these devices. Similarly, Swerdlow and colleagues[12] reported a PPV of 98% for episodes of AF detected among ICD recipients. These investigators also observed an AF duration sensitivity and specificity of 100% and 99.99%, respectively. In contrast to previous reports,[9] the RESPECT (Reducing Episodes by Septal Pacing Efficacy Confirmation Trial) investigators did not observe an interaction between the AF detection algorithm and AF prevention algorithms in the devices they analyzed.[13] Furthermore, this study demonstrated a high PPV (95%) for even very brief episodes of less than 6 minutes in duration, which underscores that there can be significant differences between manufacturers and specific devices in terms of AF detection accuracy.

AF Detection Based on Ventricular Irregularity and Incoherence

For patients who do not require brady pacing or protection against sudden cardiac death, subcutaneous devices have been developed to provide continuous arrhythmia detection and monitoring capabilities. Early versions of these ICMs were capable of detecting tachyarrhythmias based solely on ventricular rate and were not designed to be highly sensitive and specific for AF. Recently, ICMs that have dedicated and validated AF detection algorithms using ventricular irregularity and incoherence[14,15] have been designed.

The XPECT (Reveal XT Performance Trial) investigators found the sensitivity and negative predictive value for identifying patients with AF using newer ICMs were 96.1% and 97.4%, respectively.[16] In both this study and the Discerning Symptomatic and Asymptomatic Episodes Pre and Post Radiofrequency Ablation of Atrial Fibrillation (DISCERN) study,[17] AF burden was quantified with greater than 98% accuracy even though false positive detections of AF occasionally occurred. Because false positives tend to be very brief in duration, they consequently have little impact on the overall AF burden measurement. Future monitoring devices should preserve the electrocardiogram record of the longest AF episode, which has a greater probability of being a true AF episode[16] and will aid in confirming the presence of AF.

Summary

AF detection in modern CIEDs has been shown to be highly accurate. However, it is important to recognize certain devices may have interactions between AF detection algorithms and other device algorithms (such as AF suppression algorithms), which can result in a high rate of false positive AF detection. Because occasional undersensing has the potential to "chop" longer episodes into multiple short episodes, the duration of individual episodes may not be the most robust metric available for correlation with stroke risk. In contrast, the cumulative time spent in AF (AF burden) is much less susceptible to errors introduced by brief periods of undersensing and has been shown to have greater than 98% accuracy.[6,7,12,16,17]

PART 2: EVIDENCE: DEVICE-DETECTED AF IS ASSOCIATED WITH THROMBOEMBOLIC EVENTS

One of the first articles to highlight the stroke risk of episodes of device-detected AF was an ancillary study of the MOST (MOde Selection Trial) trial published in 2003.[18] A subgroup of 312 patients was selected to evaluate the clinical consequences of AF episodes detected by the pacemakers. Analysis of this subgroup showed patients who had at least one AHRE detected by their pacemaker (defined as lasting more than 5 consecutive minutes in duration with an atrial rate $\geq$220 bpm) had a 6.7-fold increased risk of stroke, a 2.48-fold increased risk of death, a 5.93-fold increased risk of developing permanent AF, and a 2.79-fold increase in the combined endpoint of death and nonfatal stroke (**Fig. 1**).[18] The absolute stroke rate in the overall study group was 3.2%; 5% in the AHRE group and 1.3% in the group with no AHREs (**Table 1**). The finding that a minimum 5-minute episode of AF detected by pacemaker diagnostics could have such significant clinical impact was novel and surprising.

In 2005, the Italian AT500 Registry Investigators published a study of 725 patients with pacemakers and a history of symptomatic AT/AF to study the implications of AT/AF detected by pacemaker diagnostics.[19] The overall annual arterial embolic rate in the study group was 1.2% (see **Table 1**). This study showed a 3.1-fold higher arterial embolic rate (after adjusting for known risk factors) in patients who had 24 hours or more of AF detected by their pacemaker diagnostics, and a significantly lower rate for those who had no AF or episodes shorter than 1 day (**Fig. 2**).

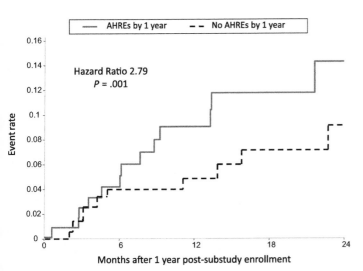

Hazard Ratio 2.79
$P = .001$

Event rate — Months after 1 year post-substudy enrollment

—— AHREs by 1 year   – – No AHREs by 1 year

Fig. 1. MOST ancillary study: Kaplan-Meier plot of death or nonfatal stroke after 1 year of follow-up in patients with AHREs versus those without AHREs, $P = .001$. (*From* Glotzer TV, Hellkamp AS, Zimmerman J, et al. Atrial high rate episodes detected by pacemaker diagnostics predict death and stroke: report of the atrial diagnostics sub-study of MOST. Circulation 2003;107:1617; with permission.)

Table 1
Summary of studies presented

Year	Study	Number of Patients	Duration of Follow-Up	Atrial Rate Cutoff	AF Burden Cut Point	Hazard Ratio for TE Event	TE Event Rate AF Burden Below Cut Point vs AF Burden Above Cut Point
2003	Ancillary MOST	312	27 mo (median)	>220 bpm	5 min	6.7 $P = .020$	3.2% overall 1.3% vs 5%
2005	Italian AT500 Registry	725	22 mo (median)	>174 bpm	24 h	3.1 $P = .044$	1.2% annual rate
2009	Botto et al	568	1 y (mean)	>174 bpm	CHADS$_2$ + AF burden	n/a	2.5% overall 0.8% vs 5%
2009	TRENDS	2486	1.4 y (mean)	>175 bpm	5.5 h	2.2 $P = .060$	1.2% overall 1.1% vs 2.4%
2012	Home monitor CRT	560	370 d (median)	>180 bpm	3.8 h	9.4 $P = .006$	2.0% overall
2012	ASSERT	2580	2.5 y (mean)	>190 bpm	6 min	2.5 $P = .007$	0.69% vs 1.69%

Data from Refs.[9,18–20,23,25]

The subsequent TRENDS trial was designed to evaluate the relationship between comprehensive AT/AF burden detected by CIEDs and thromboembolic (TE) risk, and to determine if there is a threshold value of AT/AF burden that increases TE risk.[20] Patients were enrolled if they had a class 1 or 2 indication for implantation of a pacemaker, an ICD, or a cardiac resynchronization therapy (CRT) device and had at least one stroke risk factor based on the 2001 guidelines in effect at the time this study began (including history of congestive heart failure, hypertension, age >65 years, diabetes mellitus, or prior stroke/transient ischemic attack [TIA]).[21] There was no specification regarding prior history of AF or anticoagulation use. The primary endpoint was the occurrence of an adjudicated TE event defined as an ischemic stroke, TIA, or a systemic embolism.

The TRENDS study used a novel technique to evaluate the TE risk associated with atrial arrhythmias that occurred in the proximate 30 days by analyzing atrial arrhythmia burden during 30-day rolling windows.[22] Thirty-day windows were selected to maintain a reasonable balance between too short a timeframe, whereby the likelihood of observing any AT/AF is low, and too long a timeframe, whereby observed AT/AF may not be temporally related to a TE. Thirty-day windows also allow comparison between patients who had different lengths of follow-up. AT/AF burden was classified as high burden (greater than or equal to the median of the maximum daily AT/AF burden value among 30-day windows with nonzero burden) and low burden (less than this median value). The calculated median value for maximum daily AT/AF burden in all 30-day

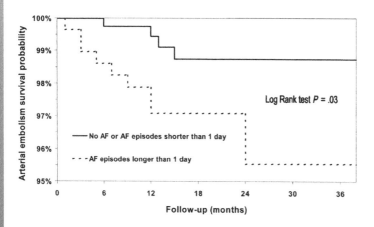

Fig. 2. Italian AT500 Registry: Kaplan-Meier cumulative survival from embolic events for patients with AF episodes longer than 1 day and for patients without AF recurrences or with AF episodes shorter than 1 day, $P = .03$. (From Capucci A, Santini M, Padeletti L, et al, Italian AT500 Registry Investigators. Monitored atrial fibrillation duration predicts arterial embolic events in patients suffering from bradycardia and atrial fibrillation implanted with antitachycardia pacemakers. J Am Coll Cardiol 2005; 46:1917; with permission.)

windows with nonzero AT/AF in the TRENDS trial was 5.5 hours.

The annualized TE rate in the overall study population was remarkably low at 1.2%. The annualized TE rate was 1.1% for both the group with zero AT/AF burden and the low AT/AF burden group. For the high burden group, the TE rate was more than double at 2.4% per year (see **Table 1**). The hazard ratio for TE events for the low burden group compared with zero AT/AF burden was 0.98. The hazard ratio for the high burden group compared with zero AT/AF burden was 2.2, which means that if a patient has ≥5.5 hours of AT/AF on a single day in the preceding 30 days, they are 2.2 times more likely to have a TE than if they had no AT/AF detected.[22]

In 2009, Botto and colleagues[23] evaluated a combination of the duration of device-detected atrial arrhythmia episodes and CHADS$_2$ score to predict TE events. In the CHADS$_2$ scheme, one point is assigned for each risk factor (history of congestive heart failure, hypertension, age >75 years, diabetes mellitus, or prior stroke/TIA, which is assigned 2 points).[24] Five hundred sixty-eight patients with pacemakers and a history of symptomatic AF were enrolled. AT/AF burden was evaluated with the following cut points: none, greater than 5 minutes, or greater than 24 hours of continuous AT/AF. The TE event rate for the entire cohort over 1 year of follow-up was 2.5% (see **Table 1**). The analysis showed if a patient's CHADS$_2$ score was zero, they were part of a group that had an extremely low TE rate of 0.8%, regardless of the

amount of AT/AF detected by the device. Conversely, if the CHADS$_2$ score was 3 or greater, these patients were part of a group that had a very high TE rate of 5%, also regardless of the amount of AT/AF detected by the device (see **Table 1**). However, in the patients with intermediate CHADS$_2$ scores (1 and 2), the combined risk markers (AT/AF duration and CHADS$_2$ score) had a significant predictive value. In patients with a CHADS$_2$ score of 1, a minimum of 24 hours of device-detected AT/AF was required to move them from a group that had a stroke risk of 0.6% to a group that had a stroke risk of 4%. In patients with a CHADS$_2$ score of 2, a minimum duration of only 5 minutes of device-detected AT/AF was required to move them from the low-risk group to the high-risk group (**Fig. 3**). Botto and colleagues introduced a unique method of analyzing AT/AF burden duration in combination with CHADS$_2$ score to predict TE risk with very meaningful results.

In 2012, there were 2 important studies published that looked at the association of device-detected AT/AF and stroke risk. Shanmugam and colleagues[25] published a study using remote home monitoring to identify AT/AF episodes in 560 patients with heart failure and implanted CRT devices. Patients were divided into 4 groups: patients with no prior history of AF and newly detected AT/AF by the device (1A), patients with no prior history of AF and no device-detected AT/AF (1B), patients with a prior history of AF and new device-detected AT/AF (2A), and patients with a prior history of AF and no device-detected

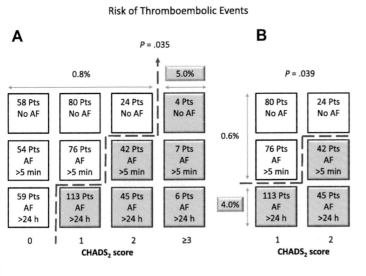

Fig. 3. Botto and colleagues: Combining the data on AF presence/absence, AF duration, and CHADS$_2$ score enabled the whole population to be subdivided into 2 subpopulations with significantly different risks of TE events (0.8% vs 5%, A). The color separates the 2 subgroups. The results show that patients with CHADS$_2$ score = 0 are at low risk, even if they have long-lasting AF episodes; by contrast, patients with CHADS$_2$ score ≥3 should be considered at high risk even when AF is no longer detected. (B) The same analysis restricted to patients with moderate risk; combining AF presence/duration with CHADS$_2$ score still yields a significantly different risk in the subgroups identified (0.6% vs 4%). This figure also shows the number of patients in each subgroup, according to the AF classification assigned and CHADS$_2$ score. Columns correspond to CHADS$_2$ score and rows to AF classification. (*From* Botto GL, Padeletti L, Santini M, et al. Presence and duration of atrial fibrillation detected by continuous monitoring: crucial implications for the risk of thromboembolic events. J Cardiovasc Electrophysiol 2009;20:245; with permission.)

AT/AF (2B). For the purposes of this study, patients were classified as having device-detected AT/AF when an AHRE lasted at least 1% of a day, which equates to a cumulative duration of 14 minutes, the limit of the remote monitoring technology.

Over a mean follow-up of 370 days, the overall thromboembolism rate was 2% (see **Table 1**). The risk of TE events was greatest among patients with device-detected AHRE over the follow-up period, irrespective of whether they had a prior history of AF (group 2A, 4.1%) or not (group 1A, 4.0%). Patients with a prior history of AF and no AHRE detected during the study had an intermediate risk of TE (group 2B, 2.5%), whereas the group with no prior history of AF and no device-detected AHRE had the lowest TE risk (group 1B, 0%). The survival free from TE for all 4 groups is presented in **Fig. 4**.

The authors performed an additional analysis of the median daily value of AT/AF burden detected via remote monitoring similar to the analysis conducted in the TRENDS trial; the median daily value in this study was 3.8 hours. The hazard ratio for the low burden group (less than 3.8 hours on a given day) compared with zero burden was not statistically significant. The hazard ratio for the high burden group (more than 3.8 hours on a given day) compared with the zero burden group was 9.4 (P<.006) (see **Table 1**).[25] The conclusion of this study was that patients with no prior history of AF but with newly detected AT/AF lasting at least 14 minutes by an implanted device have a markedly increased stroke risk. In addition, episodes lasting more than 3.8 hours on a given day increase the TE risk more than 9-fold.

The results of a prospective cohort design study (ASSERT) to determine if device-detected atrial arrhythmias are associated with an increased risk of stroke was also published in 2012.[26] Patients with hypertension and age greater than 65 years (n = 2580) were enrolled after implantation of a first pacemaker or ICD. Patients were excluded if they were on oral anticoagulants or had a history of AF. After enrollment, patients were monitored for 3 months to classify the patients as having AHRE or not. An AHRE was defined as an episode with an atrial rate greater than 190 bpm lasting for at least 6 minutes. Patients remained fixed in these categories for the remainder of the trial even if atrial tachyarrhythmias were subsequently detected in those without early episodes.[27]

Over 2.5 years mean follow-up, the stroke rate in the 261 patients with AHRE detected in the initial 3 months (10% of the patients) was 1.69% per year, whereas the stroke rate in the 2319 patients without AHRE detected in the initial 3 months (90% of patients) was 0.69% per year, resulting in a relative risk of 2.49 (P = .007) (**Fig. 5**, see **Table 1**).[26] AHRE patients also had a 5.56 times greater likelihood of being diagnosed with clinical AF or flutter via surface electrocardiogram (6.29 vs 1.22% per year, P<.001) during follow-up. At present, the outcome of the patients (an additional 633 patients or 24.5% of the entire cohort) who developed subsequent 6-minute episodes of atrial arrhythmias is not known, as they were analyzed together with the patients who experienced no atrial arrhythmias as per the initial trial design.[27] One could hypothesize that the patients who had 6-minute episodes detected in the initial 3 months are the patients with the highest AHRE burden and that is why both the AF was detected early and the TE rates were the highest.

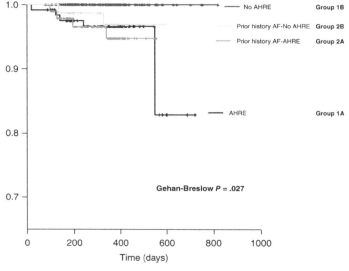

AHRE defined as 14 min = 1% of a day, A rate > 180

Fig. 4. Shanmugam and colleagues: Kaplan-Meier cumulative survival free from TE events for 4 groups of patients with implantable defibrillators. Patients with no prior history of AF and NDAF by the device (1A), patients with no prior history of AF and no device-detected AF (1B), patients with a prior history of AF and new device-detected AF (2A), and patients with a prior history of AF and no device-detected AF (2B). An episode of device-detected AF was defined as lasting 1% of a day, which is a cumulative duration of 14 minutes. (*From* Shanmugam N, Boerdlein A, Proff J, et al. Detection of atrial high-rate events by continuous home monitoring: clinical significance in the heart failure—cardiac resynchronization therapy population. Europace 2012;14:234; with permission.)

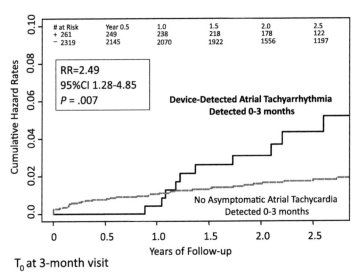

Fig. 5. ASSERT trial: The risk of ischemic stroke or systemic embolism after the 3-month visit, according to whether subclinical atrial tachyarrhythmias were or were not detected between enrollment and the 3-month visit, *P* = .007. (*Data from* Healey JS, Connolly SJ, Gold MR, et al; ASSERT Investigators. Subclinical atrial fibrillation and the risk of stroke. N Engl J Med 2012;366:128.)

T_0 at 3-month visit

PART 3: TEMPORAL PROXIMITY OF DEVICE-DETECTED AF EPISODES TO TE EVENTS

The subgroup of 40 patients enrolled in the TRENDS study who experienced a TE event and for whom at least 30 days of monitoring data before the TE was available were evaluated to determine the temporal proximity of AT/AF episodes to the TE event.[28] AT/AF (lasting at least 5 minutes) was detected by the device, at any time, before the TE event in only 20 patients and was not detected by the device before the TE in the remaining 20 patients. Of the 20 patients with AT/AF before the TE event, 9 (45%) did not have any AT/AF within 30 days prior to the TE (**Fig. 6**). Among the 20 patients in whom AT/AF was *not* detected before the TE, 6 (30%) had AT/AF recorded 181 ± 143 days after the TE. One caveat is that the duration of preevent monitoring was significantly shorter in the patients *without* AT/AF detected prior (251 ± 221 days) compared with the patients *with* AT/AF detected prior (485 ± 273 days). Thus, most TE patients (29/40 [73%]) had zero AT/AF episodes within the 30 days before the TE event.

For those patients in the home monitoring CRT study who had a documented AHRE before their TE event, the mean interval between the embolic event and the most recent AF episode was 46.7 ± 71.9 days with a range of 0–194 days. In addition, more than a third of the patients who developed a TE event had no prior AHRE recorded.[25]

These data imply a proximate temporal relationship does *not* always exist between AT/AF episodes and TE. Therefore, the mechanism of stroke in patients with an implantable device often is not solely related to the AT/AF episodes.

PART 4: NEWLY DETECTED AF IN PATIENTS WITH NO PRIOR HISTORY OF AF

Previous studies have shown the probability of detecting AT/AF using intermittent monitoring decreases as the amount of AT/AF decreases.[29,30] Therefore, to find brief episodes of "silent AF," an implanted monitor is essential to provide complete, comprehensive data on the detection of atrial arrhythmias. An analysis of the TRENDS study population to quantify the incidence and duration of newly detected AF (NDAF) in patients who had no prior history of AF, no previous stroke/TIA, and no warfarin or antiarrhythmic drug use was reported in 2012.[31] NDAF was defined as device-detected atrial arrhythmias lasting at least 5 minutes on any day of the study.

Thirty percent of patients in the substudy experienced NDAF. The incidence of NDAF was consistent across patients with intermediate (virtual $CHADS_2$ score of 1) (30%), high (virtual $CHADS_2$ score of 2) (31%), and very high (virtual $CHADS_2$ score of ≥3) (31%) stroke risk factors (*P* = .92). Interestingly, a significant increase was seen in the proportion of patients having days with greater than 6 hours of AT/AF as the virtual $CHADS_2$ score increased; 12%, 15%, and 18% for intermediate, high, and very high risk, respectively; *P* = .04 (**Fig. 7**). Just more than half of NDAF patients (55%) with ≥2 stroke risk factors exceeded 5.5 hours of NDAF on a given day, a cut point that was established in the main TRENDS trial to elevate TE risk.

In another analysis from the TRENDS trial, NDAF was analyzed in patients who had a prior history of stroke or TIA.[32] Patients with a documented history of AF, warfarin use, or antiarrhythmic drug use were excluded from analysis. NDAF was again

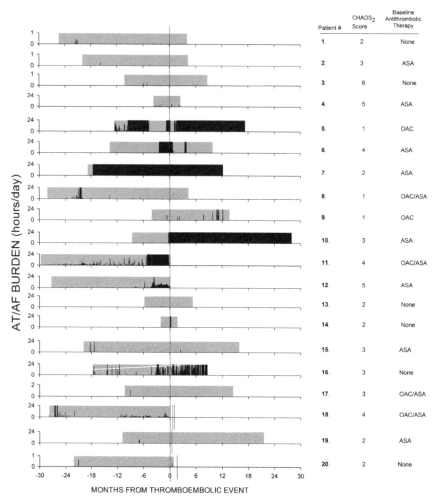

Fig. 6. TRENDS trial: Summary of AT/AF burden per day relative to onset of cerebrovascular events/systemic emboli (CVE/SE). Each row in the graph represents the data extracted from the implanted device for each of the 20 patients with AT/AF detected by the device before CVE/SE. Gray-shaded areas depict the period of continuous monitoring when the device was implanted. Each day of CVE/SE(s) is represented by the vertical red line (some patients had more than one CVE/SE). All monitoring is aligned with the first CVE/SE. The number of hours of AT/AF per day is represented by the height of each black vertical line. For some patients, the y-axis scale is 0–1 or 0–2 hours rather than 0–24 hours. Each patient's CHADS₂ score and antithrombotic therapy at the time of enrollment is summarized on the right. ASA, aspirin. (*From* Daoud EG, Glotzer TV, Wyse DG, et al, TRENDS Investigators. Temporal relationship of atrial tachyarrhythmias, cerebrovascular events, and systemic emboli based on stored device data: a subgroup analysis of TRENDS. Heart Rhythm 2011;8:1417; with permission.)

defined as device-detected atrial arrhythmias lasting at least 5 minutes on any day of the study. NDAF was identified by the implantable device in 45 of 163 patients (28%) with a prior history of stroke/TIA over a mean follow-up of 1.1 years.[32] Of those patients who had NDAF, 58% of them had at least 1 day with NDAF that lasted more than 5.5 hours, a value shown in the main trial to increase risk of TE. The median time from enrollment in the study to identification of NDAF was 1.7 (interquartile range, 0.4–6.7) months among patients with a history of previous TE and 2.0

(interquartile range, 0.3–5.4) months among patients with no prior history of TE (*P* = .56).

In the ASSERT trial, NDAF (defined as lasting at least 6 minutes in duration) was detected at least once in patients with no prior history of AF in 34.7% of the patients over a mean follow-up of 2.5 years.[26] As stated above, only 10% of the patients (1/3 of those who ultimately developed NDAF) had the NDAF detected in the first 3 months of the study.

Taken together, these 2 large studies show remarkably similar results: in patients with CIEDs,

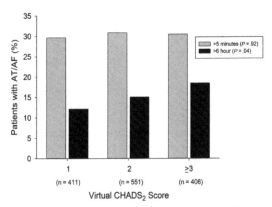

Fig. 7. TRENDS trial: Incidence of NDAF (>5 minutes) and days with greater than 6 hours of NDAF as a function of virtual CHADS$_2$ scores. (*From* Ziegler PD, Glotzer TV, Daoud EG, et al. Detection of previously undiagnosed atrial fibrillation in patients with stroke risk factors and usefulness of continuous monitoring in primary stroke prevention. Am J Cardiol 2012;110:1311; with permission.)

stroke risk factors, and no prior history of AF (regardless of TE history), NDAF is identified in approximately 30% of patients. Future studies are required to determine if the benefits of oral anticoagulation (OAC) outweigh the risks of bleeding in this patient population. In patients with CHADS$_2$ scores ≥ 2 and NDAF, OAC may be indicated for stroke prevention.

PART 5: THE FUTURE

Several current studies have been designed to answer the question: "Can outcomes be improved by continuously, remotely monitoring episodes of AF detected by modern implanted devices, and adjusting treatment according to the monitoring results?" IMPACT was a multicenter randomized trial of remote surveillance in patients who had implanted ICD and cardiac resynchronization therapy-defibrillator devices.[33] A combination of AF duration and CHADS$_2$ score was used to determine thresholds for initiation and discontinuation of anticoagulation therapy. An analysis of 75% of the events resulted in premature termination of the study due to futility.

TACTIC-AF (Tailored Anticoagulation for non-Continuous AF; clincaltrials.gov identifier NCT01650298) is a prospective, randomized, multicenter study of continuous remote monitoring in patients with CIEDs who are already on an NOAC, to determine if discontinuation of the NOAC, in patients with very low or no AF burden, can improve outcomes with regard to stroke and major bleeding.

The REACT.COM (Rhythm Evaluation for Anticoagulation with Continuous Monitoring) study (clincaltrials.gov identifier NCT01706146) is a 75-patient multicenter pilot study evaluating the feasibility of device-tailored anticoagulation using the Reveal XT device for continuous rhythm surveillance.

These studies are important because they will address whether it is safe to discontinue OAC in high-risk patients who have been free of AT/AF episodes for prolonged periods of time. One could infer that if AF is temporally responsible for increased stroke risk, these studies should prove positive. However, if AF is merely a marker for increased risk of stroke, it may not be prudent to discontinue OAC at any time following diagnosis of the arrhythmia in patients with concomitant stroke risk factors, and these studies may have negative results.

In the area of primary stroke prevention, the REVEAL AF[34] and ASSERT II[35] trials are being conducted to explore the incidence of NDAF in patients at high risk of stroke (with high virtual CHADS$_2$ scores) using ICMs. The studies do not mandate interventions when AF is detected by the implanted monitor, and REVEAL AF will examine actions physicians take in the face of AF detected by the device. These primary prevention studies offer the possibility of providing a new view into the temporal relationship between AF and stroke in the broader population of "at-risk" patients.

LIMITATIONS

All of the studies presented in this review have limitations that must be taken into consideration when using the results to make therapeutic recommendations for patients. The main limitation is that most of the studies had unexpectedly low stroke rates.[19,22,25,26] Because of the low overall stroke rates and the requirement to preserve statistical significance, more precise evaluation of multiple AT/AF burden cut points could not be performed in most studies. In addition, endpoints used in the trials were not consistent: some reported stroke, some included TIAs, and some included peripheral embolism. Second, even in the studies where strokes were adjudicated, it cannot be certain all strokes were embolic in origin because some may have been lacunar infarcts or emboli from the vasculature and not the atrium. Third, although it is generally accepted that device-detected AF episodes have greater than 95% sensitivity and specificity for being true AF,[11] not all AHREs discussed in these studies were adjudicated. Finally, although use of OACs is accounted for in regression models, international normalized ratio values were not systematically recorded.

SUMMARY

It is well established that the presence of AF is associated with an almost 5-fold increased risk of stroke.[36] However, the precise role AF plays in increasing the risk of stroke is less well understood, and this is especially true for the implanted device population. Is AF merely a marker for other disease processes that predispose a patient to an increased risk of stroke, or does a patient's risk of stroke increase primarily during, and shortly following, the occurrence of AF?

The major studies regarding the TE risk of device-detected AHREs are summarized in **Table 1**.[37] All of these studies show increases in stroke rate associated with device-detected AF episodes. As previously discussed, current CIEDs have a very high sensitivity and specificity for true AF detection. A minimum of 5 minutes of AF was found to have clinical relevance first in 2003. Alternative burden cut points have been explored over the last 10 years, ranging from 5 minutes to 24 hours, coming back full circle to the clinical significance of 6 minutes of AHRE burden in 2012. It does not seem to matter if the AF episode is proximal to the stroke event, and risk seems to be increased by relatively brief AF episodes. What does seem to be consistent is the finding that the appearance of new AHREs increases TE event rates. AHREs occur in about 50% of unselected patients with pacemakers[18,38] and NDAF occurs in approximately 30% of patients with CIEDs, stroke risk factors, and no prior history of AF.[26,31,32]

Perhaps it will be learned in the future that device-detected AF is not directly causative of the TE events, but rather these brief, silent episodes are simply markers of increased TE risk. Perhaps the finding of device-detected AF will be one more risk factor to add to a $CHADS_2$ score or CHA_2DS_2-VASc score to make a determination of the risk-benefit ratio of OAC therapy. Ongoing studies will shed more light on these dilemmas. Until larger trials or registries are conducted, it is important to follow established guidelines regarding anticoagulation.

REFERENCES

1. Page RL, Wilkinson WE, Clair WK, et al. Asymptomatic arrhythmias in patients with symptomatic paroxysmal atrial fibrillation and paroxysmal supraventricular tachycardia. Circulation 1994;89:224–7.
2. Strickberger SA, Ip J, Saksena S, et al. Relationship between atrial tachyarrhythmias and symptoms. Heart Rhythm 2005;2:125–31.
3. Quirino G, Giammaria M, Corbucci G, et al. Diagnosis of paroxysmal atrial fibrillation in patients with implanted pacemakers: relationship to symptoms and other variables. Pacing Clin Electrophysiol 2009;32:91–8.
4. Orlov MV, Ghali JK, Araghi-Niknam M, et al. Asymptomatic atrial fibrillation in pacemaker recipients: incidence, progression, and determinants based on the Atrial High Rate Trial. Pacing Clin Electrophysiol 2007;30:404–11.
5. Israel CW. Analysis of mode switching algorithms in dual chamber pacemakers. Pacing Clin Electrophysiol 2002;25:380–93.
6. Passman RS, Weinberg KM, Freher M, et al. Accuracy of mode switch algorithms for detection of atrial tachyarrhythmias. J Cardiovasc Electrophysiol 2004; 15:773–7.
7. de Voogt WG, van Hemel NM, van de Bos AA, et al. Verification of pacemaker automatic mode switching for the detection of atrial fibrillation and atrial tachycardia with Holter recording. Europace 2006; 8:950–61.
8. Pakarinen S, Toivonen L. Performance of atrial tachyarrhythmia-sensing algorithms in dual-chamber pacing using a fixed long AV delay in patients with sinus node dysfunction. J Interv Card Electrophysiol 2012;35:207–13.
9. Kaufman ES, Israel CW, Nair GM, et al, ASSERT Steering Committee and Investigators. Positive predictive value of device-detected atrial high-rate episodes at different rates and durations: an analysis from ASSERT. Heart Rhythm 2012;9: 1241–6.
10. Pollak WM, Simmons JD, Interian A Jr, et al. Clinical utility of intra-atrial pacemaker stored electrograms to diagnose atrial fibrillation and flutter. Pacing Clin Electrophysiol 2001;24:424–9.
11. Purerfellner H, Gillis AM, Holbrook R, et al. Accuracy of atrial tachyarrhythmia detection in implantable devices with arrhythmia therapies. Pacing Clin Electrophysiol 2004;27:983–92.
12. Swerdlow CD, Schoels W, Dijkman B, et al. Detection of atrial fibrillation and flutter by a dual-chamber implantable cardioverter-defibrillator. Circulation 2000;101: 878–85.
13. Ziegler PD, Curwin JH, Kremers MS, et al. Accuracy of atrial fibrillation detection in implantable pacemakers. Heart Rhythm 2013;10:S147.
14. Sarkar S, Ritscher D, Mehra R. A detector for a chronic implantable atrial tachyarrhythmia monitor. IEEE Trans Biomed Eng 2008;55:1219–24.
15. Lian J, Wang L, Muessig D. A simple method to detect atrial fibrillation using RR intervals. Am J Cardiol 2011;107:1494–7.
16. Hindricks G, Pokushalov E, Urban L, et al, XPECT Trial Investigators. Performance of a new leadless implantable cardiac monitor in detecting and quantifying atrial fibrillation: results of the XPECT trial. Circ Arrhythm Electrophysiol 2010;3:141–7.

17. Verma A, Champagne J, Sapp J, et al. Discerning the incidence of symptomatic and asymptomatic episodes of atrial fibrillation before and after catheter ablation (DISCERN AF): a prospective, multicenter study. JAMA Intern Med 2013;173:149–56.

18. Glotzer TV, Hellkamp AS, Zimmerman J, et al. Atrial high rate episodes detected by pacemaker diagnostics predict death and stroke: report of the atrial diagnostics sub-study of MOST. Circulation 2003; 107:1614–9.

19. Capucci A, Santini M, Padeletti L, et al, Italian AT500 Registry Investigators. Monitored atrial fibrillation duration predicts arterial embolic events in patients suffering from bradycardia and atrial fibrillation implanted with antitachycardia pacemakers. J Am Coll Cardiol 2005;46:1913–20.

20. Glotzer TV, Daoud EG, Wyse DG, et al. Rationale and design of a prospective study of the clinical significance of atrial arrhythmias detected by implanted device diagnostics: TRENDS. J Interv Card Electrophysiol 2006;15:9–14.

21. Fuster V, Ryden LE, Asinger AW, et al. ACC/AHA/ESC guidelines for the management of patients with atrial fibrillation: executive summary. Circulation 2001;104:2118–50.

22. Glotzer TV, Daoud EG, Wyse DG, et al, TRENDS Investigators. The relationship between daily atrial tachyarrhythmia burden from implantable device diagnostics and stroke risk: the TRENDS study. Circ Arrhythm Electrophysiol 2009;2:474–80.

23. Botto GL, Padeletti L, Santini M, et al. Presence and duration of atrial fibrillation detected by continuous monitoring: crucial implications for the risk of thromboembolic events. J Cardiovasc Electrophysiol 2009;20:241–8.

24. Gage BF, Waterman AD, Shannon W, et al. Validation of clinical classification schemes for predicting stroke: results from the National Registry of Atrial Fibrillation. JAMA 2001;285:2864–70.

25. Shanmugam N, Boerdlein A, Proff J, et al. Detection of atrial high-rate events by continuous home monitoring: clinical significance in the heart failure-cardiac resynchronization therapy population. Europace 2012;14:230–7.

26. Healey JS, Connolly SJ, Gold MR, et al, ASSERT Investigators. Subclinical atrial fibrillation and the risk of stroke. N Engl J Med 2012;366:120–9.

27. Hohnloser SH, Capucci A, Fain E, et al. ASymptomatic atrial fibrillation and stroke evaluation in pacemaker patients and the atrial fibrillation reduction atrial pacing trial (ASSERT). Am Heart J 2006;152:442–7.

28. Daoud EG, Glotzer TV, Wyse DG, et al, TRENDS Investigators. Temporal relationship of atrial tachyarrhythmias, cerebrovascular events, and systemic emboli based on stored device data: a subgroup analysis of TRENDS. Heart Rhythm 2011;8:1416–23.

29. Hanke T, Charitos EI, Stierle U, et al. Twenty-four-hour Holter monitor follow-up does not provide accurate heart rhythm status after surgical atrial fibrillation ablation therapy. Up to 12 months experience with a novel permanently implantable heart rhythm monitor device. Circulation 2009;120(Suppl 11):S177–84.

30. Ziegler PD, Koehler JL, Mehra R. Comparison of continuous versus intermittent monitoring of atrial arrhythmias. Heart Rhythm 2006;3:1445–52.

31. Ziegler PD, Glotzer TV, Daoud EG, et al. Detection of previously undiagnosed atrial fibrillation in patients with stroke risk factors and usefulness of continuous monitoring in primary stroke prevention. Am J Cardiol 2012;110:1309–14.

32. Ziegler PD, Glotzer TV, Daoud EG, et al. Incidence of newly detected atrial arrhythmias via implantable devices in patients with a prior history of thromboembolic events. Stroke 2010;41:256–60.

33. Ip J, Waldo AL, Lip GY, et al. Multicenter randomized study of anticoagulation guided by remote rhythm monitoring in patients with implantable cardioverter-defibrillator and CRT-D devices: rationale, design, and clinical characteristics of the initially enrolled cohort. The IMPACT study. Am Heart J 2009;158: 364–70.

34. Reiffel J, Verma A, Halperin JL, et al. Rationale and design of Reveal AF: A prospective study of previously undiagnosed atrial fibrillation as documented by an insertable cardiac monitor in high risk patients. Am Heart J 2014;167:22–7.

35. Prevalence of sub-clinical atrial fibrillation using an implantable cardiac monitor (ASSERT-II). Available at: http://www.clinicaltrials.gov/ct2/show/NCT01694394. Accessed January 2, 2013.

36. Wolf PA, Abbott RD, Kannel WB. Atrial fibrillation as an independent risk factor for stroke: the Framingham study. Stroke 1991;22:983–8.

37. Glotzer TV, Zeigler PD. Silent AF as a stroke risk factor and anticoagulation indication. Can J Cardiol 2013;29:S14–23.

38. Healey JS, Martin JL, Duncan A, et al. Pacemaker-detected atrial fibrillation in patients with pacemakers: prevalence, predictors, and current use of oral anticoagulation. Can J Cardiol 2013;29: 224–8.

Newer Algorithms in Bradycardia Management

Daniel Sohinki, MD[a],*, Owen A. Obel, MD[a,b]

KEYWORDS

- Automated threshold testing • Right ventricular pacing • Pacemaker-mediated tachycardia
- Mode switching • Rate modulation • Remote monitoring • Atrioventricular search hysteresis

KEY POINTS

- Automated threshold testing algorithms have been shown to be effective in maintaining myocardial capture in the right ventricle and, more recently, in the right atrium and left ventricle.
- Atrioventricular search hysteresis algorithms and the managed ventricular pacing algorithm are aimed at the maximum reduction of unnecessary right ventricular pacing.
- Extension of the postventricular atrial refractory period (PVARP) remains the cornerstone of prevention and treatment of pacemaker-mediated tachycardia.
- Most rate-responsive permanent pacemaker systems in the United States are accelerometer based, although alternatives such as closed-loop stimulation and, to a lesser extent, minute ventilation both offer alternatives for patients in whom rate response is required but where there is no acceleration.
- Advances in arrhythmia storage and remote monitoring improve patient follow-up and allow tailoring of drug and device therapies on a day-to-day basis.

INTRODUCTION

Since the inception of cardiac pacing more than 50 years ago, use of permanent pacemakers (PPMs) has been steadily increasing. In the United States between 1993 and 2009, 2.9 million patients (mean age at implant 75.4 years) received PPMs, while the annual rate of PPM implantation increased by 55.6%. The majority (nearly 80%) of all new PPM implants in the United States are dual-chamber devices, irrespective of pacing indication.[1]

Significant improvements in PPM design and functionality have allowed for the development of an advanced set of algorithms aimed at allowing physicians to tailor device-based therapies for bradyarrhythmias. Modern PPMs more are able to respond in a dynamic fashion to fluctuations in patients' intrinsic rhythm, pacing, and sensing thresholds, and level of activity.

This review seeks to highlight newer device algorithms that serve to optimize PPM functionality, including those used in: (1) automated threshold testing; (2) the prevention of right ventricular (RV) pacing; (3) prevention and treatment of pacemaker-mediated tachycardia (PMT); (4) mode switching in response to atrial tachyarrhythmias; (5) methods of rate modulation in response to exercise; and (6) advances in arrhythmia storage and remote monitoring capability. There are other important newer algorithms that are not

Disclosures: D. Sohinki: None; O.A. Obel: Speaker for Medtronic (Minneapolis, MN), St. Jude Medical (St. Paul, MN), Biotronik (Berlin, Germany).
a Division of Internal Medicine, University of Texas Southwestern Medical Center, 5323 Harry Hines Boulevard, Dallas, TX 75390-9047, USA; b Division of Cardiology, Veterans Health Administration (VA) North Texas Healthcare System, 4500 South Lancaster Road, Dallas, TX 75216, USA
* Corresponding author. Internal Medicine, Parkland Health and Hospital System, 5201 Harry Hines Boulevard, Dallas, TX 75235.
E-mail address: daniel.sohinki@phhs.org

mentioned owing to space constraints. Where possible, generic terminology is used; however, where appropriate, specific manufacturers' algorithms are mentioned. This review largely addresses standard PPM function. However, many patients who have indications for an implantable cardioverter-defibrillator (ICD) or biventricular (BiV) device also have a bradycardia pacing indication, and this article is also relevant to these devices.[2]

AUTOMATED THRESHOLD TESTING

The threshold at which myocardial capture consistently occurs, changes with differing physiologic and pathologic conditions. In the first 90 days after lead insertion the threshold often rises, thereafter falling to a steady state, coinciding with resolution of local inflammation associated with lead implantation.[2,3] Subsequently, there is sometimes a later rise in threshold known as exit block.[4,5] Metabolic and electrolyte abnormalities, changes in autonomic tone, myocardial ischemia, and antiarrhythmic drugs may influence pacing threshold,[5,6] and necessitate a means by which the PPM can optimize its pacing output to reliably capture myocardium while preserving battery life.[7,8]

Automated threshold testing (ATT) algorithms involve the use of a closed-loop feedback system allowing for dynamic assessment of pacing threshold and adjustment of pacing output. Most RV lead algorithms function by periodically affecting a stepwise reduction in voltage until loss of the evoked response (ER) is detected. When this occurs, a backup pulse is delivered to avoid a prolonged pause in ventricular pacing, following which the output is increased to factor in a safety margin of approximately 2 to 3 times the measured threshold.

Device companies vary with respect to voltage and pulse-width of the backup pulse, the frequency that threshold testing occurs, and functionality in single-chamber versus dual-chamber devices. For example, Medtronic's (MDT; Minneapolis, MN) and Boston Scientific (BOS; Natick, MA) PPMs deliver a programmable backup pulse after each pacing pulse during threshold testing, whereas St Jude (SJM; St Paul, MN) PPMs deliver a backup pulse only in the event of noncapture.[9]

Until recently ATT in the atrium has been challenging, owing to the small ER.[10] Several newer algorithms have been developed to address this issue. MDT's Atrial Capture Management (ACM) algorithm does not involve ER testing, but rather determines the patient's intrinsic rhythm, and analyzes the response to a pacing stimulus in 1 of 2 potential ways depending on whether the patient has intrinsic atrially sensed (As) or atrially paced (Ap) rhythm. In As rhythm, atrial chamber reset (ACR) is activated, which functions on the assumption that a captured atrial test pace will reset the sinus node (and thus will not be followed by a sensed intrinsic event), whereas a noncapturing test pace will not reset atrial rate. After the atrium is paced for 5 beats at normal settings, voltage is decreased until loss of capture (LOC) occurs. Conversely, if the rhythm is Ap, the Atrioventricular Conduction (AVC) algorithm is activated. Once a stable Ap-V-sense (Vs) pattern is established the device delivers an premature test Ap followed by a higher-output backup Ap 70 milliseconds later, and 2 ventricular sensing windows are set up. If the test pace captures the atrium, the conducted Vs event will occur during the earlier window, and capture is confirmed. If the test pace does not capture atrium, the Vs event will later occur in the second window in response to the backup pulse (**Fig. 1**).[11,12] AVC requires intact atrioventricular (AV) conduction whereas ACR requires As rhythm and, therefore, ACM cannot operate for patients who both require atrial pacing and do not have intact AV conduction. SJM's "A cap confirm" senses an atrial ER by comparing the morphology of the ER with a LOC morphology template. The algorithm first determines whether this morphology comparison is

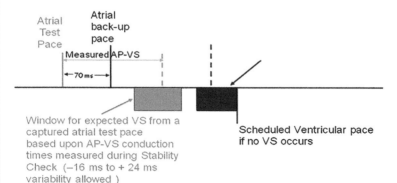

Atrial Test Pace

Atrial back-up pace

Measured AP-VS

←70 ms→

Window for expected VS from a captured atrial test pace based upon AP-VS conduction times measured during Stability Check (−16 ms to + 24 ms variability allowed)

Scheduled Ventricular pace if no VS occurs

Fig. 1. Function of Medtronic atrial capture management. Two windows are dynamically defined, the first for detection of a ventricular event in response to an atrial test pace, the second for detection of a ventricular event in response to a backup atrial pace. AP, atrial pace event; VS, ventricular sense event. (*Courtesy of* Medtronic, Langhorne, PA.)

possible (94% of cases). Once the device determines a threshold, an additional safety margin is added to ensure consistent capture.[13]

BiV PPMs also raise the possibility of left ventricular (LV) automatic threshold testing. MDT has developed LV capture management, which involves 3 stages: (1) a stability check monitors 12 cycles to ensure a stable rhythm; (2) conduction testing, whereby the LVp-RVs and Ap-to-RVs intervals are measured so that the two can be distinguished; (3) the LV pacing threshold search delivers a series of test paces from the LV lead over a range of pulse widths. The capture-detection window on the RV channel is initiated for 30 milliseconds before and 20 milliseconds after the longest LV-RV conduction time measured during conduction testing, and if RV sense occurs during this window, LV capture is confirmed.[14] Once the threshold has been determined, the device sets device output, with an added safety margin (**Fig. 2**).[15,16]

ALGORITHMS AIMED AT AVOIDING RV PACING

Recent data have shown that excessive RV pacing can be physiologically and clinically detrimental as a result of asynchronous LV activation and iatrogenic left bundle branch block (LBBB). Unwanted effects include an increase in heart failure (HF)-related hospitalizations, reduced LV ejection fraction (EF), increased electrical and mechanical interventricular dyssynchrony, and an increased risk of atrial fibrillation (AF).[17] Other studies have shown alterations in myocardial perfusion and workload, ventricular size and geometry, and increasing degrees of mitral regurgitation as a result of RV pacing.[18–21]

Therefore, several algorithms aimed at the avoidance of unnecessary RV pacing have been developed. The most widely used algorithm is AV search hysteresis (AVSH), which periodically and incrementally extends the AV delay to a programmed maximum from the baseline, searching for intrinsic AV conduction. If intrinsic conduction is not found, the device returns to the baseline programmed AV delay. If intrinsic conduction is detected, the AV delay is left at the value at which intrinsic conduction occurred, and the device monitors for ventricular pacing. SJM's Ventricular Intrinsic Preference (VIP) and BOS's AV Search+ function in this way, although they differ with respect to interval between searches and number of cycles allowed at the prolonged AV delay (**Fig. 3A**).

AVSH offers the advantage of a prespecified defined maximum AV delay, which allows the avoidance of nonphysiologic AV delays but is limited by not being able to distinguish fusion or pseudofusion (which are preferable to pure RV pacing) from full RV capture, and in such cases will revert to a shorter AV delay and resultant pure RV pacing. In addition, patients with intermittent AV block may experience an inappropriately high percentage of RV pacing, although newer algorithms can now be programmed

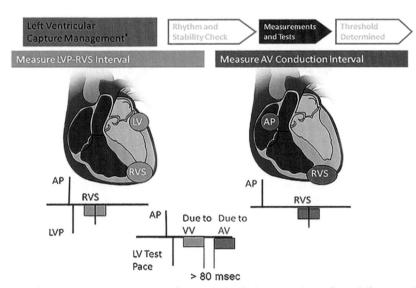

Fig. 2. Left-ventricular capture management. Left ventricular (LV) capture is confirmed if a sensed right ventricular (RV) event occurs in the capture detection window after the test pace. The length of the detection window is determined by conduction times measured during LV-RV conduction testing. AP, atrial pace; LVP, left ventricular pace; RVS, right ventricular sense. (*Courtesy of* Medtronic, Langhorne, PA.)

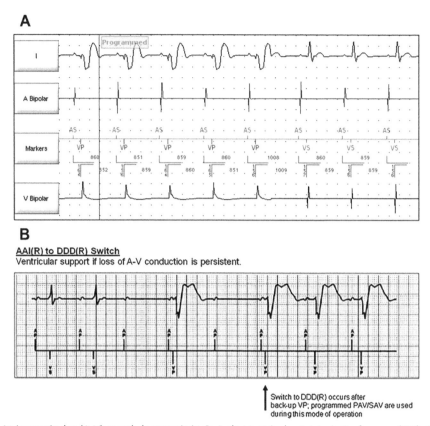

Fig. 3. (*A*) Atrioventricular (A-V) search hysteresis in St Jude Ventricular Intrinsic Preference (VIP). These traces show expiration of VIP's search timer, causing extension of the AV delay and subsequent R-wave sensing. (*B*) AAI(R) to DDD(R) mode switch in Medtronic Managed Ventricular Pacing (MVP) algorithm. A mode switch occurs if 2 of the last 4 atrial events have no corresponding sensed ventricular event. The device continuously checks for restoration of AV conduction to return to atrial tracking mode. AS, atrial sense; PAV, paced AV delay; SAV, sensed AV delay; VP, ventricular pace; VS, ventricular sense. (*Courtesy of* [*A*] St. Jude Medical, St. Paul, MN; with permission; and [*B*] Medtronic, Langhorne, PA.)

to wait for consistent loss of AV conduction over consecutive atrial cycles before returning from the extended to the basic AV-delay settings.[22–25]

MDT's Managed Ventricular Pacing (MVP) offers a different method for maximizing intrinsic conduction that was, until recently, the only algorithm of its kind. As opposed to AVSH, MVP includes a mode switch. At baseline, only the atrium is paced and the device is in AAI mode (although because ventricular activity is still being sensed, the mode is best described as ADI). If an atrial event (sensed or paced) does not conduct to the ventricle (ie, there are 2 consecutive atrial events without a Vs event), a backup V pace (Vp) is delivered. Following this, if any of the following 5 A-A intervals do not have an intervening Vs event, the device mode switches to DDD. When in DDD mode, the algorithm checks for intrinsic conduction by allowing for intrinsic conduction (in which case AAI will resume) at 4 minutes, then 8 minutes, constantly doubling the check time until 16 hours has been reached, and thence every 16 hours.[26] The MVP algorithm is effective in reducing the percentage of RV pacing.[26–28] In one study comparing MVP with AVSH, the MVP group had 16.4% RV pacing compared with 91.9% of patients with AVSH, over a 1-month period.[28] In the SAVE PACe study, patients with MVP had 9.1% RV pacing compared with 99.0% in a conventional arm. In addition, patients with devices using MVP had a significant reduction in AF.[29,30] Just as with AVSH, MVP may result in nonphysiologic AV-delay settings. In addition, some patients are highly sensitive to the ventricular pauses inherently associated with this algorithm, and MVP has been shown to have the potential to result in ventricular arrhythmias caused by abrupt changes in ventricular cycle length (see **Fig. 3**B).[30,31]

PACEMAKER-MEDIATED TACHYCARDIA: PREVENTION AND INTERVENTION

PMT refers to any situation whereby the device paces the heart inappropriately fast, and has several variants. Classic PMT is a device-dependent, endless-loop tachycardia in DDD mode whereby paced ventricular impulses conduct retrogradely through the AV node, resulting in atrial depolarizations that are tracked to the ventricle.[32] Classic PMT initiates after a premature ventricular complex (PVC) with retrograde conduction, although atrial LOC or undersensing may also act as triggers.[33,34] A key requirement for PMT is intact V-A conduction, which may be even present in the presence of antegrade AV block.[34,35] Classic PMT also requires that the retrograde atrial sensed event (As) is sensed after the postventricular atrial refractory period (PVARP), to trigger V pacing. Because the upper tracking rate (UTR) cannot be violated, most PMTs occur near the UTR.

The most commonly used algorithm for PMT prevention is automatic extension of the PVARP following a PVC (defined as a Vs event without a preceding atrial event). If V-A conduction occurs as a result of the PVC, this will likely occur in the extended PVARP.[36] In SJM's "A-pace on PVC," the device searches for atrial activity in the extended PVARP. If sensed the PVARP is terminated, and a paced atrial beat is delivered 330 milliseconds thereafter to avoid atrial noncapture, which can cause reinitiation of PMT.

If PMT does occur, the PPM must first detect and then attempt to terminate the arrhythmia (by PVARP extension). In MDT's PMT Termination, PMT is detected when the device records 8 consecutive Vp-As events with a V-A interval of less than 400 milliseconds. On the ninth beat, the PVARP is extended and PMT intervention is then disabled for 90 seconds, preventing unnecessary intervention in the event of an intrinsic fast atrial rate. SJM's method of PMT intervention begins once 10 consecutive As-Vp events occur faster than a programmable PMT detection rate, and the PVARP is extended for 1 beat. SJM devices also use an algorithm known as auto-detect to distinguish fast atrial rhythms from PMT. When the intrinsic atrial rate is greater than the PMT detection rate, the Vp-As interval is averaged over 8 cycles. If each individual interval is within 16 milliseconds of the average interval, the rhythm is assumed to be PMT (**Fig. 4**).

MODE-SWITCH ALGORITHMS

Dual-chamber PPMs programmed to DDD mode have the capacity to track pathologic atrial arrhythmias (ATA) and inappropriately pace the ventricle at the UTR. Mode-switching algorithms (MSA) reprogram the PPM from a tracking (DDD) to a nontracking mode, thus avoiding rapid pacing in response to ATAs. Optimal mode switching requires: (1) rapid detection of ATAs with the highest possible sensitivity and specificity; (2) avoiding a sudden rate change at mode switch; and (3) rapid and accurate mode-switch reversion to DDD mode. Details of the number and duration of mode-switch episodes are part of the interrogation report, and are often used as a surrogate for AF burden.[37]

As indicated, the MSA must first sense the onset of ATAs accurately. ATA detection algorithms are designed largely to account for the possibility of the intermittent atrial undersensing, which can

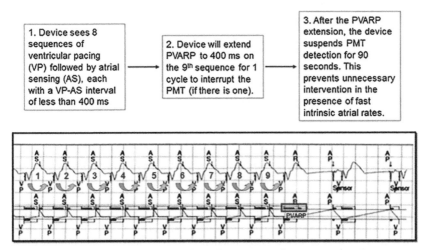

| 1. Device sees 8 sequences of ventricular pacing (VP) followed by atrial sensing (AS), each with a VP-AS interval of less than 400 ms | 2. Device will extend PVARP to 400 ms on the 9th sequence for 1 cycle to interrupt the PMT (if there is one). | 3. After the PVARP extension, the device suspends PMT detection for 90 seconds. This prevents unnecessary intervention in the presence of fast intrinsic atrial rates. |

Fig. 4. Function of Medtronic PMT Intervention algorithm. AP, atrial pace; AS, atrial sense; PMT, pacemaker-mediated tachycardia; PVARP, postventricular atrial refractory period; VP, ventricular pace. (*Courtesy of* Medtronic, Langhorne, PA.)

cause a delay in mode switch as well as inappropriate reversion back to DDD mode.[38,39] The potential effects of such errors include an erratic cardiac rhythm, battery drainage, and inaccurate estimation of AF burden. Detection algorithms for ATA vary between the different device companies. For example, most current MDT devices use a probabilistic counter within a sliding window, analogous to algorithms in ICDs for the detection of ventricular fibrillation. ATA is declared when "x of y" A-A intervals fall below the ATA-detection cycle length. In addition to using a probabilistic counter, Biotronik's (BTK; Berlin, Germany) algorithm has an additional option, automatic mode conversion, whereby mode switching occurs when the A-A interval falls below the atrial refractory period. Selected MDT dual-chamber PPMs (those based on ICD platforms) are also equipped to use an "AF evidence counter," which "advances by 1" if 2 or more atrial sensed events fall without an intervening V-V interval, and "decrements by 1" when atrial signals are sensed within the V-V interval.[39] SJM's mode switch is activated when atrial rate, defined through a continuously updated average, the filtered atrial rate interval (FARI), surpasses an atrial tachycardia detection rate (ADTR). The use of the FARI as opposed to the detected A-A interval allows the PPM to distinguish between sustained and nonsustained ATAs.[40,41]

Atrial flutter conducted 2:1 may be underdetected by MSAs if one of the flutter beats falls within the postventricular atrial blanking period (PVAB). To circumvent this, MDT PPMs use a "blanked flutter search," which examines atrial cycle length to detect if it is: (1) less than 2 times functional the atrial blanking period (sum of the AV interval and PVAB); and (2) less than or equal to 2 times the mode-switch detection interval for 8 consecutive cycles. If these criteria are fulfilled, the PVARP is extended for 1 cycle, allowing the device to scan the blanking period for an A-A interval below the detect rate, and effect a mode switch (**Fig. 5**).[39,42]

MSAs cause a device to revert from a tracking mode (DDD) to one of a variety of nontracking modes including VVI, DDI, or VDI (with or without rate response), depending on the device. Although device companies vary with regard to which nontracking mode becomes active, the net result is the same, namely, demand ventricular pacing. MSAs usually takes at least a few seconds (depending on the MSA) to change from DDD mode, during which time the ATA will track ventricular pacing close to the UTR. After reversion to the nontracking mode, there is significant potential for precipitous rate drop, and several strategies have been developed to minimize this: (1) most devices have a mode-switch base rate, which is usually programmed higher than the lower rate in DDD mode; (2) BOS's recent PPMs include rate-smoothing at the time of mode switch, which enables a gradual rate reduction over several cardiac cycles; (3) the nontracking mode in MDT devices defaults to one that includes rate response (ie, DDIR), which will usually result in a faster rate and more dynamic heart-rate response.

When ATAs terminate, the device must effect an accurate and timely reversion to tracking mode. For example, in SJM PPMs, the devices change back to atrial tracking when the FARI falls below the maximum tracking rate (MTR). In MDT devices, atrial tracking resumes when 7 atrial cycles fall below the MTR, or when 5 atrial paces occur.[40]

RATE-RESPONSIVE PACING

To accommodate the physiologic demands imposed by physical activities ranging from

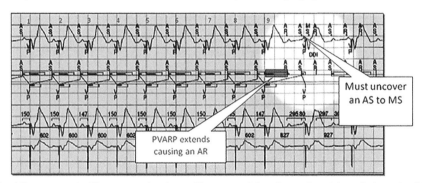

Fig. 5. Blanked flutter search. The pacemaker is tracking an atrial tachycardia with cycle length of 600 milliseconds, which is less than 660 milliseconds (twice the total atrial blanking period) and 686 milliseconds (twice the mode-switch detection interval). PVARP is extended after 8 cycles, making the normally tracked atrial sense refractory, and revealing an atrial sense that has been decreasing in pacemaker blanking period. The device then mode switches. AR, atrial refractory event; AS, atrial sense; MS, mode switch; PVARP, postventricular atrial refractory period. (*Courtesy of* Medtronic, Langhorne, PA.)

activities of daily living to vigorous exercise, heart rate in healthy patients varies by up to 3-fold from resting values.[43] Rate-responsiveness algorithms (RRA) in PPMs were therefore specifically developed to mimic the physiologic chronotropic response for patients such as those with significant sinus bradycardia (with or without AV block), or those in AF with high-degree AV block. Since the advent of rate-responsive PPMs, several reports have demonstrated their superior effect on increased exercise capacity and cardiac output in comparison with fixed-rate PPMs.[44,45] The letter R on the standard code indicates that rate response is active. A variety of physiologic and nonphysiologic parameters have been investigated to estimate heart-rate requirements for RRAs, including, but not limited to, oxygen saturation, venous pH, QT interval, central venous temperature, and vibration sensors. Nevertheless, only 3 methods have endured: (1) accelerometer; (2) minute ventilation; and (3) closed-loop stimulation (CLS).

The most widely used RRAs use an accelerometer coupled with a piezoelectric material. As the patient moves or accelerates, the coupling mass applies mechanical pressure to the piezoelectric material, producing a proportionate electric charge, which is translated into a heart-rate requirement.[46,47] Accelerometer-based systems have the advantage of being able to respond promptly to increased activity, but are limited in situations where acceleration does not occur and yet increased heart rate is required (eg, stationary bike, mental exertion, heart failure, and other physiologic stressors).

Certain PPMs (almost exclusively those made by BOS) have the capacity to estimate minute ventilation (MV), which is the product of tidal volume and respiratory rate, by measuring transthoracic impedance from a rapid, low-amplitude current impulse applied between the lead tip and pulse generator. Impedance varies proportionately with MV, which activates this RRA and is dependent on respiratory drive.[46,47] It should be noted that MV is always used in combination with an accelerometer (blended sensing) and therefore does not become active unless at least some acceleration takes place, and to that extent may be limited in certain situations.

CLS is available exclusively in BTK devices, and is an RRA that estimates cardiac sympathetic activation by measuring intracardiac impedance. It works on the valid assumption that patients with chronotropic incompetence have an intact sympathetic response to exercise in terms of enhanced cardiac contractility. During situations of high sympathetic tone contractility increases, causing increased cardiac ejection and an increase in intracardiac impedance. The opposite occurs during situations of reduced sympathetic tone. Thus CLS can act as an autoregulating algorithm, because once metabolic demands of stress are met, sympathetic tone responds by falling.[48] Several studies have illustrated the effectiveness of CLS in appropriately modulating pacing output in response to both physical and mental stress[49,50] for both patients in sinus rhythm and those with AF.[48] BTK devices offer the option of CLS as well as an accelerometer-based RRA.

All of the aforementioned RRAs have programmability, allowing PPM therapy to be tailored to the individual patient. Programmable features include maximum sensor-driven rate (SDR), threshold, slope, response time, and recovery time. Threshold refers to the amount of sensed exertion required to activate the system. Slope refers to the relationship between sensed exertion level and degree of heart-rate response. Response and recovery indicate the times required to get from baseline to sensor-indicated rate, and vice versa. SJM PPMs offer the option of using an "auto" setting, which measures activity level with the accelerometer over the preceding 18 hours to model appropriate threshold, slope, response, and recovery times.[48] In MDT systems, the device employs 2 separate rate-response profiles based on the assumption that most of the time, patients require chronotropic response for activities of daily living, for which there is a separate curve and SDR. A second exertion response is activated when more intense exertion is detected.

Programming of these features begins at the time of PPM implantation, often requiring optimization at follow-up, particularly when patients who require chronotropic support do not respond ideally to PPM therapy. Such follow-up includes careful history and PPM interrogation, and may include a hall-walk test or even a treadmill test. Some PPMs include algorithms whereby a practitioner chooses a simulated optimal rate profile after a patient performs a hall-walk or treadmill test. The PPM then suggests a proposed set of programmable values to achieve the rate optimal profile.

ARRHYTHMIA STORAGE AND REMOTE MONITORING

The basic utility of PPMs remains the treatment of bradyarrhythmias; however, PPMs also offer significant diagnostic capability. This ability enables PPMs to report important statistics such as arrhythmia occurrences; maximum, minimum, and mean heart rate; PVC burden; number of mode switches; percentage of pacing; and other metrics. Stored intracardiac electrograms (IE) from separate atrial and ventricular leads in dual-chamber and BiV PPM systems allow for the detailed analysis of individual tachyarrhythmia episodes with a high degree of accuracy.[51]

Storage capacity varies significantly between devices, ranging from less than 1 minute to more than 30 minutes in newer devices. The utility of stored atrial IEs allows the device to report atrial tachyarrhythmia (in particular AF) burden, and detailed information regarding ventricular rate burden during AF.[51,52] In the Vitatron Selection AFm Registry Study, investigators examined the impact of stored IE data on clinical decision making in patients with paroxysmal AF. Of 282 patients, 119 had 311 therapeutic interventions including alterations in rate and rhythm-controlling medications, use of anticoagulation, and PPM reprogramming, based on analysis of stored IE data.[53] Certain devices allow for the storage of IE data from before an arrhythmia episode begins (eg, MDT's "prearrhythmia" option). These data sometimes offer important information on arrhythmia onset, for example, AF driven by a simple trigger such as atrial tachycardia or AV nodal reentrant tachycardia. It should be noted that although such utility is potentially very useful, it imposes a significant burden on battery life in many PPMs. However, in SJM's most recent iteration of PPMs, IEs are stored using "on-chip RAM," which means that IE storage occurs via the hard drive and not the PPM battery, and pre-episode arrhythmia IE storage does not impose significant battery drain.

Remote monitoring of PPMs was previously performed exclusively via a technology known as transtelephonic monitoring (TTM), which gave limited information regarding battery status, sensing, intrinsic rhythm and, sometimes, information regarding thresholds. The recent introduction of remote monitoring over either cellular networks or land lines allows the PPM to transmit full interrogation data including details on heart rate and arrhythmia burden and relevant IEs, in addition to lead sensing, impedance, and automatic threshold data, battery longevity, and other data. Such transmissions can occur at scheduled times or on demand should patients have symptoms or concerns. Recent studies have demonstrated that home monitoring systems reduce the frequency of device clinic visits, and improve patient adherence to scheduled follow-up without compromising safety.[54–56] In a study using BTK's remote monitoring system, the mean interval between last follow-up and event recorded remotely was 26 days, which translated to physician notification occurring 154 days earlier than routine follow-up at 6 months.[57] Remote monitoring systems can be tailored to interact seamlessly with hospital-based electronic medical record systems.

SUMMARY

The utility of pacing systems continues to grow significantly. The unique ways in which these devices interact with a patient's intrinsic conduction system has necessitated the development of algorithms that can minimize the detrimental effects of pacing on a patient's heart, while maintaining and amplifying its benefits. Algorithms aimed at preventing RV pacing and PMT, and performing mode switching, have significantly decreased some of the morbidity associated with these devices. As PPM technology has advanced, device manufacturers have been able to further customize their devices to more closely mimic normal cardiac electrophysiology with rate-responsive pacing. The ability of PPMs to store and transmit information has allowed them to provide information to the clinician that can be used to guide diagnostic and treatment decisions.

REFERENCES

1. Greenspon AJ, Patel JD, Lau E, et al. Trends in permanent pacemaker implantation in the united states from 1993 to 2009: increasing complexity of patients and procedures. J Am Coll Cardiol 2012;60:1540–5.
2. Epstein AE, DiMarco JP, Ellenbogen KA, et al. ACC/AHA/HRS 2008 guidelines for device-based therapy of cardiac rhythm abnormalities: executive summary a report of the American College of Cardiology/American Heart Association Task Force on practice guidelines (Writing Committee to Revise the ACC/AHA/NASPE 2002 Guideline Update for implantation of cardiac pacemakers and Antiarrhythmia devices): developed in Collaboration with the American Association for Thoracic Surgery and Society of Thoracic Surgeons. Circulation 2008;117:2820–40.
3. Thalen HJ, Meere CC. Fundamentals of cardiac pacing. Hingham (MA): Martinus Nijhoff Publishers; 1979.
4. Sung RJ, Lauer MR. Fundamental approaches to the management of cardiac arrhythmias. Dordrecht (The Netherlands): Kluwer Academic Publishers; 2000.
5. Sambelashvili AT, Nikolski VP, Efimov IR. Virtual electrode theory explains pacing threshold increase caused by cardiac tissue damage. Am J Physiol Heart Circ Physiol 2004;286:H2183–94.
6. Timperley J, Leeson P, Mitchell A, et al. Pacemakers and ICDs. New York: Oxford University Press; 2008.

7. Preston TA, Fletcher RD, Lucchesi BR, et al. Changes in myocardial threshold. physiologic and pharmacologic factors in patients with implanted pacemakers. Am Heart J 1967;74:235–42.

8. Dohrmann ML, Goldschlager NF. Myocardial stimulation threshold in patients with cardiac pacemakers: effect of physiologic variables, pharmacologic agents, and lead electrodes. Cardiol Clin 1985;3:527–37.

9. Lau C, Siu C. Pacing technology: advances in pacing threshold management. J Zhejiang Univ Sci B 2010;11:634–8.

10. Gelvan D, Crystal E, Dokumaci B, et al. Effect of modern pacing algorithms on generator longevity. Pacing Clin Electrophysiol 2003;26:1796–802.

11. Kam R. Automatic capture verification in pacemakers (autocapture)-utility and problems. Indian Pacing Electrophysiol J 2004;4:73.

12. Rey JL, Quenum S, Hero M. Automatic assessment of atrial pacing threshold in current medical practice. Europace 2012;14:1615–9.

13. Sperzel J, Milasinovic G, Smith TW, et al. Automatic measurement of atrial pacing thresholds in dual-chamber pacemakers: clinical experience with atrial capture management. Heart Rhythm 2005;2:1203–10.

14. Biffi M, Sperzel J, Martignani C, et al. Evolution of pacing for bradycardia: autocapture. Eur Heart J Suppl 2007;9:I23–32.

15. Tsiperfal A, Ottoboni L, Beheiry S, et al. Cardiac arrhythmia management: a practical guide for nurses and allied professionals. Ames (IA): Wiley-Blackwell; 2011.

16. Crossley GH, Mead H, Kleckner K, et al. Automated left ventricular capture management. Pacing Clin Electrophysiol 2007;30:1190–200.

17. Albertsen AE, Mortensen PT, Jensen HK, et al. Adverse effect of right ventricular pacing prevented by biventricular pacing during long-term follow-up: a randomized comparison. Eur J Echocardiogr 2001;12:767–72.

18. Sweeney MO, Hellkamp AS, Ellenbogen KA, et al. Adverse effect of ventricular pacing on heart failure and atrial fibrillation among patients with normal baseline QRS duration in a clinical trial of pacemaker therapy for sinus node dysfunction. Circulation 2003;107:2932–7.

19. Leclercq C, Gras D, Le Helloco A, et al. Hemodynamic importance of preserving the normal sequence of ventricular activation in permanent cardiac pacing. Am Heart J 1995;129:1133–41.

20. Vanderheyden M, Coethals M, Ancuera I, et al. Hemodynamic deterioration following radiofrequency ablation of the atrioventricular conduction system. Pacing Clin Electrophysiol 1997;20:2422–8.

21. Kolb C, Schmidt R, Dietl JU, et al. Reduction of right ventricular pacing with advanced atrioventricular search hysteresis: results of the PREVENT study. Pacing Clin Electrophysiol 2011;34:975–83.

22. Melzer C, Sowelam S, Sheldon TJ, et al. Reduction of right ventricular pacing in patients with sinus node dysfunction using an enhanced search AV algorithm. Pacing Clin Electrophysiol 2005;28:521–7.

23. Olshansky B, Day J, McGuire M, et al. Reduction of right ventricular pacing in patients with Dual-Chamber ICDs. Pacing Clin Electrophysiol 2006;29:237–43.

24. Simantirakis EN, Arkolaki EG, Vardas PE. Novel pacing algorithms: do they represent a beneficial proposition for patients, physicians, and the health care system? Europace 2009;11:1272–80.

25. Pakarinen S, Toivonen L. Minimizing ventricular pacing by a novel atrioventricular (AV) delay hysteresis algorithm in patients with intact or compromised intrinsic AV conduction and different atrial and ventricular lead locations. Ann Med 2013;45(5–6):1–8.

26. Quesada A, Botto G, Erdogan A, et al. Managed ventricular pacing vs. conventional dual-chamber pacing for elective replacements: the PreFER MVP study: clinical background, rationale, and design. Europace 2008;10:321–6.

27. Murakami Y, Tsuboi N, Inden Y, et al. Difference in percentage of ventricular pacing between two algorithms for minimizing ventricular pacing: results of the IDEAL RVP (Identify the Best Algorithm for Reducing Unnecessary Right Ventricular Pacing) study. Europace 2010;12:96–102.

28. Gillis AM, Puererfellner H, Israel CW, et al. Reducing unnecessary right ventricular pacing with the managed ventricular pacing mode in patients with sinus node disease and AV block. Pacing Clin Electrophysiol 2006;29:697–705.

29. Sweeney MO, Bank AJ, Nsah E, et al. Minimizing ventricular pacing to reduce atrial fibrillation in sinus-node disease. N Engl J Med 2007;357:1000–8.

30. Vavasis C, Slotwiner DJ, Goldner BG, et al. Frequent recurrent polymorphic ventricular tachycardia during sleep due to managed ventricular pacing. Pacing Clin Electrophysiol 2010;33:641–4.

31. Sweeney MO, Ruetz LL, Belk P, et al. Bradycardia pacing-induced short-long-short sequences at the onset of ventricular tachyarrhythmias: a possible mechanism of proarrhythmia? J Am Coll Cardiol 2007;50:614–22.

32. Ullah W, Stewart A. Pacemaker-mediated tachycardia. Heart 2010;96:1062.

33. Calfee RV. Pacemaker-mediated tachycardia: engineering solutions. Pacing Clin Electrophysiol 1988;11:1917–28.

34. Hayes DL, Levine PA. Pacemaker timing cycles. In: Ellenbogen KA, Wood M, editors. Cardiac pacing and ICDs. 4th edition. Malden (MA): Blackwell Publishing; 2002. p. 265–321.

35. Dulk K, Lindemans FW, Wellens HJ. Merits of various antipacemaker circus movement tachycardia features. Pacing Clin Electrophysiol 1986; 9:1055–62.

36. Lloyd MS, El Chami MF, Langberg JJ. Pacing features that mimic malfunction: a review of current programmable and automated device functions that cause confusion in the clinical setting. J Cardiovasc Electrophysiol 2009;20:453–60.

37. Israel CW. Analysis of mode switching algorithms in dual chamber pacemakers. Pacing Clin Electrophysiol 2002;25:380–93.

38. Marshall H, Kay G, Hess M, et al. Mode switching in dual chamber pacemakers effect of onset criteria on arrhythmia-related symptoms. Europace 1999;1:49–54.

39. Goethals M, Timmermans W, Geelen P, et al. Mode switching failure during atrial flutter: the '2: 1 lock-in' phenomenon. Europace 2003;5:95–102.

40. Santomauro M, Duilio C, Riganti C, et al. Different automatic mode switching in DDDR pacemakers. In: Das MR, editor. Modern pacemakers—present and future. Rijeka (Croatia): InTech; 2011. p. 25–36.

41. de Voogt WG, van Hemel NM, van de Bos AA, et al. Verification of pacemaker automatic mode switching for the detection of atrial fibrillation and atrial tachycardia with Holter recording. Europace 2006;8:950–61.

42. Chang H, Huang H, Yeh K. Ventricular tachycardia triggered by blanked flutter search-mediated cycle length alternation. Europace 2011;13:875.

43. Furman S. Rate-modulated pacing. Circulation 1990;82:1081–94.

44. Candinas RA, Gloor HO, Amann FW, et al. Activity-sensing rate responsive versus conventional fixed-rate pacing: a comparison of rate behavior and patient well-being during routine daily exercise. Pacing Clin Electrophysiol 1991;14:204–13.

45. Greco E, Guardini S, Citelli L. Cardiac rehabilitation in patients with rate responsive pacemakers. Pacing Clin Electrophysiol 1998;21:568–75.

46. Kaszala K, Ellenbogen KA. Device sensing sensors and algorithms for pacemakers and implantable cardioverter defibrillators. Circulation 2010;122: 1328–40.

47. Lau C, Tse H, Camm AJ, et al. Evolution of pacing for bradycardias: sensors. Eur Heart J Suppl 2007; 9:I11–22.

48. Proietti R, Manzoni G, Di Biase L, et al. Closed loop stimulation is effective in improving heart rate and blood pressure response to mental stress: report of a single-chamber pacemaker study in patients with chronotropic incompetent atrial fibrillation. Pacing Clin Electrophysiol 2012;35:990–8.

49. Chandiramani S, Cohorn LC, Chandiramani S. Heart rate changes during acute mental stress with closed loop stimulation: report on two single-blinded, pacemaker studies. Pacing Clin Electrophysiol 2007;30:976–84.

50. Coenen M, Malinowski K, Spitzer W, et al. Closed loop stimulation and accelerometer-based rate adaptation: results of the PROVIDE study. Europace 2008;10:327–33.

51. Pollak WM, Simmons JD, Interian A, et al. Clinical utility of intraatrial pacemaker stored electrograms to diagnose atrial fibrillation and flutter. Pacing Clin Electrophysiol 2001;24:424–9.

52. Cabrera S, Mercé J, de Castro R, et al. Pacemaker clinic: an opportunity to detect silent atrial fibrillation and improve antithrombotic treatment. Europace 2011;13:1574–9.

53. Kim MH, Reiter MJ, Canby R, et al. The impact of stored atrial rhythm diagnostics in permanent pacemakers and the management of atrial fibrillation: the Vitatron Selection AFm Registry study. J Interv Card Electrophysiol 2010;28:227–34.

54. Brugada P. What evidence do we have to replace in-hospital implantable cardioverter defibrillator follow-up? Clin Res Cardiol 2006;95:iii3–9.

55. Heidbüchel H, Lioen P, Foulon S, et al. Potential role of remote monitoring for scheduled and unscheduled evaluations of patients with an implantable defibrillator. Europace 2008;10:351–7.

56. Burri H, Senouf D. Remote monitoring and follow-up of pacemakers and implantable cardioverter defibrillators. Europace 2009;11:701–9.

57. Nielsen JC, Kottkamp H, Zabel M, et al. Automatic home monitoring of implantable cardioverter defibrillators. Europace 2008;10:729–35.

Indications for Cardiac Resynchronization Therapy

Thomas M. O'Brien, MD, Edward J. Schloss, MD,
Eugene S. Chung, MD*

KEYWORDS

- Heart failure • Biventricular pacing • Cardiac resynchronization therapy • Dyssynchrony

KEY POINTS

- CRT indications are evolving.
- EF less than 35% remains a cornerstone of indication.
- LBBB and QRS greater than 150 ms appear important criteria for favorable response.
- EKG remains most important indicator of dyssynchrony.

PACING FOR HEART FAILURE

The concept of using pacing to treat heart failure (HF) symptoms predates the development of techniques for left ventricular (LV) pacing and cardiac resynchronization therapy (CRT). There was hope that dual-chamber pacing techniques would improve HF outcomes by optimizing heart rate, atrioventricular (AV) timing, and cardiac output. Noting the adverse hemodynamic consequences of VVI pacing, dual-chamber pacing algorithms were developed that mimicked the natural AV interval with changing heart rates. Small, uncontrolled studies in the early 1990s suggested benefit of standard right atrial and right ventricular (RV) DDD pacing in HF patients.[1–3] When subjected to a randomized controlled trial,[4] however, DDD pacing failed to confirm positive outcomes. The deleterious effects of RV pacing and attendant left bundle branch block (LBBB) only became fully appreciated with the reporting of the Dual Chamber and VVI Implantable Defibrillator (DAVID) trial in 2002.[5] DAVID enrolled 506 patients with LV ejection fraction (LVEF) less than or equal to 40%, randomized to VVI at 40 beats per minute (bpm) versus DDD pacing at 70 bpm, with death or HF hospitalization as the primary endpoint.

This trial showed that those in the DDD arm were approximately 40% more likely to achieve the primary endpoint compared with controls at 1 year. Data from the Mode Selection Trial in Sinus Node Dysfunction (MOST) highlighted the potential of RV pacing to cause HF; a substudy from MOST that demonstrated an RV pacing threshold of approximately 40% was identified as putting patients at 3-fold increased risk of HF hospitalization.[6] The presumed mechanism by which RV pacing led to an apparent increase in HF was the LBBB and resulting mechanical dyssynchrony. In the general HF population, approximately 30% of patients with systolic HF have wide QRS intervals, also correlated with adverse outcomes.[7,8] In mechanistic support of this association, intraventricular conduction delay has been linked to a wide array of hemodynamic derangements, including reduced pulse pressure, impaired diastolic function, and functional mitral regurgitation.[9]

Early attempts to address this clinical problem by performing biventricular pacing (CRT) in the 1990s showed improvements in acute hemodynamics and medium-term functional measures.[10,11] In 1996, Cazeau and colleagues[12] reported a series of 8 advanced HF patients with

Disclosures: E.S. Chung, consulting (Medtronic, Boston Scientific); E.J. Schloss, consulting (Medtronic, Boston Scientific); and T.M. O'Brien, none.
The Heart and Vascular Center, The Christ Hospital, 2139 Auburn Ave, Cincinnati, OH 45219, USA
* Corresponding author. 2123 Auburn Avenue, Suite 137, Cincinnati, OH 45219.
E-mail address: chunge@ohioheart.org

widened QRS intervals. All received atrial-triggered biventricular pacemakers. Four died in the perioperative period, but of the 4 who survived, HF class improved from IV to II. CHF worsened when pacing was deactivated. These and other favorable early experiences set the stage for large-scale CRT trials.

INITIAL INDICATIONS

Presented in 1999, and later published in 2002, the PATH-CHF trial investigated pacing in patients with advanced HF.[13] Enrolled patients had 2 pulse generators implanted, then randomized to either univentricular (LV) or biventricular pacing. Both modes of pacing demonstrated improved oxygen consumption parameters and exercise capacity.

In 2001, the MUSTIC study[14] reported a convincingly positive impact of CRT in 67 randomized patients with reduced LVEF (mean 23%), New York Heart Association (NYHA) class 3 HF, Left LV end-diastolic diameter (LVEDD) greater than 60 mm, and QRS greater than 150 ms. The mean distance walked in 6 minutes was 23% greater with active pacing, the quality-of-life score improved by 32%, peak oxygen uptake increased by 8%, and hospitalizations decreased by more than 60% (P<.05).

In the same year, results of the MIRACLE trial[15] were presented. It was the largest multicenter, prospective, randomized clinical trial to date, enrolling 453 patients with QRS greater than or equal to 130 ms, LVEF less than or equal to 35%, LVEDD greater than or equal to 55 mm, and NYHA class 3–4. Compared with controls, CRT improved functional class, 6-minute hall walk distance, maximum oxygen consumption, and quality of life. Improvement was seen in 67% of CRT patients versus 39% of controls. In the years afterwards, the CARE-HF[16] and COMPANION[17] trials showed a reduction in the primary composite endpoint (all-cause mortality or hospitalization for MACE) from CRT compared with standard medical therapy alone. A further meta-analysis reported approximately a 30% reduction in both hospitalization and mortality.[18] Based on these trials, guidelines incorporated CRT as a treatment option for those with LVEF less than or equal to 35%, QRS greater than or equal to 120 ms, and NYHA 3–4.

In the current era, 3 separate expert groups have generated guidelines for utilization of CRT, each synthesizing their interpretation of the aforementioned landmark trials, coupled with expert opinion. The American Heart Association together with the American College of Cardiology and the Heart Rhythm Society,[19] the Heart Failure Society of America,[20] and the European Society of Cardiology[21] have recently published relevant guidelines. Although there are a few distinctions among the guidelines, a vast majority of recommendations put forth are concordant. The initial indications for CRT have evolved to incorporate the degree of QRS prolongation, QRS morphology, presence of atrial fibrillation, and lower NYHA class to provide a more nuanced approach to patient selection. **Fig. 1** summarizes these adjustments and **Box 1** attempts to incorporate and simplify these recommendations into a more practical approach.

In the past few years, the guidelines have been updated in such a way as to improve patient selection according to their likelihood of improvement with CRT. These adjustments arose from evolving evidence that QRS duration greater than or equal to 150 ms and an LBBB pattern seem to correlate with the most favorable outcomes after CRT.[22] Attempts to further refine selection criteria beyond ECG evidence of electrical dyssynchrony have largely involved echocardiographic assessments of mechanical dyssynchrony.[23–25] The largest multicenter trial to test the hypothesis,

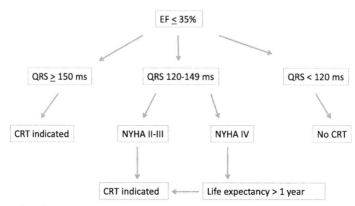

Fig. 1. Practical algorithm for CRT indication.

<table>
<tr><td>

Box 1
Summary of guidelines

Class I—LVEF ≤35%, LBBB with QRS ≥150 ms; NYHA class 2–4a

Class IIa—LVEF ≤35%, NYHA class 2–4a, plus 1 of the following:

　　LBBB with QRS 120–149 ms,

　　Non-LBBB with QRS ≥150, or

　　Ventricular pacing expected >40%

Class IIb—LVEF ≤35%, non-LBBB, plus 1 of the following:

　　QRS 120–149 ms with NYHA class 3–4a

　　QRS ≥150 ms with NYHA class 2

　　AFIB, QRS ≥120 ms with NYHA 2–3

Class IIb—LVEF ≤30%, LBBB with QRS ≥150 ms, NYHA class 1

</td></tr>
</table>

PROSPECT, however, did not identify any clinically useful predictors of a favorable response.[26] Therefore, patient selection criteria for CRT remain based on measurement of LV systolic function, QRS duration and morphology, and functional class.

EVOLUTION OF CRT

The rationale for CRT in the landmark clinical trial patients was based on selecting a patient population that had the highest likelihood of benefit from therapy. The distinctions drawn by NYHA and LVEF, however, are fairly arbitrary. Both NYHA class and LVEF can change frequently, and the same putative abnormality that underlies CRT in the clinical trial populations (ie, mechanical dyssynchrony) can exist in patients with lower NYHA and higher LVEF. This section reviews and summarizes the recent efforts to refine and extend the application of CRT.

Earlier Timing of CRT: REVERSE and MADIT-CRT

As discussed previously, initial indications for CRT based on landmark trials included patients with NYHA 3–4 functional status. The concept of earlier intervention in patients with NYHA 1–2 status and those who might have transiently improved to less than NYHA status 3 at time of evaluation, however, warranted further study. In this regard, the Resynchronization Reverses Remodeling in Systolic Left Ventricular Dysfunction (REVERSE)[27] study and Multicenter Automatic Implanted Defibrillator Trial with Cardiac Resynchronization

Therapy (MADIT-CRT)[28] were conducted. REVERSE evaluated 610 patients with NYHA 1–2 functional class, LVEF less than or equal to 40%, and QRS greater than or equal to 120 ms in a randomized, prospective, double-blinded study design. Although the primary endpoint of clinical composite score was not met ($P = .10$), there were benefits seen in echocardiographic and HF hospitalization parameters. The MADIT-CRT trial evaluated 1820 patients with LVEF less than or equal to 30%, QRS greater than or equal to 130 ms, and NYHA 1–2, with the primary endpoint of death or nonfatal HF event. There was a 36% reduction in the primary endpoint, largely driven by a large reduction in HF hospitalizations in those with QRS greater than 150 ms. The RAFT[29] trial studied 1798 patients with NYHA 2–3 HF symptoms, LVEF less than or equal to 30, and QRS greater than or equal to 120 ms and found a 27% relative reduction in death or HF hospitalization in the subgroup with NYHA functional class 2 on enrollment (n = 1438). Based on the results of these studies, guidelines have incorporated CRT for those with less severe NYHA functional status.

Narrow QRS Duration: EchoCRT

The QRS duration has been interpreted as a surrogate for LV mechanical dyssynchrony. Wider QRS duration is associated with worse outcomes in HF patients, and existing data suggest a positive relationship between wider baseline QRS and improvement after CRT.[16,28] There are, however, other measures of mechanical dyssynchrony in the imaging arena, particularly using echocardiography. Using direct assessment of LV mechanical properties, echocardiographic methods of measuring dyssynchrony have been used to establish the presence of dyssynchrony in some HF patients with narrow QRS duration (<120 ms).[30,31] Furthermore, single-center studies have shown the potential for symptomatic and structural improvement in HF patients with a narrow QRS.[32–34] Based on these data, the Cardiac Resynchronization Therapy in Patients with Heart Failure and Narrow QRS (RethinQ)[35] and the Echocardiography Guided Cardiac Resynchronization Therapy (EchoCRT)[36] trials have been conducted. RethinQ randomized 172 patients to CRT or control. Entry criteria were LVEF less than or equal to 35%, QRS less than or equal to 130 ms, NYHA 3 functional class, and evidence of mechanical dyssynchrony based on echocardiographic criteria (primarily tissue Doppler and few M-mode based). The primary endpoint was percentage of patients with at least 1 mg/kg/min improvement in peak oxygen consumption at 6 months. Although there was a signal for CRT benefit in the subgroup of patients with QRS greater than 120 to 130 ms, no benefit was seen in the overall group. The EchoCRT trial was a larger study of 809 patients with similar entry criteria to those of RethinQ (NYHA 3–4, QRS $\leq$130 ms, and LVEF $\leq$35%) but using more robust echocardiographic markers of dyssynchrony. Later-generation methods using speckle tracking or tissue Doppler measurements were performed on every potential patient by a central core laboratory, which determined study eligibility. The primary endpoint of all-cause death or HF-related hospitalization, however, was not different between the CRT and control groups, and there was a worrisome signal for increased mortality in the CRT group. Based on these studies, the concept of using more sensitive methods of detecting dyssynchrony to select patients for CRT in narrow QRS patients has proved ineffective. Therefore, a cornerstone of patient selection remains an increased QRS duration.

Higher LVEF: MIRACLE EF

The current indications for CRT include an LVEF less than or equal to 35%. Those with higher LVEF, however, may still manifest significant mechanical dyssynchrony whose treatment may improve HF status. Furthermore, there are preliminary[37] and post hoc[38] data to suggest that the benefit of CRT may not be limited to those with LVEF less than or equal to 35%. Fung and colleagues[37] showed that in 15 patients with HF symptoms, QRS greater than 130 ms, and LVEF between 35% and 45%, echocardiographic parameters and NYHA class improved significantly with CRT. In a subanalysis of the PROSPECT trial, those with a core laboratory measured LVEF greater than 35% were compared with those with LVEF less than 35%.[38] CRT effects on the clinical composite score and LV end-systolic volume were found similar between the 2 groups. In this light, the MIRACLE EF trial was conceived (clinicaltrials.gov: NCT01735916). With the primary endpoint of all-cause death or an HF urgent care event, patients with HF symptoms, LBBB with QRS duration greater than 130 ms, and LVEF between 36% and 50% will be randomized 2:1 to CRT versus control. As an event-driven trial, up to 2300 patients are expected to be enrolled.

AV Block Requiring Ventricular Pacing: BLOCK HF

In those patients who require ventricular pacing for AV block, data from DAVID and MOST have demonstrated a deleterious effect of RV pacing on LV function, with the presumed mechanism of mechanical dyssynchrony arising from the iatrogenic LBBB. In this setting, biventricular pacing rather than the traditional RV pacing may prevent the onset of HF detected in the DAVID and MOST populations. In this light, the BLOCK HF trial enrolled 691 patients with LVEF less than or equal to 50% and indication for ventricular pacing due to AV block, randomizing them to conventional RV pacing versus biventricular pacing. Biventricular pacing led to a significant 27% relative reduction in the primary endpoint of all cause death, HF urgent care event, or a greater than or equal to 15% reduction in LV end-systolic volume.[39] As of this writing, the expanded indication for biventricular pacing to include this population is under Food and Drug Administration regulatory assessment.

Post–Myocardial Infarction HF: PROMPT

After a large ST-elevated myocardial infarction (MI), the development of HF remains a significant concern.[40,41] The onset of HF post MI is heralded by progressive LV remodeling that occurs very early after an MI and continues for years despite optimal therapy.[42,43] Given the relationship between LV dilation and mortality in HF, LV remodeling is an attractive target for potential therapies. A potential application of biventricular pacing, in particular, the LV lead, is to place the pacing location near the infarct to pre-excite the vulnerable region and reduce the local stress and external work.[44,45] In the chronic setting, this therapy may lead to attenuation of the progressive LV remodeling that marks the natural history after a large MI. After an initial feasibility study (OPIS),[46] a pilot trial was performed to test the hypothesis (MENDMI).[47] Although the primary endpoint (echocardiography biplane LV end-diastolic volume at 1 year) was not met, there were signals of improvement in the 4 chamber volumes and LV wall motion. The PROMPT trial (clinicaltrials.gov: NCT01213251) was, therefore, designed to further test the hypothesis by enrolling patients with higher peak creatine kinase levels, receiving earlier device implantation (within 7 days of MI), longer follow-up (18 months), and larger enrollment target. Furthermore, one third of the patients will be control, another third treated with biventricular pacing, and the final third treated with LV pacing only. The study completed enrollment in October 2013 and is currently in the follow-up phase.

SUMMARY

CRT is firmly established as standard of care for a substantial portion of patients with HF. Current practice guidelines for patient selection have evolved from the initial landmark studies to further improve the chance of a favorable outcome. These guidelines are sure to change, however, as more data become available. The decision to apply CRT should be based on patients' clinical profile as well as the balance of risk tolerance and likelihood of benefit.

REFERENCES

1. Hochleitner M, Hortnagl H, Ng CK, et al. Usefulness of physiologic dual-chamber pacing in drug-resistant idiopathic dilated cardiomyopathy. Am J Cardiol 1990;66(2):198–202.

2. Hochleitner M, Hortnagl H, Hortnagl H, et al. Long-term efficacy of physiologic dual-chamber pacing in the treatment of end-stage idiopathic dilated cardiomyopathy. Am J Cardiol 1992;70(15):1320–5.

3. Auricchio A, Sommariva L, Salo RW, et al. Improvement of cardiac function in patients with severe congestive heart failure and coronary artery disease by dual chamber pacing with shortened AV delay. Pacing Clin Electrophysiol 1993;16(10):2034–43.

4. Gold MR, Feliciano Z, Gottlieb SS, et al. Dual-chamber pacing with a short atrioventricular delay in congestive heart failure: a randomized study. J Am Coll Cardiol 1995;26(4):967–73.

5. Wilkoff BL, Cook JR, Epstein AE, et al. Dual-chamber pacing or ventricular backup pacing in patients with an implantable defibrillator: the Dual Chamber and VVI Implantable Defibrillator (DAVID) Trial. JAMA 2002;288(24):3115–23.

6. Sweeney MO, Hellkamp AS, Ellenbogen KA, et al. Adverse effect of ventricular pacing on heart failure and atrial fibrillation among patients with normal baseline QRS duration in a clinical trial of pacemaker therapy for sinus node dysfunction. Circulation 2003;107(23):2932–7.

7. Aaronson KD, Schwartz JS, Chen TM, et al. Development and prospective validation of a clinical index to predict survival in ambulatory patients referred for cardiac transplant evaluation. Circulation 1997; 95(12):2660–7.

8. Baldasseroni S, Opasich C, Gorini M, et al. Left bundle-branch block is associated with increased 1-year sudden and total mortality rate in 5517 outpatients with congestive heart failure: a report from the Italian network on congestive heart failure. Am Heart J 2002;143(3):398–405.

9. Stellbrink C, Nowak B. The importance of being synchronous: on the prognostic value of ventricular conduction delay in heart failure. J Am Coll Cardiol 2002;40(11):2031–3.

10. Foster AH, Gold MR, McLaughlin JS. Acute hemodynamic effects of atrio-biventricular pacing in humans. Ann Thorac Surg 1995;59(2):294–300.

11. Leclercq C, Cazeau S, Le Breton H, et al. Acute hemodynamic effects of biventricular DDD pacing in patients with end-stage heart failure. J Am Coll Cardiol 1998;32(7):1825–31.

12. Cazeau S, Ritter P, Lazarus A, et al. Multisite pacing for end-stage heart failure: early experience. Pacing Clin Electrophysiol 1996;19(11 Pt 2):1748–57.

13. Auricchio A, Stellbrink C, Sack S, et al. Long-term clinical effect of hemodynamically optimized cardiac resynchronization therapy in patients with heart failure and ventricular conduction delay. J Am Coll Cardiol 2002;39(12):2026–33.

14. Cazeau S, Leclercq C, Lavergne T, et al. Effects of multisite biventricular pacing in patients with heart failure and intraventricular conduction delay. N Engl J Med 2001;344(12):873–80.

15. Abraham WT, Fisher WG, Smith AL, et al. Cardiac resynchronization in chronic heart failure. N Engl J Med 2002;346(24):1845–53.

16. Cleland JG, Daubert JC, Erdmann E, et al. The effect of cardiac resynchronization on morbidity and mortality in heart failure. N Engl J Med 2005;352(15): 1539–49.

17. Bristow MR, Saxon LA, Boehmer J, et al. Cardiac-resynchronization therapy with or without an implantable defibrillator in advanced chronic heart failure. N Engl J Med 2004;350(21):2140–50.

18. Stellbrink C, Breithardt OA, Franke A, et al. Impact of cardiac resynchronization therapy using hemodynamically optimized pacing on left ventricular remodeling in patients with congestive heart failure and ventricular conduction disturbances. J Am Coll Cardiol 2001;38(7):1957–65.

19. Writing Group M, Tracy CM, Epstein AE, et al. 2012 ACCF/AHA/HRS focused update of the 2008 guidelines for device-based therapy of cardiac rhythm abnormalities: a report of the American College of Cardiology Foundation/American Heart Association Task Force on Practice Guidelines. J Thorac Cardiovasc Surg 2012;144(6):e127–45.

20. Stevenson WG, Hernandez AF, Carson PE, et al. Indications for cardiac resynchronization therapy: 2011 update from the Heart Failure Society of America Guideline Committee. J Card Fail 2012;18(2): 94–106.

21. Brignole M, Auricchio A, Baron-Esquivias G, et al. 2013 ESC Guidelines on cardiac pacing and cardiac resynchronization therapy: the Task Force on cardiac pacing and resynchronization therapy of the European Society of Cardiology (ESC). Developed in collaboration with the European Heart Rhythm Association (EHRA). Eur Heart J 2013; 34(29):2281–329.

22. Stavrakis S, Lazzara R, Thadani U. The benefit of cardiac resynchronization therapy and QRS duration: a meta-analysis. J Cardiovasc Electrophysiol 2012;23(2):163–8.

23. Yu CM, Fung WH, Lin H, et al. Predictors of left ventricular reverse remodeling after cardiac resynchronization therapy for heart failure secondary to idiopathic dilated or ischemic cardiomyopathy. Am J Cardiol 2003;91(6):684–8.

24. Bax JJ, Marwick TH, Molhoek SG, et al. Left ventricular dyssynchrony predicts benefit of cardiac resynchronization therapy in patients with end-stage heart failure before pacemaker implantation. Am J Cardiol 2003;92(10):1238–40.

25. Pitzalis MV, Iacoviello M, Romito R, et al. Cardiac resynchronization therapy tailored by echocardiographic evaluation of ventricular asynchrony. J Am Coll Cardiol 2002;40(9):1615–22.

26. Chung ES, Leon AR, Tavazzi L, et al. Results of the Predictors of Response to CRT (PROSPECT) trial. Circulation 2008;117(20):2608–16.

27. Linde C, Abraham WT, Gold MR, et al. Randomized trial of cardiac resynchronization in mildly symptomatic heart failure patients and in asymptomatic patients with left ventricular dysfunction and previous heart failure symptoms. J Am Coll Cardiol 2008; 52(23):1834–43.

28. Moss AJ, Hall WJ, Cannom DS, et al. Cardiac-resynchronization therapy for the prevention of heart-failure events. N Engl J Med 2009;361(14):1329–38.

29. Tang AS, Wells GA, Talajic M, et al. Cardiac-resynchronization therapy for mild-to-moderate heart failure. N Engl J Med 2010;363(25):2385–95.

30. Yu CM, Lin H, Zhang Q, et al. High prevalence of left ventricular systolic and diastolic asynchrony in patients with congestive heart failure and normal QRS duration. Heart 2003;89(1):54–60.

31. Hawkins NM, Petrie MC, MacDonald MR, et al. Selecting patients for cardiac resynchronization therapy: electrical or mechanical dyssynchrony? Eur Heart J 2006;27(11):1270–81.

32. Achilli A, Sassara M, Ficili S, et al. Long-term effectiveness of cardiac resynchronization therapy in patients with refractory heart failure and "narrow" QRS. J Am Coll Cardiol 2003;42(12):2117–24.

33. Bleeker GB, Holman ER, Steendijk P, et al. Cardiac resynchronization therapy in patients with a narrow QRS complex. J Am Coll Cardiol 2006;48(11):2243–50.

34. Yu CM, Chan YS, Zhang Q, et al. Benefits of cardiac resynchronization therapy for heart failure patients with narrow QRS complexes and coexisting systolic asynchrony by echocardiography. J Am Coll Cardiol 2006;48(11):2251–7.

35. Beshai JF, Grimm RA, Nagueh SF, et al. Cardiac-resynchronization therapy in heart failure with narrow QRS complexes. N Engl J Med 2007;357(24):2461–71.

36. Ruschitzka F, Abraham WT, Singh JP, et al. Cardiac-resynchronization therapy in heart failure with a narrow QRS complex. N Engl J Med 2013;369(15): 1395–405.

37. Fung JW, Zhang Q, Yip GW, et al. Effect of cardiac resynchronization therapy in patients with moderate left ventricular systolic dysfunction and wide QRS complex: a prospective study. J Cardiovasc Electrophysiol 2006;17(12):1288–92.

38. Chung ES, Katra RP, Ghio S, et al. Cardiac resynchronization therapy may benefit patients with left ventricular ejection fraction >35%: a PROSPECT trial substudy. Eur J Heart Fail 2010;12(6):581–7.

39. Curtis AB, Worley SJ, Adamson PB, et al. Biventricular pacing for atrioventricular block and systolic dysfunction. N Engl J Med 2013;368(17):1585–93.

40. Velagaleti RS, Pencina MJ, Murabito JM, et al. Long-term trends in the incidence of heart failure after myocardial infarction. Circulation 2008;118(20): 2057–62.

41. Ezekowitz JA, Kaul P, Bakal JA, et al. Declining in-hospital mortality and increasing heart failure incidence in elderly patients with first myocardial infarction. J Am Coll Cardiol 2009;53(1):13–20.

42. Giannuzzi P, Temporelli PL, Bosimini E, et al. Heterogeneity of left ventricular remodeling after acute myocardial infarction: results of the Gruppo Italiano per lo Studio della Sopravvivenza nell'Infarto Miocardico-3 Echo Substudy. Am Heart J 2001; 141(1):131–8.

43. Bolognese L, Neskovic AN, Parodi G, et al. Left ventricular remodeling after primary coronary angioplasty: patterns of left ventricular dilation and long-term prognostic implications. Circulation 2002;106(18): 2351–7.

44. Prinzen FW, Hunter WC, Wyman BT, et al. Mapping of regional myocardial strain and work during ventricular pacing: experimental study using magnetic resonance imaging tagging. J Am Coll Cardiol 1999;33(6):1735–42.

45. Kass DA, Chen CH, Curry C, et al. Improved left ventricular mechanics from acute VDD pacing in patients with dilated cardiomyopathy and ventricular conduction delay. Circulation 1999;99(12):1567–73.

46. Chung ES, Menon SG, Weiss R, et al. Feasibility of biventricular pacing in patients with recent myocardial infarction: impact on ventricular remodeling. Congest Heart Fail 2007;13(1):9–15.

47. Chung ES, Dan D, Solomon SD, et al. Effect of peri-infarct pacing early after myocardial infarction: results of the prevention of myocardial enlargement and dilatation post myocardial infarction study. Circ Heart Fail 2010;3(6):650–8.

MRI for Patients with Cardiac Implantable Electrical Devices

Grant V. Chow, MD[a], Saman Nazarian, MD, PhD[a,b],*

KEYWORDS

• MRI • Pacemaker • Defibrillator • Cardiac implantable electrical device

KEY POINTS

• The clinical utility of MRI scans may outweigh the risk of performing the study in patients with a cardiac implantable electrical device (CIED).
• MRI evaluations can be performed safely in patients with certain pacemaker and implantable cardioverter-defibrillator (ICD) systems, using a protocol based on device selection, appropriate device reprogramming, and close monitoring during the scan.
• MRI should only be performed in cases where the potential benefit clearly outweighs the risks and with adequate subspecialty supervision and monitoring equipment.
• A Food and Drug Administration (FDA)-approved, magnetic resonance (MR)-conditional pacemaker system is now available for use in the United States, with all major device companies in the process of refining their technology.
• MR-conditional systems is needed to ensure that complication rates remain reasonable in comparison with the benefit attained.

INTRODUCTION

The use of MRI for the diagnosis of soft tissue and bony abnormalities is increasing as scanners have become more available throughout the United States. MR scans yield higher spatial resolution than CT images, without the need for ionizing radiation or iodinated contrast injection.[1] At present, approximately 2 million Americans have CIEDs,[2] and an estimated 50% to 75% of these individuals will have an indication for MRI during the lifetime of their device.[3,4] The body of evidence reporting successful use of MRI in patients with CIEDs is growing.[5–8] This article reviews the risks and recent literature on the use of MRI in patients with CIEDs and reports the Johns Hopkins safety protocol.

KNOWN RISKS ASSOCIATED WITH MRI

Current guidelines from the American Heart Association discourage MRI scanning in non–pacemaker-dependent patients, except in cases of a strong clinical indication (highly compelling) where benefits clearly outweigh the risks and an alternative diagnostic modality is unavailable.[4] There are 3 major sources of risk associated with MRI with regard to implantable devices. First, CIED components are subject to potential magnetic field–induced force and torque that might result in system dislodgement or internal reed switch activation (in older devices), the latter of which could permanently disable tachycardia therapies or result in asynchronous pacing.[9,10] Second, electrical current may be induced by the

Disclosures and Financial Support: Dr S. Nazarian is a scientific advisor to and principal investigator for research support to Johns Hopkins from Biosense Webster Inc. Dr S. Nazarian is also funded by NIH grants K23HL089333 and R01HL116280.
a Section for Cardiac Electrophysiology, Department of Medicine, Johns Hopkins University School of Medicine, Carnegie 592A, 600 North Wolfe Street, Baltimore, MD 21287, USA; b Department of Epidemiology, Johns Hopkins Bloomberg School of Public Health, 615 North Wolfe Street, Baltimore, MD 21205, USA
* Corresponding author. Carnegie 592A, 600 North Wolfe Street, Baltimore, MD 21287.
E-mail address: snazarian@jhmi.edu

magnetic field and result in myocardial capture and, rarely, ventricular or atrial arrhythmia induction. Third, device leads can act as an antenna and amplify local energy deposition, resulting in lead heating, tissue damage, and resultant sensing or capture threshold changes.[11,12] Radiofrequency noise may also result in inappropriate inhibition of demand pacing, tachycardia therapies, or programming changes. Early use of MRI in patients with CIEDs resulted in suboptimal outcomes or even death in a small number of patients[13]; therefore, several institutions initiated MRI protocols to evaluate the safety of this imaging modality for strong clinical indications.

THE HOPKINS PROTOCOL

The authors' institution initiated a protocol for both noncardiac and cardiac MRI more than 10 years ago in patients with either permanent pacemakers or ICDs.[10] Since its inception, the authors' program has successfully performed more than 1500 MRI examinations under an institutional review board–approved research protocol (**Fig. 1**).[2] Imaging at the authors' institution was performed using 1.5-T scanners. Patients with newly implanted (<6 weeks), abandoned, or epicardial leads were excluded as were those who were pacemaker dependent with ICD devices. All patients signed an informed consent form that delineated potential risks (discussed previously).

In its first stage, the authors' protocol assists the provider by screening out devices that have no significant data supporting their safe use with MRI technology. Subsequent stages include device reprogramming to minimize both inappropriate device activation of tachycardia therapies and inhibition of bradycardia therapies, prescan and postscan lead parameter checks, and restoration of original programming settings. For most patients, an inhibited pacing mode is programmed for the duration of the MRI scan, and, if the device is an ICD, tachycardia therapies are disabled. In pacemaker-dependent patients, an asynchronous mode is chosen to minimize risks of inappropriate pacing inhibition. After the scan, the authors' institution strongly encourages long-term follow-up 6 months after MRI to ensure no significant chronic changes in device parameters.

In the first 555 MRI studies performed at the authors' institution in patients with CIEDs,[2] the median age of patients undergoing the scan was 68 years. Approximately half of patients had pacemakers (54%), whereas the other half (46%) had ICDs. Most scans were performed for brain (40%) or spine (22%) imaging, with indications, including abscess or infection, mental status changes, stroke, seizure, and radiculopathy. A smaller number of scans (16%) were used to evaluate cardiac viability and/or cardiomyopathy. When comparing immediate changes after MRI with prescan values, the authors observed small changes in right ventricular sensing and various lead impedances. Although statistically significant, no changes were clinically significant enough to require system revision or device reprogramming.

Three patients in the authors' cohort experienced power-on-reset episodes. In 1 patient (who had a single-chamber ICD), a pulling sensation was noted and the MRI scan was stopped. In the other 2 patients (who both had pacemakers and were not pacemaker dependent), the scan was continued. Occasional pacing inhibition was noted with reversion to an inhibited pacing mode, but no immediate or long-term adverse events were seen in follow-up in any of these 3 individuals.

In addition to the authors' expanding experience, the MagnaSafe Registry is an ongoing, multicenter, prospective cohort study of up to 1500 MRI examinations in patients with either pacemakers or ICDs undergoing nonthoracic MRI.[14] As of August 2012, 701 MRI scans had been performed. The registry uses a safety protocol similar to the authors', in that patients with an ICD who are pacemaker dependent are referred for a different imaging modality, whereas those who are not dependent undergo reprogramming to a monitoring-only mode (ventricular sensing without pacing/dual chamber sensing without pacing [OVO/ODO]). Patients with pacemakers are also divided into 2 groups: those who are device dependent (with reprogramming to an asynchronous mode, ventricular asynchronous pacing/dual-chamber asynchronous pacing [VOO/DOO]) and those who are not (set to monitoring-only). All patients then undergo MRI examination, followed by restoration of initial programming and evaluation of parameter changes. Follow-up interrogation is planned at 7 days, 3 months, and 6 months, if postscan parameters have significantly changed, or at 3 and 6 months, if no significant changes are detected. Results of the MagnaSafe Registry are expected to add to the body of literature regarding the safety profile of MRI scanning in patients with devices implanted after 2001.

MRI WITHIN 6 WEEKS OF DEVICE IMPLANTATION

The protocol previously reported from the authors' institution excludes patients who have newly implanted leads. A recent publication by Friedman and colleagues,[15] however, reported outcomes from 171 patients who underwent MRI scanning

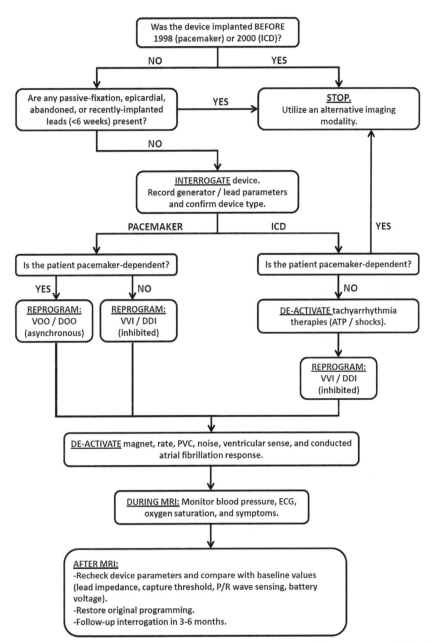

Fig. 1. Hopkins safety protocol for MRI use with a cardiac implantable electrical device. DDI, dual-chamber inhibited pacing without atrial tracking; DOO, dual-chamber asynchronous pacing; P/R wave sensing, atrial/ventricular sensing amplitude; PVC, premature ventricular contraction; VOO, ventricular asynchronous pacing; VVI, ventricular inhibited pacing. (*Adapted from* Nazarian S, Hansford R, Roguin A, et al. A prospective evaluation of a protocol for magnetic resonance imaging of patients with implanted cardiac devices. Ann Intern Med 2011;155:417.)

with CIEDs, including 8 patients who received an MRI scan within 42 days of new lead implantation. All studies were performed in a 1.5-T MRI scanner, and patients were excluded if they were pacemaker dependent or had more than 1 implanted generator. An asynchronous pacing mode (AOO, VOO, or DOO), programmed to 20 beats above the intrinsic rate, was used if the intrinsic rate was less than 90 beats per minute. If the intrinsic rate was greater than 90 beats per minute, a monitor-only mode (OAO, OVO, or ODO) was programmed.

Of the 8 patients in the early cohort, 1 had a permanent-temporary system in place, using an active fixation right ventricular lead (5076, Medtronic, Mounds View, Minnesota) attached to an externalized pacemaker generator (Sensia, Medtronic) secured to the patient's skin. In a different individual, right ventricular lead impedance increased from 550 to 950 Ω after MRI scanning, but there were no significant changes in sensing or capture thresholds. Overall, there were no clinically significant complications for any patient in the early cohort, suggesting that recent lead implantation (within 6 weeks) is not an absolute contraindication to MRI scanning. The authors have also performed MRI in 2 patients with acutely implanted systems and another 2 patients with temporary systems with active fixation right ventricular leads and an externalized permanent pacemaker in the setting of absolute urgency for imaging. All examinations were completed uneventfully without significant changes in system parameters.

STATE OF THE ART: MRI-CONDITIONAL DEVICES

At present, medical devices are categorized into 1 of 3 groups by the American Society for Testing and Materials: (1) MR-safe: an item that poses no known hazards in an MR environment; (2) MR-conditional: an item that has been demonstrated to pose no known hazards in a specified MR environment with specified conditions of use; and (3) MR-unsafe: an item that is known to pose hazards in all MR environments.[16] Although a recent review[17] of 1400 pacemaker recipients with non–MR-conditional devices revealed no fatalities associated with MRI in the modern era, the use of this technology cannot be considered safe in all settings. Device manufacturers are now addressing the need for MRI-compatible devices with several different MR-conditional systems in varying stages FDA approval (several prominent studies described later).

Initial safety and efficacy studies regarding MR-conditional devices were performed largely in European centers, with the first clinical report by Forleo and colleagues[18] in 2010. During an 11-month study period, 107 patients (34% female, mean age 73) were implanted with either an MR-conditional Revo system (n = 50), consisting of an EnRhythm MRI pulse generator and CapSureFix model 5086 MRI leads (Medtronic), or a standard dual-chamber pacemaker (n = 57). In this system, the leads were modified to reduce radiofrequency lead tip heating, internal circuits were changed to reduce the potential for cardiac stimulation, ferromagnetic materials used for construction were limited, and internal circuits were protected to prevent disruption of the internal power supply. Furthermore, the reed switch was replaced by a Hall sensor to allow improved

predictability in a static magnetic field. Study results found that on serial follow-up, lead and pacing parameters were stable in both study groups. Neither group experienced clinically significant complications or lead dislodgement.

In 2011, Wilkoff and colleagues[19] published the results of a prospective, randomized controlled trial using the same MR-conditional dual-chamber pacemaker system (Revo/EnRhythm) with the addition of randomization to MRI scanning versus no scan. A total of 484 patients were enrolled, and 258 were randomized to an MRI scan 9 to 12 weeks postimplant in a 1.5-T scanner. All patients were seen and evaluated at 3 and 4 months postimplant. Overall, the study found no MRI-related complications at the time of the scan, with minimal changes in capture threshold or sensed electrogram amplitude between study groups. Furthermore, MRI scanning with the Revo system was not associated with any major or minor complications through the end of the study period.

The Advisa MRI study, a prospective, randomized controlled trial, enrolled 269 subjects (with 263 implants) from 35 centers internationally.[20] The protocol used the second-generation Advisa SureScan MRI pacemaker system, consisting of an Advisa MRI implantable pulse generator and 2 CapSureFix 5086 MRI leads (Medtronic). Patients were randomized in a 2:1 fashion to 16 chest and head MRI evaluations in a 1.5-T scanner 9 to 12 weeks postimplant, versus no scan. The system passed both primary endpoints, demonstrating no significant increase in MRI-related complications or capture threshold from pre-MRI versus 1 month post-MRI scan in the intervention group. The Advisa pacemaker system was FDA approved for scanning from above C1 and below T12 in February 2013. The authors have safely performed thoracic MRI in patients with Medtronic MR-conditional systems using their safety protocol for standard pacemakers. The Revo and Advisa systems and their leads include a distinctive radiographic device label and lead appearance to allow identification by chest radiograph. Similar studies are under way to evaluate pacing systems from other major device manufacturers, including

- The Accent MRI pacemaker with Tendril MRI lead (St. Jude Medical, St. Paul, Minnesota).[21] The Accent MRI system also has distinct radiopaque markers for quick radiographic identification of the system.
- The ImageReady pacemaker system comprised of an Ingenio MRI pulse generator with the Ingevity lead platform (Boston Scientific, Natick, Massachusetts).[22]

- The Evia/Entovis ProMRI pacemaker with Safio S pacing leads (Biotronik, Berlin, Germany).[23]

Thus far, however, none of these 3 systems has been FDA approved for use in the United States.

EARLY CLINICAL EXPERIENCES WITH LEAD-RELATED COMPLICATIONS

As of the writing of this article, there have been 2 recent publications[24,25] that did find an increased incidence of clinically significant adverse events in patients receiving MR-conditional pacemaker leads. In a retrospective case-control study of 65 consecutive patients implanted with two 5086 MRI leads compared with 92 consecutive control patients implanted with two 5076 leads over a 14-month period, Elmouchi and colleagues[25] identified a significantly higher complication rate (including lead dislodgement, cardiac perforation, tamponade, or death) within 30 days in 8 of 65 cases (12.3%) versus 2 of 92 controls (2.2%), yielding an odds ratio of 6.3 (95% CI, 1.3–30.8; $P = .02$) for an adverse event. Four patients receiving 5086 MRI leads experienced lead dislodgement, whereas none was seen in the 5076 group ($P<.03$).

When evaluating a larger cohort of 466 patients enrolled prospectively in the EnRhythm MRI study (each receiving two 5086 MRI leads) versus 316 patients receiving two 5076 leads in previous clinical studies, Rickard and colleagues[24] also identified a higher lead dislodgement rate (3.8%) with the 5086 MR-conditional lead, when followed over a mean 30.8-month period, compared with the 5076-lead (0.6%; $P = .05$), when followed for a mean 9.6 months. In this study, the overall rate of cardiac perforation was not significantly different between groups (0.6% for the 5086 MRI group vs 0.9% for control), and there were otherwise no clinically significant differences in lead performance.

SUMMARY

In many situations, the clinical utility of MRI scans may outweigh the risk of performing the study in patients with a CIED. MRI evaluations can be performed safely in patients with certain pacemaker and ICD systems, using a protocol based on device selection, appropriate device reprogramming, and close monitoring during the scan. MRI should be performed only in cases of the potential benefit clearly outweighing the risks and with adequate subspecialty supervision and monitoring equipment. At present, a vast majority of available data have been obtained in closed-bore scanners

with a magnetic strength of 1.5 T; thus, results of these studies should not be generalized to all MRI scanners. An FDA-approved, MR-conditional pacemaker system is now available for use in the United States, with all major device companies in the process of refining their technology. Continued monitoring of MR-conditional leads is needed to ensure that complication rates remain reasonable in comparison with the benefit attained.

REFERENCES

1. Marcu CB, Beek AM, van Rossum AC. Clinical applications of cardiovascular magnetic resonance imaging. Can Med Assoc J 2006;175:911–7.
2. Nazarian S, Hansford R, Roguin A, et al. A prospective evaluation of a protocol for magnetic resonance imaging of patients with implanted cardiac devices. Ann Intern Med 2011;155:415–24.
3. Kalin R, Stanton MS. Current clinical issues for MRI scanning of pacemaker and defibrillator patients. Pacing Clin Electrophysiol 2005;28:326–8.
4. Levine GN, Gomes AS, Arai AE, et al. Safety of magnetic resonance imaging in patients with cardiovascular devices: An American Heart Association scientific statement from the Committee on Diagnostic and Interventional Cardiac Catheterization, Council on Clinical Cardiology, and the Council on Cardiovascular Radiology and Intervention: Endorsed by the American College of Cardiology Foundation, the North American Society for Cardiac Imaging, and the Society for Cardiovascular Magnetic Resonance. Circulation 2007;116:2878–91.
5. Martin ET, Coman JA, Shellock FG, et al. Magnetic resonance imaging and cardiac pacemaker safety at 1.5-Tesla. J Am Coll Cardiol 2004;43:1315–24.
6. Gimbel JR, Johnson D, Levine PA, et al. Safe performance of magnetic resonance imaging on five patients with permanent cardiac pacemakers. Pacing Clin Electrophysiol 1996;19:913–9.
7. Sommer T, Vahlhaus C, Lauck G, et al. MR imaging and cardiac pacemakers: in-vitro evaluation and in-vivo studies in 51 patients at 0.5 T. Radiology 2000; 215:869–79.
8. Vahlhaus C, Sommer T, Lewalter T, et al. Interference with cardiac pacemakers by magnetic resonance imaging: are there irreversible changes at 0.5 Tesla? Pacing Clin Electrophysiol 2001;24:489–95.
9. Roguin A, Zviman MM, Meininger GR, et al. Modern pacemaker and implantable cardioverter/defibrillator systems can be magnetic resonance imaging safe: In vitro and in vivo assessment of safety and function at 1.5 T. Circulation 2004;110:475–82.
10. Nazarian S, Roguin A, Zviman MM, et al. Clinical utility and safety of a protocol for noncardiac and cardiac magnetic resonance imaging of patients with permanent pacemakers and implantable

cardioverter defibrillators at 1.5 Tesla. Circulation 2006;114:1277–84.

11. Sommer T, Naehle CP, Yang A, et al. Strategy for safe performance of extrathoracic magnetic resonance imaging at 1.5 Tesla in the presence of cardiac pacemakers in non-pacemaker-dependent patients: a prospective study with 115 examinations. Circulation 2006;114:1285–92.

12. Vahlhaus C. Heating of pacemaker leads during magnetic resonance imaging. Eur Heart J 2005;26: 1243–4.

13. Roguin A, Schwitter J, Vahlhaus C, et al. Magnetic resonance imaging in individuals with cardiovascular implantable electronic devices. Europace 2008; 10:336–46.

14. Russo RJ. Determining the risks of clinically indicated nonthoracic magnetic resonance imaging at 1.5 T for patients with pacemakers and implantable cardioverter-defibrillators: rationale and design of the MagnaSafe Registry. Am Heart J 2013;165: 266–72.

15. Friedman HL, Acker N, Dalzell C, et al. Magnetic resonance imaging in recently implanted pacemakers. Pacing Clin Electrophysiol 2013;36:1090–5.

16. American Society for Testing and Materials (ASTM) International. ASTM F2503–13: standard practice for marking medical devices and other items for safety in the magnetic resonance environment. West Conshohocken (PA): ASTM International; 2013. Available at: http://www.astm.org. Accessed October 6, 2006.

17. Zikria JF, Machnicki S, Rhim E, et al. MRI of patients with cardiac pacemakers: a review of the medical literature. Am J Roentgenol 2011;196:390–401.

18. Forleo GB, Santini L, Della Rocca DG, et al. Safety and efficacy of a new magnetic resonance imaging-compatible pacing system: early results of a prospective comparison with conventional dual-chamber implant outcomes. Heart Rhythm 2010;7: 750–4.

19. Wilkoff BL, Bello D, Taborsky M, et al. Magnetic resonance imaging in patients with a pacemaker system designed for the magnetic resonance environment. Heart Rhythm 2011;8:65–73.

20. Gimbel JR, Bello D, Schmitt M, et al. Randomized trial of pacemaker and lead system for safe scanning at 1.5 Tesla. Heart Rhythm 2013;10:685–91.

21. Safety and efficacy of the Accent Magnetic Resonance Imaging (MRI) pacemaker and Tendril MRI lead. Available at: ClinicalTrials.gov, http://clinicaltrials.gov/show/NCT01576016. Accessed October 6, 2013.

22. ImageReady MR Conditional Pacing System Clinical Study (SAMURAI). Available at: ClinicalTrials.gov, http://clinicaltrials.gov/show/NCT01781078. Accessed October 6, 2013.

23. ProMRI AFFIRM study of the EVIA/ENTOVIS pacemaker system with Safio S pacemaker leads (ProMRIAFFIRM). Available at: ClinicalTrials.gov, http://clinicaltrials.gov/show/NCT01460992. Accessed October 6, 2013.

24. Rickard J, Taborsky M, Bello D, et al. Short and long term electrical performance of the 5086 MRI pacing lead. Heart Rhythm 2013. [Epub ahead of print].

25. Elmouchi DA, Rosema S, Vanoosterhout SM, et al. Cardiac perforation and lead dislodgement after implantation of a MR-conditional pacing lead: a single-center experience. Pacing Clin Electrophysiol 2013. [Epub ahead of print].

Implantable Defibrillators in Long QT Syndrome, Brugada Syndrome, Hypertrophic Cardiomyopathy, and Arrhythmogenic Right Ventricular Cardiomyopathy

Mustafa Dohadwala, MD, Mark S. Link, MD*

KEYWORDS

- Long QT syndrome • Hypertrophic cardiomyopathy • Brugada syndrome
- Arrhythmogenic right ventricular cardiomyopathy • Channelopathy • Sudden death
- Genetic syndrome

KEY POINTS

- Sudden death is often the first manifestation in inherited cardiac arrhythmia syndromes.
- Patients with long QT syndrome who have an episode of syncope while on beta-blockade should be offered an implantable cardioverter-defibrillator (ICD).
- In Brugada syndrome and hypertrophic cardiomyopathy, ICDs are often the most effective treatment of primary and secondary prevention of cardiac arrest.
- Risk stratification is crucial in identifying those at greatest risk to provide lifesaving therapy while avoiding complications in those unlikely to receive benefit.

INTRODUCTION

Sudden cardiac death (SCD) has an overall incidence of 0.1% to 0.2% per year with 300,000 to 350,000 deaths annually in the United States. Depending on the patient population, up to 20% of SCDs are attributable to primary genetic disorders.

Prevention of SCD in these inherited syndromes often requires implantable cardioverter-defibrillators (ICDs). However, implantation of ICDs has short-term and long-term risks, especially in a young person. This article reviews the role of ICDs and adjunctive treatments in 4 major inherited syndromes that lead to sudden death;

namely long QT syndrome (LQTS), Brugada syndrome (BrS), hypertrophic cardiomyopathy (HCM), and arrhythmogenic right ventricular cardiomyopathy (ARVC).

LQTS

Overview, Clinical Presentation, and Pathophysiology

Since the initial description of the LQTS, 13 genetic LQTSs have been delineated.[1,2] Because of variable penetrance and geographic differences, the prevalence ranges from 1 in 2000 to 1 in 10,000[3,4] with a slight female preponderance.[5,6] The initial presentation in LQTS may include

Department of Medicine, The Cardiac Arrhythmia Center, Tufts Medical Center, 800 Washington Street, Box #197, Boston, MA 02111, USA
* Corresponding author. Tufts Medical Center, 800 Washington Street, Box #197, Boston, MA 02111.
E-mail address: mlink@tuftsmedicalcenter.org

Cardiol Clin 32 (2014) 305–318
http://dx.doi.org/10.1016/j.ccl.2013.11.003
0733-8651/14/$ – see front matter © 2014 Elsevier Inc. All rights reserved.

palpitations, presyncope, syncope, or even cardiac arrest. LQTS type 1 (LQT1), LQTS type 2 (LQT2), and LQTS type 3 (LQT3) account for approximately 75% of LQTS.

In an observational study of 193 consecutive genotype-proven families with more than 600 patients over almost 3 decades, 13% (n = 81) had cardiac arrest or death before 40 years of age.[7] LQT1 is caused by a mutation (KCNQ1) of the IKs channel. Although cardiac events are more frequent, the risk of sudden death remains similar to that with LQT2 and LQT3. Emotional and physical stress and activities such as swimming and diving classically trigger events. LQT2 is caused by a mutation (KCNH2) of the IKr channel. Common triggers include emotional stress, sudden arousal, and auditory stimulation. LQT3, unlike LQT1 and LQT2, is characterized by the SCN5A mutation in the INa channel. Events are less frequent in this group, but events tend to be more dangerous.[8] Early afterdepolarizations (EADs) caused by reactivation of L-type calcium channels and, less frequently, from late INa or Na-Ca exchange trigger polymorphic ventricular tachycardia (VT). Transmural heterogeneity in repolarization, particularly in the M cells, provides substrate for block and reentry leading to perpetuation of torsades de pointes (TDP).[9]

Diagnosis

Diagnosis of LQTS relies on a combination of clinical presentation, personal history, family history, and electrocardiogram (ECG). Coexistent factors, such as congenital deafness, can be a clue for syndromic LQTS. Depending on clinical suspicion, the ECG should be repeated frequently because the QT interval can be dynamic.[10,11] The 2 clinical scoring systems, Schwartz and Keating, combine ECG and clinical findings for diagnosis. Both are hindered by a high false-negative rate. In response, it has been suggested to use a QTc cutoff of 430 milliseconds with gene testing to provide better sensitivity.[2,12–14] The recently published expert consensus recommendations from the Heart Rhythm Society (HRS)/European Heart Rhythm Association (EHRA)/Asia Pacific Heart Rhythm Society (APHRS) for diagnosis of LQTS are available (**Box 1**).[15]

Risk Stratification

QTc is a strong predictor for cardiac events and sudden death. A QTc greater than 470 milliseconds is a risk predictor for symptoms, whereas QTc greater than 500 milliseconds is a risk predictor for life-threatening events.[2,7,8] In the

second decade of life, a QTc greater than 530 milliseconds increases risk for an event by a hazard ratio of 2.3 (95% confidence interval, 1.6–3.3).[16] Because the QTc can change by 47 ± 40 milliseconds on repeated ECGs,[17] it should be repeated and interpreted cautiously for risk stratification. The strongest clinical predictor for cardiac arrest remains recent syncope. Recent syncope in children, adolescents, and young adults can increase the likelihood of sudden death or cardiac arrest by 10-fold to 20-fold.[17–19] Even a remote syncopal episode increases the likelihood by 2.7.[16] If syncope is present while on β-blockers, the risk of death is the same as if not on a β-blocker.[19] In childhood, boys, especially with LQT1, are at a higher risk of sudden death and cardiac arrest.[20] By adolescence, the risk of life-threatening events equalizes between the genders. After the second decade of life, women, especially with LQT2, have higher risk of cardiac arrest and sudden death.[21–23] Gender differences are less exaggerated with LQT3. Programmed electrical stimulation[24] and family history[25] do not predict events.

Beta-Blockade and Adjunctive Therapies for Sudden Death Prevention

Beta-blockade is most effective in LQT1 and β-blockers decrease the sudden cardiac arrest rate to 1% over the course of 5 years.[26,27] Patients with LQTS1 who are compliant with β-blockers and are off all QT-prolonging drugs did not have recurrent events in one study.[28] The response to β-blockers is not as assured with LQT2 and LQT3.[26,27] Even with beta-blockade, the aborted cardiac arrest rate has been reported to be 6.6% over 5 years and 14% over 5 years.[27]

Defibrillator Therapy for Sudden Death Prevention

A collection of small studies in the early 2000s and larger studies more recently have began to clarify the role of ICD in the LQTS. In 27 patients with LQTS who received ICD for aborted arrest (n = 17), syncope on β-blockers (n = 9), and family history of SCD (n = 1), 10 of 17 patients with history of cardiac arrest had a total of 169 appropriate shocks. None of the 9 patients with syncope on β-blockers required a shock. Those with prior cardiac arrest have a particularly malignant course, because 19% of patients had appropriate shocks despite being started on β-blockers.[29] In a study of 459 patients with LQTS; 51 had an ICD. Of these, 24% had appropriate, ventricular fibrillation (VF)–terminating therapy during follow-up of 7.3 years. Women with LQTS2 were most likely to receive appropriate therapy. The likelihood of appropriate ICD therapy correlated with secondary prevention indication, non-LQT3 genotype, QTc greater than 500 milliseconds, syncope, history of Torsades, and negative family history. None of the patients without an ICD implanted died.[30] The largest experience of ICDs in LQTS was the European LQTS registry. Of 233 patients followed for 4.6 ± 3.2 years, 28% of patients had an appropriate shock. Predictors of appropriate therapy included age less than 20 years at implantation, QTc greater than 500 milliseconds, prior arrest, and cardiac events despite β-blocker therapy. No patients without an aforementioned risk factor had an appropriate shock. Risk factors were additive; if a patient had all of the risk factors, 70% had a shock.[31]

Thus, ICD implantation seems reasonable in the following patients: (1) those who have survived a cardiac arrest, (2) patients with syncope despite b-blocker, and (3) asymptomatic patients with QTc greater than or equal to 550 milliseconds with electrical instability (ie, T-wave alternans) or other long sinus pauses that may favor early afterdepolarizations.[32] ICD implantation may be considered in women with LQT2 with QTc greater than 500 milliseconds who either have symptoms or cannot tolerate β-blockers. Routine use of ICDs in LQT3 does not seem to be appropriate. The recently published expert consensus recommendations from the HRS/EHRA/APHRS for therapeutic interventions in LQTS are available **(Box 2)**.[15]

ICD Considerations Specific to LQTS

If an ICD is implanted, permanent pacing can be considered to reduce bradycardia-dependent QT prolongation and short-long-short sequences. Beta-blockade should be prescribed to prevent events.

BRS
Overview, Clinical Presentation, and Pathophysiology

BrS is an autosomal dominant condition that disproportionately affects men with an 8:1 ratio. Prevalence of Brugada, from ECG, varies markedly based on population studied. In the United States 0.012% to 0.43% of individuals show the ECG pattern, whereas in endemic areas of southeast Asia the pattern may be present in up to 3% of patients.[33,34] In the seminal article by Brugada and colleagues,[35] 547 patients with either spontaneous (n = 408) or antiarrhythmic-induced (n = 156) Brugada pattern ECG were followed over 24 ± 32 months. None had preceding cardiac arrest, the mean age of patients was 41 ± 15 years, and 408 were men. During the follow-up period, 45 patients (8%) sustained SCD or VF. In endemic areas, it is the leading cause of death in men less than 40 years of age and frequently is the cause of sudden infant death syndrome. Sudden death is the initial manifestation of Brugada in 30%, so diagnosis and primary prevention are paramount.

The first mutation linked to BrS was the SCN5A, accounting for 15% to 30% of genotyped Brugada, which is a loss-of-function mutation leading to diminished Na inward current. Over time, other mutations in the Na channel, along with mutations that reduce Ca current or enhance transient inward K current, have been discovered. Patients with BrS have arrhythmic events and death in the early morning hours during sleep and bradycardia. Other triggers include fevers, large meals, alcohol, and cocaine.[36] In children, BrS can be mistaken for febrile seizures.[37] In addition to ventricular arrhythmias, 20% of patients have paroxysmal supraventricular arrhythmia (SVT) and atrial fibrillation,[38,39] which can trigger ventricular arrhythmias.

Box 2
Treatment of LQTS

Class I

1. The following lifestyle changes are recommended in all patients with a diagnosis of LQTS:

   a. Avoidance of QT-prolonging drugs (www.qtdrugs.org)

   b. Identification and correction of electrolyte abnormalities that may occur during diarrhea, vomiting, metabolic conditions, or imbalanced diets for weight loss

2. β-Blockers are recommended in patients with a diagnosis of LQTS who are:

   a. Asymptomatic with QTc greater than or equal to 470 milliseconds, and/or

   b. Symptomatic for syncope or documented VT/VF

3. Left cardiac sympathetic denervation (LCSD) is recommended in high-risk patients with a diagnosis of LQTS in whom:

   a. ICD therapy is contraindicated or refused, and/or

   b. β-Blockers are either not effective in preventing syncope/arrhythmias, not tolerated, not accepted, or contraindicated

4. ICD implantation is recommended in patients with a diagnosis of LQTS who are survivors of a cardiac arrest.

5. All patients with LQTS who wish to engage in competitive sports should be referred to a clinical expert for the evaluation of risk.

Class IIa

6. β-Blockers can be useful in patients with a diagnosis of LQTS who are asymptomatic with QTc less than or equal to 470 milliseconds.

7. ICD implantation can be useful in patients with a diagnosis of LQTS who experience recurrent syncopal events while on β-blocker therapy.

8. LCSD can be useful in patients with a diagnosis of LQTS who experience breakthrough events while on therapy with β-blockers/ICD.

9. Sodium channel blockers can be useful as add-on therapy for patients with LQT3 with a QTc of 450 milliseconds who shorten their QTc by 440 milliseconds following an acute oral drug test with one of these compounds.

Class III

10. Except under special circumstances, ICD implantation is not indicated in asymptomatic patients with LQTS who have not been tried on β-blocker therapy.

From Priori SG, Wilde AA, Horie M, et al. HRS/EHRA/APHRS expert consensus statement on the diagnosis and management of patients with inherited primary arrhythmia syndromes. Expert consensus statement on inherited primary arrhythmia syndromes: document endorsed by HRS, EHRA, and APHRS in May 2013 and by ACCF, AHA, PACES, and AEPC in June 2013. Heart Rhythm 2013:e75–106; with permission.

Patients may also have conduction disease with PR and HV prolongation.

Diagnosis

Electrocardiographic abnormalities in right precordial leads form the basis for diagnosis of BrS. ECG findings have been categorized into 3 types. Type 1, the most specific and diagnostic for BrS, represents ST elevation of greater than or equal to 2 mm with a coved (or downward convex) morphology associated with either incomplete or complete right bundle branch pattern followed by descending negative T wave with little or no isoelectric separation. Type II and III patterns are characterized by saddleback appearance of the ST segment, with type II having greater ST elevation than type III. Both are nonspecific.[40] The ECG pattern may be dynamic and/or elicited by Na channel blocking antiarrhythmics. A more cephalad placement of the right precordial leads (up to the second intercostal space above normal) increases the sensitivity without decreasing specificity.[41] Other strategies to unmask the ECG pattern include nighttime monitoring of ST segments and documenting ECG at times of any stress.[33]

Aside from the classic findings, QT interval prolongation and QRS fragmentation along the right precordium may be present.[42,43] Signal average ECG may show late potentials in 60% to 70% of patients with Brugada.[33,40] Particularly with SCN5A mutation, patients may have depolarization abnormalities with increased P-wave duration, prolonged PR interval, and increased QRS duration. To make BrS diagnosis, a patient should have spontaneous or pharmacologically inducible type 1 pattern in greater than or equal to 1 right precordial lead (ie, V1–V3) with 1 of the following: (1) history of VF, (2) history of polymorphic VT, (3) family history of SCD at less than 45 years of age, (4) coved-type ECG in another family member, (5) inducibility of VT with programmed electrical stimulation, (6) history of syncope, or (7) nocturnal agonal respirations. Despite low sensitivity, genetic testing for SCN5A is a useful adjunct with type I ECG pattern for family members.[14] The recently published expert consensus recommendations from the HRS/EHRA/APHRS for diagnosis of BrS are available (**Box 3**).[15]

Risk Stratification

There has been controversy regarding risk predictors for cardiac arrest. Patients with aborted

---

Box 3
Diagnosis of BrS

1. BrS is diagnosed in patients with ST-segment elevation with type I morphology greater than or equal to 2 mm in greater than or equal to 1 lead among the right precordial leads V1 and V2 positioned in the second, third, or fourth intercostal space occurring either spontaneously or after provocative drug test with intravenous administration of class I antiarrhythmic drugs.

2. BrS is diagnosed in patients with type 2 or type 3 ST-segment elevation in greater than or equal to 1 lead among the right precordial leads V1 and V2 positioned in the second, third, or fourth intercostal space when a provocative drug test with intravenous administration of class I antiarrhythmic drugs induces a type I ECG morphology.

From Priori SG, Wilde AA, Horie M, et al. HRS/EHRA/APHRS expert consensus statement on the diagnosis and management of patients with inherited primary arrhythmia syndromes. Expert consensus statement on inherited primary arrhythmia syndromes: document endorsed by HRS, EHRA, and APHRS in May 2013 and by ACCF, AHA, PACES, and AEPC in June 2013. Heart Rhythm 2013:e75–106; with permission.

---

sudden death have a recurrence rate of up to 11%/y.[44] For asymptomatic patients and those with syncope, the event rate is lower.[35,45] Finding higher risk patients within this group becomes crucial. Brugada and colleagues[35] suggested electrophysiological (EP) study, but recent data have caused this to be questioned.[37,45–48] Although controversial,[35,45,49] a spontaneous type I ECG pattern seems to confer risk compared with a drug-induced pattern.[35,37,45,46,50,51] In a meta-analysis of 1545 patients with Brugada ECG, the overall event rate (sudden cardiac arrest, syncope, or ICD shock) at 32 months was 10%. Predictors included previous cardiac arrest or syncope (relative risk [RR], 3.24), male gender (RR, 3.47), and spontaneous type I pattern (RR, 4.65). Family history, SCN5A mutation, and inducibility during programmed electrical stimulation were not predictors of risk.[46] In the more recently published European FINGER registry, 1029 consecutive patients (72% male, median age 42 years, range 35–55 years) with spontaneous or inducible BrS were followed over 31.9 months (range, 14–54.4 months). The ICD event rate was 7.7%, 1.9%, and 0.5% in patients with history of aborted sudden death, syncope, and without symptoms, respectively. Presence of spontaneous type 1 ECG predicted events, whereas gender, family history, inducibility via EP study, and SCN5A mutation were not predictive.[52] In another study of 320 (54% spontaneous, 46% inducible) patients with BrS with prior syncope or no symptoms, major events occurred in patients with 2 or more of prior syncope, family history of sudden death, or a positive EP study. Those with 2 or more risk factors and spontaneous type I ECG had a 30% event rate.[51] From these data, major risk predictors include prior cardiac arrest, prior syncope, and spontaneous type I ECG. Inducibility on programmed electrical stimulation remains controversial.

Defibrillator and Adjunctive Therapies for Sudden Death Prevention

Medications (ie, β-blocker) have not proved useful for either primary or secondary prevention; an ICD is the only proven therapy for Brugada. Thus, patients with type I Brugada who have history of cardiac arrest or syncope should receive an ICD. There is no consensus for asymptomatic patients. Experts argue for (1) close follow-up; (2) ICD implantation in those with positive EP study, especially if there is a family history of sudden death; and (3) ICD implantation in all spontaneous type 1 patterns. Pharmacologic therapies in Brugada are adjunctive, to decrease risk of recurrent events and ICD storm. These therapies include Ito blockers or ICaL augmenting agents that can restore the right ventricular (RV) epicardial action potential dome and normalize ST segments.[40] Such medications include quinidine, denopamine, cilostazol, bepridil, tedisamil, mexiletine, disopyramide, and isoproterenol. More recently, there has been success in ablating areas within the RV outflow tract (RVOT) that could be responsible for phase 2 reentry and initiation of VT/VF in BrS.[53] The recently published expert consensus recommendations from the HRS/EHRA/APHRS for therapeutic interventions in BrS are available (**Box 4**).[15]

HCM

Overview, Clinical Presentation, and Pathophysiology

HCM is the most common genetic cardiac disease, affecting 1 in 500 people. It is an autosomal dominant disease with variable clinical penetrance; half of the cases are familial and the remaining sporadic. More than 900 mutations in 24 genes encoding sarcomeric proteins have been reported, leading to thickening of the left ventricle with myocyte disarray. There are several forms, including asymmetric hypertrophy of the septum, symmetric hypertrophy, and apical hypertrophy. Between 5%

Box 4
Treatment of BrS

Class I

1. The following lifestyle changes are recommended in all patients with diagnosis of BrS:

   a. Avoidance of drugs that may induce or aggravate ST-segment elevation in right precordial leads (eg, Brugadadrugs.org)

   b. Avoidance of excessive alcohol intake

   c. Immediate treatment of fever with antipyretic drugs

2. ICD implantation is recommended in patients with a diagnosis of BrS who:

   a. Are survivors of a cardiac arrest, and/or

   b. Have documented spontaneous sustained VT with or without syncope

Class IIa

3. ICD implantation can be useful in patients with a spontaneous diagnostic type I ECG who have a history of syncope judged likely to be caused by ventricular arrhythmias.

4. Quinidine can be useful in patients with a diagnosis of BrS and history of arrhythmic storms defined as more than 2 episodes of VT/VF in 24 hours.

5. Quinidine can be useful in patients with a diagnosis of BrS who:

   a. Qualify for an ICD but present a contraindication to the ICD or refuse it, and/or

   b. Have a history of documented supraventricular arrhythmias that require treatment

6. Isoproterenol infusion can be useful in suppressing arrhythmic storms in patients with BrS.

Class IIb

7. ICD implantation may be considered in patients with a diagnosis of BrS who develop VF during programmed electrical stimulation (inducible patients).

8. Quinidine may be considered in asymptomatic patients with a diagnosis of BrS with a spontaneous type I ECG.

9. Catheter ablation may be considered in patients with a diagnosis of BrS and history of arrhythmic storms or repeated appropriate ICD shocks.

Class III

10. ICD implantation is not indicated in asymptomatic patients with BrS with a drug-induced type I ECG and a family history of SCD alone.

From Priori SG, Wilde AA, Horie M, et al. HRS/EHRA/APHRS expert consensus statement on the diagnosis and management of patients with inherited primary arrhythmia syndromes. Expert consensus statement on inherited primary arrhythmia syndromes: document endorsed by HRS, EHRA, and APHRS in May 2013 and by ACCF, AHA, PACES, and AEPC in June 2013. Heart Rhythm 2013:e75–106; with permission.

and 10% may progress to end-stage or burnt-out HCM with left ventricular (LV) dysfunction. HCM manifests in a myriad of ways including dyspnea, chest pain, palpitations, dizziness, presyncope, syncope, and cardiac arrest. These symptoms are related to diastolic dysfunction, LV outflow tract (LVOT) obstruction, LV dysfunction, atrial fibrillation, and ventricular arrhythmias.

In the United States, HCM is the leading cause of sudden death in athletes. Early studies overestimated the rate of SCD in HCM,[54] because more recent studies show sudden death to be closer to 1% per year in the general HCM population.[55,56] The seemingly low 1% per year rate of sudden death is significant when viewed in the context of accumulated risk in a young patient with HCM. The cumulative lifetime increased risk for sudden death from VT/VF may be 10% to 20%, and, for high-risk patients, risk may be up to 5% per year.[55–57] Aborted cardiac arrest and sudden death in HCM is classically attributed to polymorphic VT or VF. However, monomorphic VT occurs more frequently than has been appreciated based on intracardiac electrogram data in patients with ICDs.[57] This is not surprising given that myofibrillar disarray, interstitial fibrosis, and perhaps focal ischemia provide arrhythmogenic substrate leading to reentrant ventricular arrhythmias.[58]

Risk Stratification

Over the past 2 decades, 5 clinical markers for sudden death in the primary prevention population have been identified: (1) family history of premature sudden death in at least 1 relative, (2) unexplained syncope (in young patients and/or on exertion), (3) nonsustained ventricular arrhythmias (NSVT) on Holter, (4) massive LV hypertrophy greater than or equal to 30 mm, and (5) hypotensive response to exercise. In the 2011 ACCF/AHA HCM guidelines, family history, syncope, and massive LV hypertrophy are major risk factors. However, NSVT and hypotensive blood pressure should be considered significant only if associated with one of the emerging risk factors.[59] Data from the Maron ICD registries showed an 11% per year risk of appropriate ICD therapy for those patients previously resuscitated from SCD.[60,61] The yearly risk of appropriate ICD therapy in those patients without a prior cardiac arrest was 3.6%. In these studies there was no difference in risk of appropriate ICD therapy in those with a single risk factor compared with multiple risk factors. In a pediatric population, similar results were observed. There was a 14%/y risk of appropriate ICD therapy for those resuscitated

from SCD, and a 3.1%/y risk in those implanted for primary prophylaxis.[62] In this population it was also observed that there was no difference in the occurrence of appropriate ICD intervention between those with a single risk factor or multiple risk factors. In contrast, data from the United Kingdom suggest that a single risk factor may not place an patient with HCM at greater risk of an event.[63]

Emerging risk factors, such as presence and extent of late gadolinium enhancement on magnetic resonance imaging, may prove useful.[64,65] Other less validated risk factors include ischemia, atrial fibrillation, LVOT obstruction, competitive sports, and certain genetic mutations. Those with end-stage HCM awaiting heart transplant or LV apical aneurysm have up to a 10%/y risk of death.[66,67] Because older patients are at low risk for sudden death even with risk factors, they should not be stratified in the same manner as younger patients.[68]

Defibrillator and Adjunctive Therapy for Sudden Death Prevention

Antiarrhythmics such as amiodarone and sotalol have not proved to be effective in preventing sudden death or VT.[61,69,70] Thus, ICDs are central for sudden death prevention. The 5-year cumulative appropriate discharge rate in HCM is almost 39% in the secondary population and 17% in the primary prevention population.[61] ICDs are thus indicated for patients with HCM with prior cardiac arrest and high-risk primary prevention patients. High-risk primary prevention patients should be selected by having at least one risk factor from the 2011 ACCF/AHA guidelines (**Box 5**)[59] because 35% of appropriate ICD interventions for VT/VF occur in patients with a single risk factor.[61]

ICD Considerations Specific to HCM

In the late 1990s, dual-chamber pacing to decrease LVOT gradient was promising based on observational trials. However, randomized trials have not proved long-term benefit but individuals more than 65 years of age may have some benefit.[71–73] Thus, older individuals with LVOT obstruction and heart failure symptoms may benefit from a dual-chamber system. Moreover, when implanting an ICD, clinicians must be mindful that defibrillation thresholds (DFTs) are on average higher compared with a non-HCM population.[74] Thus, DFTs should be routinely checked and, if a safety margin greater than or equal to 10 J is not present, adding an superior vena cava coil or subcutaneous array may be necessary.

Box 5
Defibrillator treatment of HCM

Class I

1. The decision to place an ICD in patients with HCM should include application of individual clinical judgment, as well as a thorough discussion of the strength of evidence, benefits, and risks to allow the informed patient's active participation in decision making.

2. ICD placement is recommended for patients with HCM with prior documented cardiac arrest, VF, or hemodynamically significant VT.

Class IIa

1. It is reasonable to recommend an ICD for patients with HCM with:

   a. Sudden death presumably caused by HCM in 1 or more first-degree relatives

   b. A maximum LV wall thickness greater than or equal to 30 mm

   c. One or more recent, unexplained syncopal episodes

2. An ICD can be useful in select patients with NSVT (particularly those <30 years of age) in the presence of other SCD risk factors or modifiers.

3. An ICD can be useful in select patients with HCM with an abnormal blood pressure response with exercise in the presence of other SCD risk factors or modifiers.

4. It is reasonable to recommend an ICD for high-risk children with HCM, based on unexplained syncope, massive LV hypertrophy, or family history of SCD, after taking into account the high complication rate of long-term ICD implantation (level of evidence: C).

Class IIb

1. The usefulness of an ICD is uncertain in patients with HCM with isolated bursts of NSVT in the absence of any other SCD risk factors or modifiers.

2. The usefulness of an ICD is uncertain in patients with HCM with an abnormal blood pressure response with exercise when in the absence of any other SCD risk factors or modifiers, particularly in the presence of significant outflow obstruction.

Class III

1. ICD placement as a routine strategy in patients with HCM without an indication of increased risk is potentially harmful.

2. ICD placement as a strategy to permit patients with HCM to participate in competitive athletics is potentially harmful.

3. ICD placement in patients who have an identified HCM genotype in the absence of clinical manifestations of HCM is potentially harmful.

From Gersh BJ, Maron BJ, Bonow RO, et al. 2011 ACCF/AHA guideline for the diagnosis and treatment of hypertrophic cardiomyopathy: a report of the American College of Cardiology Foundation/American Heart Association Task Force on Practice Guidelines. Circulation 2011;124(24):e783–831; with permission.

Use of antitachycardia pacing is reasonable because it terminates ventricular arrhythmias in HCM with high frequency.[75] ATP may reduce the number of appropriate shocks.[57] Small observational trials have shown some improvement in patients with HCM with cardiac resynchronization by decreasing LVOT gradient, affecting LV electrical activation, decreasing outflow tract gradient, and leading to positive remodeling.[76–78] Cardiac resynchronization therapy thus may be considered in patients with left bundle branch block in the setting of worsening LV dysfunction. There are limited data on the subcutaneous defibrillator in patients with HCM.

ARVC
Overview, Clinical Presentation, and Pathophysiology

ARVC is an inherited disease primarily of the RV myocardium with associated ventricular pump dysfunction and arrhythmias and structural abnormalities. It affects 1 in 1000 to 1 in 5000 individuals[79] with prevalence varying in different communities. It is diagnosed at mean age of 31 years and is more common in men. Approximately 30% to 50% of ARVC is familial,[80] generally with an autosomal dominant type inheritance and incomplete penetrance. Sudden death may be the first manifestation of disease in 50% of patients.

Diagnosis

Diagnosis is a challenge given phenotypic variation with incomplete and low penetrance. The 1994 Task Force criteria defined major and minor criteria for diagnosis of ARVC that were revised in 2010.[81,82] There are major and minor criteria for global or regional dysfunction, tissue characterization of the wall, repolarization abnormalities, depolarization/conduction abnormalities, arrhythmias, and family history. Increased number of major and minor criteria makes the diagnosis of ARVC more likely.

Risk Stratification

Although a risk prediction model is not well defined, several markers may predict arrhythmic events, including previous cardiac arrest, unexplained syncope, extensive RV disease, LV involvement, family history of cardiac arrest, increased QRS dispersion, increased S-wave upstroke, Naxos disease, VT during EP testing, NSVT on monitoring, male gender, young age at presentation, and ARVC type 5.[83,84]

Defibrillator and Adjunctive Therapy for Sudden Death Prevention

Defibrillators are the most effective method of sudden death prevention in the ARVC population.[85–88] In follow-up of patients with prior arrest or known ventricular arrhythmias, half of patients have appropriate therapy for VT.[86] In one study, 94% of patients with prior VT/VF and 39% of patients without a preceding event had appropriate discharges. Treatment rate for rapid VT/VF was less frequent (21%) and equivalent between the primary and secondary prevention groups.[89] Thus, patients with prior history of sustained VT/VF should receive a defibrillator. Similar to risk stratification for HCM, those with unexplained syncope, nonsustained VT on monitoring, family history of sudden death, and extensive LV disease may also be appropriate for ICD implantation.[87,88] In patients with equivocal risk, invasive EP testing may be appropriate.

ICD Considerations Specific to ARVC

ICD implantation can be challenging given lower R-wave amplitudes and associated T-wave oversensing.[90] In extensive RV disease, difficulty with lead placement or perforation may occur. A coronary sinus lead for pacing/sensing has been used in the event of low R waves.[91] β-Blockers and antiarrhythmics such as amiodarone and sotalol may have a role in reduction of shocks in patients with ARVC.[92]

GENERAL CONSIDERATIONS IN THE INHERITED SYNDROME POPULATION
Risk at Time of Implantation

These patients are at risk for typical implantation complications including lead dislodgement, tamponade, effusion, pneumothorax, and lead perforation. Device infection is a major concern, particularly because patients with inherited arrhythmias may undergo numerous device changes. For instance, in patients with HCM there has been reported to be a 3% to 5% risk of device infection.[61,93]

Reducing Shocks

High appropriate discharge rates in well-selected populations are balanced by high rates of inappropriate shocks that may exceed the appropriate discharge rate.[30,31,61,62,86,87,93–95] Inappropriate shocks may occur because of lead failure, electromagnetic interference, myopotentials, T-wave oversensing, and supraventricular tachycardia, which may be more common in inherited syndromes than in other cardiac diseases. Atrial lead implantation is controversial, because it has not been shown that SVT discrimination afforded by the atrial lead is effective[95–98] and there is an increased risk of complications with the extra lead.[98,99]

The most important intervention for avoidance of inappropriate shocks is programming the tachycardia therapy zone to a high rate cutoff. For instance, in the BrS, a single VF detection zone with cutoff of 222 beats per minute led to an inappropriate discharge rate of only 2.07%/y. No patients had syncope or died.[99] The more recent MADIT-RIT has buttressed this strategy in the general ICD population, in which a higher VT zone cutoff not only decreased inappropriate shocks by greater than 75% but also decreased mortality by greater than 40%.[100]

Device Durability

The other concern is lead longevity, which is a major concern for young patients. Prior leads have survival rates ranging from 85% to 98% at 5 years and 60% to 72% at 8 years.[101,102] It seems that newer leads that are not of small caliber have survival rates in excess of 90% at 10 years.[103,104] Moreover, even in expert hands, the risk of mortality from extraction is 0.25%.[105]

Role of Subcutaneous Device

Some of the complications and risks with the transvenous leads may make the recently US Food and Drug Administration–approved subcutaneous ICD[106] an option for many of these patients. The advantage of this system is the ability to avoid the intravascular space and possibly a more robust lead structure. The disadvantage of the subcutaneous system is inability to have anti-tachycardia pacing from the defibrillator and that it is a new technology that has not stood the test of time.

REFERENCES

1. Lu JT, Kass RS. Recent progress in congenital long QT syndrome. Curr Opin Cardiol 2010; 25(3):216–21.
2. Goldenberg I, Moss AJ. Long QT syndrome. J Am Coll Cardiol 2008;51(24):2291–300.
3. Vincent GM. The molecular genetics of the long QT syndrome: genes causing fainting and sudden death. Annu Rev Med 1998;49:263–74.
4. Schwartz PJ. The long QT syndrome. Curr Probl Cardiol 1997;22(6):297–351.
5. Modell SM, Lehmann MH. The long QT syndrome family of cardiac ion channelopathies: a HuGE review. Genet Med 2006;8(3):143–55.
6. Moss AJ, Schwartz PJ, Crampton RS, et al. The long QT syndrome. prospective longitudinal study of 328 families. Circulation 1991;84(3): 1136–44.
7. Priori SG, Schwartz PJ, Napolitano C, et al. Risk stratification in the long-QT syndrome. N Engl J Med 2003;348(19):1866–74.
8. Zareba W, Moss AJ, Schwartz PJ, et al. Influence of genotype on the clinical course of the long-QT syndrome. International Long-QT Syndrome Registry Research Group. N Engl J Med 1998;339(14): 960–5.
9. Saenen JB, Vrints CJ. Molecular aspects of the congenital and acquired long QT syndrome: clinical implications. J Mol Cell Cardiol 2008;44(4): 633–46.
10. Viskin S, Rosso R, Marquez MF, et al. The acquired Brugada syndrome and the paradox of choice. Heart Rhythm 2009;6(9):1342–4.
11. Goldenberg I, Mathew J, Moss AJ, et al. Corrected QT variability in serial electrocardiograms in long QT syndrome: the importance of the maximum corrected QT for risk stratification. J Am Coll Cardiol 2006;48(5):1047–52.
12. Hofman N, Wilde AA, Kaab S, et al. Diagnostic criteria for congenital long QT syndrome in the era of molecular genetics: do we need a scoring system? Eur Heart J 2007;28(5):575–80.
13. Rossenbacker T, Priori SG. Clinical diagnosis of long QT syndrome: back to the caliper. Eur Heart J 2007;28(5):527–8.
14. Ackerman MJ, Priori SG, Willems S, et al. HRS/EHRA expert consensus statement on the state of genetic testing for the channelopathies and cardiomyopathies this document was developed as a partnership between the Heart Rhythm Society (HRS) and the European Heart Rhythm Association (EHRA). Heart Rhythm 2011;8(8):1308–39.
15. Priori SG, Wilde AA, Horie M, et al. HRS/EHRA/APHRS expert consensus statement on the diagnosis and management of patients with inherited primary arrhythmia syndromes. Expert consensus statement on inherited primary arrhythmia syndromes: document endorsed by HRS, EHRA, and APHRS in May 2013 and by ACCF, AHA, PACES, and AEPC in June 2013. Heart Rhythm 2013;e75–106.
16. Hobbs JB, Peterson DR, Moss AJ, et al. Risk of aborted cardiac arrest or sudden cardiac death during adolescence in the long-QT syndrome. JAMA 2006;296(10):1249–54.
17. Goldenberg I, Moss AJ, Bradley J, et al. Long-QT syndrome after age 40. Circulation 2008;117(17): 2192–201.
18. Sauer AJ, Moss AJ, McNitt S, et al. Long QT syndrome in adults. J Am Coll Cardiol 2007;49(3): 329–37.
19. Jons C, Moss AJ, Goldenberg I, et al. Risk of fatal arrhythmic events in long QT syndrome patients after syncope. J Am Coll Cardiol 2010;55(8):783–8.
20. Goldenberg I, Moss AJ, Peterson DR, et al. Risk factors for aborted cardiac arrest and sudden cardiac death in children with the congenital long-QT syndrome. Circulation 2008;117(17):2184–91.
21. Goldenberg I, Bradley J, Moss A, et al. Beta-blocker efficacy in high-risk patients with the congenital long-QT syndrome types 1 and 2: implications for patient management. J Cardiovasc Electrophysiol 2010;21(8):893–901.
22. Ruan Y, Liu N, Napolitano C, et al. Therapeutic strategies for long-QT syndrome: does the molecular substrate matter? Circ Arrhythm Electrophysiol 2008;1(4):290–7.
23. Moss AJ, Goldenberg I. Importance of knowing the genotype and the specific mutation when managing patients with long QT syndrome. Circ Arrhythm Electrophysiol 2008;1(3):213–26 [discussion: 226].
24. Bhandari AK, Shapiro WA, Morady F, et al. Electrophysiologic testing in patients with the long QT syndrome. Circulation 1985;71(1):63–71.
25. Kaufman ES, McNitt S, Moss AJ, et al. Risk of death in the long QT syndrome when a sibling has died. Heart Rhythm 2008;5(6):831–6.
26. Schwartz PJ, Priori SG, Spazzolini C, et al. Genotype-phenotype correlation in the long-QT

syndrome: gene-specific triggers for life-threatening arrhythmias. Circulation 2001;103(1):89–95.

27. Priori SG, Napolitano C, Schwartz PJ, et al. Association of long QT syndrome loci and cardiac events among patients treated with beta-blockers. JAMA 2004;292(11):1341–4.

28. Vincent GM, Schwartz PJ, Denjoy I, et al. High efficacy of beta-blockers in long-QT syndrome type 1: contribution of noncompliance and QT-prolonging drugs to the occurrence of beta-blocker treatment "failures". Circulation 2009;119(2):215–21.

29. Monnig G, Kobe J, Loher A, et al. Implantable cardioverter-defibrillator therapy in patients with congenital long-QT syndrome: a long-term follow-up. Heart Rhythm 2005;2(5):497–504.

30. Horner JM, Kinoshita M, Webster TL, et al. Implantable cardioverter defibrillator therapy for congenital long QT syndrome: a single-center experience. Heart Rhythm 2010;7(11):1616–22.

31. Schwartz PJ, Spazzolini C, Priori SG, et al. Who are the long-QT syndrome patients who receive an implantable cardioverter-defibrillator and what happens to them?: data from the European Long-QT Syndrome Implantable Cardioverter-Defibrillator (LQTS ICD) registry. Circulation 2010;122(13):1272–82.

32. Schwartz PJ, Crotti L, Insolia R. Long-QT syndrome: from genetics to management. Circ Arrhythm Electrophysiol 2012;5(4):868–77.

33. Rossenbacker T, Priori SG. The Brugada syndrome. Curr Opin Cardiol 2007;22(3):163–70.

34. Patel SS, Anees S, Ferrick KJ. Prevalence of a Brugada pattern electrocardiogram in an urban population in the United States. Pacing Clin Electrophysiol 2009;32(6):704–8.

35. Brugada J, Brugada R, Brugada P. Determinants of sudden cardiac death in individuals with the electrocardiographic pattern of Brugada syndrome and no previous cardiac arrest. Circulation 2003;108(25):3092–6.

36. Campuzano O, Brugada R, Iglesias A. Genetics of Brugada syndrome. Curr Opin Cardiol 2010;25(3):210–5.

37. Probst V, Denjoy I, Meregalli PG, et al. Clinical aspects and prognosis of Brugada syndrome in children. Circulation 2007;115(15):2042–8.

38. Eckardt L, Kirchhof P, Loh P, et al. Brugada syndrome and supraventricular tachyarrhythmias: a novel association? J Cardiovasc Electrophysiol 2001;12(6):680–5.

39. Bordachar P, Reuter S, Garrigue S, et al. Incidence, clinical implications and prognosis of atrial arrhythmias in Brugada syndrome. Eur Heart J 2004;25(10):879–84.

40. Antzelevitch C, Brugada P, Borggrefe M, et al. Brugada syndrome: report of the second consensus conference: endorsed by the Heart Rhythm Society and the European Heart Rhythm Association. Circulation 2005;111(5):659–70.

41. Triedman JK. Brugada and short QT syndromes. Pacing Clin Electrophysiol 2009;32(Suppl 2):S58–62.

42. Morita H, Kusano KF, Miura D, et al. Fragmented QRS as a marker of conduction abnormality and a predictor of prognosis of Brugada syndrome. Circulation 2008;118(17):1697–704.

43. Letsas KP, Efremidis M, Weber R, et al. Epsilon-like waves and ventricular conduction abnormalities in subjects with type 1 ECG pattern of Brugada syndrome. Heart Rhythm 2011;8(6):874–8.

44. Brugada J, Brugada R, Antzelevitch C, et al. Long-term follow-up of individuals with the electrocardiographic pattern of right bundle-branch block and ST-segment elevation in precordial leads V1 to V3. Circulation 2002;105(1):73–8.

45. Eckardt L, Probst V, Smits JP, et al. Long-term prognosis of individuals with right precordial ST-segment-elevation Brugada syndrome. Circulation 2005;111(3):257–63.

46. Gehi AK, Duong TD, Metz LD, et al. Risk stratification of individuals with the Brugada electrocardiogram: a meta-analysis. J Cardiovasc Electrophysiol 2006;17(6):577–83.

47. Priori SG, Napolitano C, Gasparini M, et al. Natural history of Brugada syndrome: insights for risk stratification and management. Circulation 2002;105(11):1342–7.

48. Paul M, Gerss J, Schulze-Bahr E, et al. Role of programmed ventricular stimulation in patients with Brugada syndrome: a meta-analysis of worldwide published data. Eur Heart J 2007;28(17):2126–33.

49. Giustetto C, Drago S, Demarchi PG, et al. Risk stratification of the patients with Brugada type electrocardiogram: a community-based prospective study. Europace 2009;11(4):507–13.

50. Brugada P, Brugada J. Right bundle branch block, persistent ST segment elevation and sudden cardiac death: a distinct clinical and electrocardiographic syndrome. A multicenter report. J Am Coll Cardiol 1992;20(6):1391–6.

51. Delise P, Allocca G, Marras E, et al. Risk stratification in individuals with the Brugada type 1 ECG pattern without previous cardiac arrest: usefulness of a combined clinical and electrophysiologic approach. Eur Heart J 2011;32(2):169–76.

52. Probst V, Veltmann C, Eckardt L, et al. Long-term prognosis of patients diagnosed with Brugada syndrome: results from the FINGER Brugada syndrome registry. Circulation 2010;121(5):635–43.

53. Nademanee K, Veerakul G, Chandanamattha P, et al. Prevention of ventricular fibrillation episodes in Brugada syndrome by catheter ablation over

the anterior right ventricular outflow tract epicardium. Circulation 2011;123(12):1270–9.

54. Maron BJ, Roberts WC, Epstein SE. Sudden death in hypertrophic cardiomyopathy: a profile of 78 patients. Circulation 1982;65(7):1388–94.

55. Maron BJ. Hypertrophic cardiomyopathy: a systematic review. JAMA 2002;287(10):1308–20.

56. Maron BJ, Casey SA, Hauser RG, et al. Clinical course of hypertrophic cardiomyopathy with survival to advanced age. J Am Coll Cardiol 2003; 42(5):882–8.

57. O'Mahony C, Lambiase PD, Rahman SM, et al. The relation of ventricular arrhythmia electrophysiological characteristics to cardiac phenotype and circadian patterns in hypertrophic cardiomyopathy. Europace 2012;14(5):724–33.

58. Santangeli P, Di Biase L, Lakkireddy D, et al. Radiofrequency catheter ablation of ventricular arrhythmias in patients with hypertrophic cardiomyopathy: safety and feasibility. Heart Rhythm 2010;7(8): 1036–42.

59. Gersh BJ, Maron BJ, Bonow RO, et al. 2011 ACCF/AHA guideline for the diagnosis and treatment of hypertrophic cardiomyopathy: a report of the American College Of Cardiology Foundation/American Heart Association Task Force on Practice Guidelines. Circulation 2011;124(24):e783–831.

60. Maron BJ, Shen WK, Link MS, et al. Efficacy of implantable cardioverter-defibrillators for the prevention of sudden death in patients with hypertrophic cardiomyopathy. N Engl J Med 2000;342(6): 365–73.

61. Maron BJ, Spirito P, Shen WK, et al. Implantable cardioverter-defibrillators and prevention of sudden cardiac death in hypertrophic cardiomyopathy. JAMA 2007;298(4):405–12.

62. Maron BJ, Spirito P, Ackerman MJ, et al. Prevention of sudden cardiac death with implantable cardioverter-defibrillators in children and adolescents with hypertrophic cardiomyopathy. J Am Coll Cardiol 2013;61(14):1527–35.

63. O'Mahony C, Tome-Esteban M, Lambiase PD, et al. A validation study of the 2003 American College Of Cardiology/European Society of Cardiology and 2011 American College of Cardiology Foundation/American Heart Association risk stratification and treatment algorithms for sudden cardiac death in patients with hypertrophic cardiomyopathy. Heart 2013;99(8):534–41.

64. Adabag AS, Maron BJ, Appelbaum E, et al. Occurrence and frequency of arrhythmias in hypertrophic cardiomyopathy in relation to delayed enhancement on cardiovascular magnetic resonance. J Am Coll Cardiol 2008;51(14):1369–74.

65. Prinz C, Schwarz M, Ilic I, et al. Myocardial fibrosis severity on cardiac magnetic resonance imaging predicts sustained arrhythmic events in hypertrophic cardiomyopathy. Can J Cardiol 2013;29(3):358–63.

66. Maron MS, Finley JJ, Bos JM, et al. Prevalence, clinical significance, and natural history of left ventricular apical aneurysms in hypertrophic cardiomyopathy. Circulation 2008;118(15):1541–9.

67. Furushima H, Chinushi M, Iijima K, et al. Ventricular tachyarrhythmia associated with hypertrophic cardiomyopathy: incidence, prognosis, and relation to type of hypertrophy. J Cardiovasc Electrophysiol 2010;21(9):991–9.

68. Maron BJ, Rowin EJ, Casey SA, et al. Risk stratification and outcome of patients with hypertrophic cardiomyopathy >=60 years of age. Circulation 2013;127(5):585–93.

69. Melacini P, Maron BJ, Bobbo F, et al. Evidence that pharmacological strategies lack efficacy for the prevention of sudden death in hypertrophic cardiomyopathy. Heart 2007;93(6):708–10.

70. Maron BJ, Spirito P. Implantable defibrillators and prevention of sudden death in hypertrophic cardiomyopathy. J Cardiovasc Electrophysiol 2008; 19(10):1118–26.

71. Nishimura RA, Trusty JM, Hayes DL, et al. Dual-chamber pacing for hypertrophic cardiomyopathy: a randomized, double-blind, crossover trial. J Am Coll Cardiol 1997;29(2):435–41.

72. Gadler F, Linde C, Daubert C, et al. Significant improvement of quality of life following atrioventricular synchronous pacing in patients with hypertrophic obstructive cardiomyopathy. Data from 1 year of follow-up. PIC Study Group. Pacing in cardiomyopathy. Eur Heart J 1999;20(14):1044–50.

73. Maron BJ, Nishimura RA, McKenna WJ, et al. Assessment of permanent dual-chamber pacing as a treatment for drug-refractory symptomatic patients with obstructive hypertrophic cardiomyopathy. A randomized, double-blind, crossover study (M-PATHY). Circulation 1999;99(22):2927–33.

74. Roberts BD, Hood RE, Saba MM, et al. Defibrillation threshold testing in patients with hypertrophic cardiomyopathy. Pacing Clin Electrophysiol 2010; 33(11):1342–6.

75. Cha YM, Gersh BJ, Maron BJ, et al. Electrophysiologic manifestations of ventricular tachyarrhythmias provoking appropriate defibrillator interventions in high-risk patients with hypertrophic cardiomyopathy. J Cardiovasc Electrophysiol 2007;18(5):483–7.

76. Rogers DP, Marazia S, Chow AW, et al. Effect of biventricular pacing on symptoms and cardiac remodelling in patients with end-stage hypertrophic cardiomyopathy. Eur J Heart Fail 2008; 10(5):507–13.

77. Lenarczyk R, Wozniak A, Kowalski O, et al. Effect of cardiac resynchronization on gradient reduction in patients with obstructive hypertrophic

cardiomyopathy: preliminary study. Pacing Clin Electrophysiol 2011;34(11):1544–52.

78. Berruezo A, Vatasescu R, Mont L, et al. Biventricular pacing in hypertrophic obstructive cardiomyopathy: a pilot study. Heart Rhythm 2011;8(2):221–7.

79. Calkins H. Arrhythmogenic right-ventricular dysplasia/cardiomyopathy. Curr Opin Cardiol 2006;21(1):55–63.

80. Hermida JS, Minassian A, Jarry G, et al. Familial incidence of late ventricular potentials and electrocardiographic abnormalities in arrhythmogenic right ventricular dysplasia. Am J Cardiol 1997; 79(10):1375–80.

81. McKenna WJ, Thiene G, Nava A, et al. Diagnosis of arrhythmogenic right ventricular dysplasia/cardiomyopathy. Task force of the working group myocardial and pericardial disease of the European Society of Cardiology and of the Scientific Council on Cardiomyopathies of the International Society and Federation of Cardiology. Br Heart J 1994; 71(3):215–8.

82. Marcus FI, McKenna WJ, Sherrill D, et al. Diagnosis of arrhythmogenic right ventricular cardiomyopathy/dysplasia: proposed modification of the task force criteria. Circulation 2010;121(13):1533–41.

83. Hodgkinson KA, Parfrey PS, Bassett AS, et al. The impact of implantable cardioverter-defibrillator therapy on survival in autosomal-dominant arrhythmogenic right ventricular cardiomyopathy (ARVD5). J Am Coll Cardiol 2005;45(3):400–8.

84. Epstein AE, Dimarco JP, Ellenbogen KA, et al. ACC/AHA/HRS 2008 guidelines for device-based therapy of cardiac rhythm abnormalities. Heart Rhythm 2008;5(6):e1–62.

85. Link MS, Wang PJ, Haugh CJ, et al. Arrhythmogenic right ventricular dysplasia: clinical results with implantable cardioverter defibrillators. J Interv Card Electrophysiol 1997;1(1):41–8.

86. Wichter T, Paul M, Wollmann C, et al. Implantable cardioverter/defibrillator therapy in arrhythmogenic right ventricular cardiomyopathy: single-center experience of long-term follow-up and complications in 60 patients. Circulation 2004;109(12): 1503–8.

87. Corrado D, Calkins H, Link MS, et al. Prophylactic implantable defibrillator in patients with arrhythmogenic right ventricular cardiomyopathy/dysplasia and no prior ventricular fibrillation or sustained ventricular tachycardia. Circulation 2010;122(12): 1144–52.

88. Bhonsale A, James CA, Tichnell C, et al. Incidence and predictors of implantable cardioverter-defibrillator therapy in patients with arrhythmogenic right ventricular dysplasia/cardiomyopathy undergoing implantable cardioverter-defibrillator implantation for primary prevention. J Am Coll Cardiol 2011;58(14):1485–96.

89. Piccini JP, Dalal D, Roguin A, et al. Predictors of appropriate implantable defibrillator therapies in patients with arrhythmogenic right ventricular dysplasia. Heart Rhythm 2005;2(11):1188–94.

90. Watanabe H, Chinushi M, Izumi D, et al. Decrease in amplitude of intracardiac ventricular electrogram and inappropriate therapy in patients with an implantable cardioverter defibrillator. Int Heart J 2006;47(3):363–70.

91. Lochy S, Francois B, Hollanders G, et al. Left ventricular sensing and pacing for sensing difficulties in internal cardioverter defibrillator therapy for arrhythmogenic right ventricular cardiomyopathy. Europace 2010;12(8):1195–6.

92. Marcus GM, Glidden DV, Polonsky B, et al. Efficacy of antiarrhythmic drugs in arrhythmogenic right ventricular cardiomyopathy: a report from the North American ARVC registry. J Am Coll Cardiol 2009; 54(7):609–15.

93. Syska P, Przybylski A, Chojnowska L, et al. Implantable cardioverter-defibrillator in patients with hypertrophic cardiomyopathy: efficacy and complications of the therapy in long-term follow-up. J Cardiovasc Electrophysiol 2010;21(8):883–9.

94. Sacher F, Probst V, Bessouet M, et al. Remote implantable cardioverter defibrillator monitoring in a Brugada syndrome population. Europace 2009; 11(4):489–94.

95. Lin G, Nishimura RA, Gersh BJ, et al. Device complications and inappropriate implantable cardioverter defibrillator shocks in patients with hypertrophic cardiomyopathy. Heart 2009;95(9): 709–14.

96. Ricci RP, Quesada A, Almendral J, et al. Dual-chamber implantable cardioverter defibrillators reduce clinical adverse events related to atrial fibrillation when compared with single-chamber defibrillators: a subanalysis of the DATAS trial. Europace 2009;11(5):587–93.

97. Lee DS, Krahn AD, Healey JS, et al. Evaluation of early complications related to de novo cardioverter defibrillator implantation insights from the Ontario ICD database. J Am Coll Cardiol 2010; 55(8):774–82.

98. Dewland TA, Pellegrini CN, Wang Y, et al. Dual-chamber implantable cardioverter-defibrillator selection is associated with increased complication rates and mortality among patients enrolled in the NCDR implantable cardioverter-defibrillator registry. J Am Coll Cardiol 2011; 58(10):1007–13.

99. Veltmann C, Kuschyk J, Schimpf R, et al. Prevention of inappropriate ICD shocks in patients with Brugada syndrome. Clin Res Cardiol 2010;99(1): 37–44.

100. Moss AJ, Schuger C, Beck CA, et al. Reduction in inappropriate therapy and mortality through

ICD programming. N Engl J Med 2012;367(24): 2275–83.

101. Kleemann T, Becker T, Doenges K, et al. Annual rate of transvenous defibrillation lead defects in implantable cardioverter-defibrillators over a period of >10 years. Circulation 2007;115(19):2474–80.

102. Wollmann CG, Bocker D, Loher A, et al. Two different therapeutic strategies in ICD lead defects: additional combined lead versus replacement of the lead. J Cardiovasc Electrophysiol 2007; 18(11):1172–7.

103. Hauser RG, Kallinen LM, Almquist AK, et al. Early failure of a small-diameter high-voltage implantable cardioverter-defibrillator lead. Heart Rhythm 2007; 4(7):892–6.

104. Hauser RG, Maron BJ, Marine JE, et al. Safety and efficacy of transvenous high-voltage implantable cardioverter-defibrillator leads in high-risk hypertrophic cardiomyopathy patients. Heart Rhythm 2008;5(11):1517–22.

105. Wazni O, Epstein LM, Carrillo RG, et al. Lead extraction in the contemporary setting: The LExICon study: an observational retrospective study of consecutive laser lead extractions. J Am Coll Cardiol 2010;55(6):579–86.

106. Olde Nordkamp LR, Dabiri Abkenari L, Boersma LV, et al. The entirely subcutaneous implantable cardioverter-defibrillator: Initial clinical experience in a large Dutch cohort. J Am Coll Cardiol 2012;60(19):1933–9.

Index

Note: Page numbers of article titles are in **boldface** type.

A

AF. See Atrial fibrillation (AF)
Antitachycardia pacing (ATP)
    in ICD–related shock avoidance, 194–195
Arrhythmia storage and remote monitoring
    in bradycardia management, 289–290
Arrhythmogenic right ventricular cardiomyopathy (ARVC)
    ICDs in, 312–313
ARVC. See Arrhythmogenic right ventricular cardiomyopathy (ARVC)
ATP. See Antitachycardia pacing (ATP)
Atrial fibrillation (AF)
    CIEDs–detected, **271–281**
        clinical relevance of, **271–281**
        future of, 279
        limitations of, 279
        mode-switching in, 272
        in patients with no prior history of AF, 277–279
        rate- and pattern-based, 272
        sensitivity and specificity of, 271–273
        TE–associated, 273–276
        temporal proximity to TE events, 277
        ventricular irregularity and incoherence–related, 272–273
    management of
        CIEDs in, 243–244
Automated threshold testing
    in bradycardia management, 284–285

B

Bradycardia
    management of
        newer algorithms in, **283–292**
            algorithms aimed at avoiding RV pacing, 285–286
            arrhythmia storage and remote monitoring, 289–290
            automated threshold testing, 284–285
            introduction, 283–284
            mode-switch algorithms, 287–288
            pacemaker-mediated tachycardia, 287
            rate-response pacing, 288–289
BRS. See Brugada syndrome (BRS)
Brugada syndrome (BRS)
    ICDs in, 307–310
        clinical presentation of, 307
        defibrillator and adjunctive therapies for SCD prevention, 309–310
        diagnosis of, 308–309
        overview of, 307
        pathophysiology of, 307–308
        risk stratification in, 309

C

Cardiac implantable electronic defibrillator(s) (CIEDs), **239–252**
    AF detected by, **271–281**. See also Atrial fibrillation (AF), CIEDs–detected
    clinical trials with, 240–242
    device management, 242–243
        recalls and advisories, 242–243
    disease management, 243–244
        AF, 243–244
        HF, 244
        mega-cohort studies, 244
    future directions in, 247–250
        creating integrated remote monitoring center, 249
        remote interrogation in other health care settings, 249
        remote reprogramming, 249–250
        shared labor force model, 247–249
    introduction, 239–242
    in modern practice, **239–252**
    MRI for patients with, **299–304**
        within 6 weeks of device implantation, 300–302
        Hopkins' protocol for, 300
        introduction, 299
        lead-related complications, 303
        MRI–conditional devices, 302–303
        risks associated with, 299–300
        state of the art devices, 302–303
    remote follow-up and monitoring with, 240
        barriers to, 244–245
        follow-up clinic in era of, 246
    remote technologies, 240
Cardiac implantable electronic defibrillator (CIED) infection
    lead extraction for, 201–202
Cardiac resynchronization therapy (CRT)
    evolution of, 295–296
        AV block requiring ventricular pacing, 296
        earlier timing, 295
        higher LVEF, 296
        narrow QRS duration, 295–296
    history of, 181

Cardiac (*continued*)
   indications for, 293–298
      HF, 293–294
      initial, 294–295
      newer, **184–188**
      post–MI HF, 296
Cardiomyopathy
   recent diagnosis of
      WCD after, 262–264
Catheter ablation
   in ICD–related shock avoidance, 193
Children
   WCD in, 268
Chronic pain
   lead extraction for, 202
CIEDs. *See* Cardiac implantable electronic
   defibrillator(s) (CIEDs)
Coronary revascularization
   with LV dysfunction
      WCD after, 260–262
CRT. *See* Cardiac resynchronization therapy (CRT)

D

Defibrillation threshold (DFT)
   defined, 211–212
Defibrillation threshold (DFT) testing
   impact on mortality and arrhythmic death,
      218–219
   introduction, 211
   necessity for, **211–224**
   practice trends, 219
   randomized trial data on
      paucity of, 219–220
   reasons to avoid, 215–218
      complications can lead to morbidity or
         mortality, 216–217
      increases cost, 218
      limits expansion of device implantation, 218
      low probability of high DFTs, 215
      majority of treated events are VT, effectively
         treated with antitachycardia pacing, 215
      requires heavier sedation and additional
         personnel, 215–216
      shocks may increase mortality, 217–218
      subsequent shocks are likely to be
         successful, 215
   reasons to support, 212–215
      assessment for device–device interaction in
         patients with more than one CIED, 214–215
      assessment of lead problems that may only be
         identified with high-voltage testing, 214
      assessment of system integrity and reliable
         sensing, 212
      assurance of safety margin for testing after
         addition of antiarrhythmic drugs, 214
      assurance that device is not "lemon," 214

      discovery of high DFTs needing system
         modification, 212
      discovery of low DFTs that may allow
         programming of lower first-shock
         energies, 214
      evidence-based medicine, clinical trials, and
         standard of care, 215
      increased assurance that defibrillation of VF
         will be successful during clinical events, 214
      poor predictive value of clinical factors in
         identifying high DFTs, 212–214
DFT testing. *See* Defibrillation threshold (DFT) testing

H

HCM. *See* Hypertrophic cardiomyopathy (HCM)
Heart failure (HF)
   management of
      CIEDs in, 244
   pacing for, 293–294
   post–MI
      CRT for, 296
   severe
      WCD for, 264–265
HF. *See* Heart failure (HF)
Hypertrophic cardiomyopathy (HCM)
   ICDs in, 310–312
      clinical presentation of, 310–311
      considerations related to, 311–312
      defibrillator and adjunctive therapies in SCD
         prevention, 311, 312
      overview of, 310–311
      pathophysiology of, 310–311
      risk stratification in, 311

I

ICDs. *See* Implantable cardioverter defibrillators
   (ICDs)
Implantable cardioverter defibrillators (ICDs)
   background of, 191–192
   guideline changes related to, 184–186
   history of, 181
   indications for, **305–318**. *See also specific*
      indications, e.g., Long QT syndrome (LQTS)
      ARVC, 312–313
      BRS, 307–310
      HCM, 310–312
      inherited syndrome population, 313–314
      introduction, 305
      LQTS, 305–307
      newer, **181–184**
   introduction, 191, 211
   in primary prevention, 182–184
   in secondary prevention, 181–182
   shock avoidance with, **191–200**
      catheter ablation in, 193

device programming in, 193–197
    ATP, 194–195
    AV relationship and choosing single-
        chamber or dual-chamber ICDs, 196
    detection duration, 194
    lowest detected rate, 194
    morphology, 195–196
    remote interrogation and monitoring, 197
    stability, 195
    sudden onset, 195
    SVT discrimination, 195
    ventricular oversensing, 196–197
  management options in, 192–197
  medical therapy in, 192–193
subcutaneous, **225–237**. *See also* Subcutaneous
  implantable cardioverter defibrillator (S-ICD)
WCD as bridge to, 265
WCD *vs.*
  in primary prevention of SCD, 258
Inherited syndrome population
  ICDs in, 313–314

L

Lead(s)
  complications associated with
    MRI in CIED patients and, 303
Lead extraction, **201–210**
  complications of, 208–209
    vascular and cardiac injury
      emergency surgical management of, 208
  indications for, 201–204
    chronic pain, 202
    CIED infection, 201–202
    functional, 202–204
    nonfunctional, 204
    thrombosis, 202
    venous stenosis, 202
  introduction, 201
  outcomes of, 208–209
  prevalence of, 201
  procedural aspects, 204–208
    device pocket preparation, 206
    facilities and training requirements, 204–205
    lead extraction procedure, 206–208
    preprocedural considerations, 205
    procedure considerations, 205
Left ventricular (LV) dysfunction
  coronary revascularization with
    WCD after, 260–262
  MI with
    WCD after, 258–260
Long QT syndrome (LQTS)
  ICDs in, 305–307
    beta-blockade and adjunctive therapies for
      SCD prevention, 307
    clinical presentation of, 306

    considerations in, 307
    diagnosis of, 306
    overview of, 305–306
    pathophysiology of, 306
    risk stratification in, 306
LQTS. *See* Long QT syndrome (LQTS)
Lumos-T Safety RedUceS RouTine Office Device
  Follow-up (TRUST) trial, 197, 244

M

Magnetic resonance imaging (MRI)
  for patients with CIEDs, **299–304**. *See also*
    Cardiac implantable electrnic defibrillator(s)
    (CIEDs), MRI for patients with
MI. *See* Myocardial infarction (MI)
Mode-switch algorithms
  in bradycardia management, 287–288
Myocardial infarction (MI)
  HF after
    CRT for, 296
  with LV dysfunction
    WCD after, 258–260

P

Pacemaker-mediated tachycardia
  prevention of/intervention for, 287
Pain
  chronic
    lead extraction for, 202

R

Rate-response pacing
  in bradycardia management, 288–289
Remote interrogation and monitoring
  in ICD–related shock avoidance, 197
Right ventricular (RV) pacing
  algorithms aimed at avoiding
    in bradycardia management, 285–286
RV. *See* Right ventricular (RV)

S

S-ICD. *See* Subcutaneous implantable cardioverter
  defibrillator (S-ICD)
SCD. *See* Sudden cardiac death (SCD)
Shock(s)
  avoidance of
    ICD–related, **191–200**. *See also* Implantable
      cardioverter defibrillators (ICDs)
  inappropriate
    with WCD, 268
Subcutaneous implantable cardioverter defibrillator
  (S-ICD), **225–237**
  clinical outcomes of, 231–234
  complications of, 234

Subcutaneous (*continued*)
    concerns related to, 234
    introduction, 225–227
    patient selection for, 227–229
    perioperative management, 229–231
    specifications for, 227
    surgical technique, 229–231
Sudden cardiac death (SCD)
    prevention of
        beta-blockade in
            in LQTS, 307
        defibrillator and adjunctive therapies in
            in ARVC, 313
            in BRS, 309–310
            in HCM, 311
            in LQTS, 307
        primary
            ICD *vs.* WCD, 258
Supraventricular tachycardia (SVT) discrimination
    in ICD–related shock avoidance, 195
SVT. *See* Supraventricular tachycardia (SVT)
Syncope
    monitoring of
        WCD in, 265

T

Tachycardia
    pacemaker-mediated
        prevention of and intervention for, 287
Tachycardia therapy algorithms
    newer, **191–200**
TE events. *See* Thromboembolic (TE) events
Thromboembolic (TE) events
    CIEDs–detected AF associated with, 273–276
Thrombosis
    lead extraction for, 202

V

Venous stenosis
    lead extraction for, 202
Ventricular oversensing
    in ICD–related shock avoidance, 196–197

W

WCD. *See* Wearable cardioverter defibrillator (WCD)
Wearable cardioverter defibrillator (WCD), **253–270**
    after coronary revascularization with LV dysfunction, 260–262
    after MI with LV dysfunction, 258–260
    after recent diagnosis of cardiomyopathy, 262–264
    as bridge to indicated ICD therapy, 265
    in children, 268
    in clinical practice, 257–258
    compliance with, 265
    described, 253–254
    effectiveness of, 265–268
    efficacy of, 265–268
    guidelines and expert consensus statements on, 255–257
    in high-risk syncope monitoring, 265
    ICD *vs.*
        in primary prevention of SCD, 258
    inappropriate shocks with, 268
    indications for
        approved, 255
    limitations of, 268
    monitoring capabilities of, 255
    programming and detection with, 254–255
    for severe HF, 264–265

Moving?

Make sure your subscription moves with you!

To notify us of your new address, find your **Clinics Account Number** (located on your mailing label above your name), and contact customer service at:

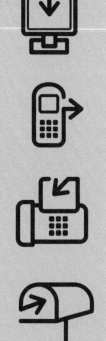

Email: journalscustomerservice-usa@elsevier.com

800-654-2452 (subscribers in the U.S. & Canada)
314-447-8871 (subscribers outside of the U.S. & Canada)

Fax number: 314-447-8029

Elsevier Health Sciences Division
Subscription Customer Service
3251 Riverport Lane
Maryland Heights, MO 63043

Printed and bound by CPI Group (UK) Ltd, Croydon, CR0 4YY

03/10/2024

01040382-0010